PUBLIC HEALTH
IN THE VICTORIAN AGE

VICTORIAN SOCIAL CONSCIENCE

A series of facsimile reprints of selected articles from *The Edinburgh Review, The Westminster Review, The Quarterly Review, Blackwood's Magazine* and *Fraser's Magazine* 1802–1870

THE SERIES INCLUDES:

Poverty 4 vols.
Urban Problems 2 vols.
The Working Classes 4 vols.
Prostitution
Emigration
Population Problems 2 vols.
Trade Unions 4 vols.
Working Conditions
Public Health 2 vols.

PUBLIC HEALTH IN THE VICTORIAN AGE

Debates on the issue from

19th century critical journals

With an introduction

by

Ruth Hodgkinson

Volume II

1973

GREGG INTERNATIONAL PUBLISHERS LIMITED

© Editorial matter Gregg International
Publishers Limited, 1973

Publishers Note.
Article entitled 'Spasmodic Cholera' *Westminster Review*
Vol 15 1831 has been abridged

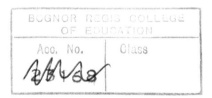
ISBN 0 576 53264 9

Republished in 1973 by Gregg International Publishers Limited
Westmead, Farnborough, Hants, England

Printed in Germany

CONTENTS

INTRODUCTION

Consideration of the health of the people on its present scale and complexity has been another product of the Industrial Revolution. If becoming 'the workshop of the world' worsened living conditions, it also gradually made amelioration possible. An increase in national wealth meant a rise in the standard of living; and the great technological and scientific advances played their part. Later came the dependence on progress in scientific medicine.

With acceleration in industrialisation, urbanisation and the increase in population, the problems of the public health, in the widest connotation, assumed an urgency never known before in history. The need for a pure water supply, sewage disposal, street paving and cleansing, for instance, had been recognised in antiquity. Overcrowding and insanitary dwellings had always existed, but not to the degree reached in the nineteenth century. Not only did the population double during the first fifty years from an estimated 9 m. to 18 m., but the imbalance of the distribution reached disturbing dimensions. As the mobility of labour increased, the settling and integration of migrants became difficult. This was augmented by the immigration of starving Irish, and later, political refugees from continental Europe. The social upheaval of the Industrial Revolution with its psychological and physical ill effects, the unhealthy environmental and working conditions, poverty, disease, epidemics, were all interrelated problems.

Agricultural areas and decaying centres of domestic industry had their health hazards. But it was in the new urban industrial areas, or extended old ones, that the most blatant abuses arose. Cheap shelter was provided in conglomerations of shoddy back-to-back houses devoid of any amenities, or in decrepit old houses in the town centre, where frequently whole families would share a room without water, sanitation or refuse disposal. Cellar dwellings, insanitary, airless and damp were common. Dark alleys and courts received all the filth and refuse thrown out, not only from private homes but from the innumerable small businesses such as bone or tripe boilers, tanneries or slaughterhouses. Blood, offal, excrement was left to decompose, until sufficiently large heaps had accumulated to make removal a profitable business proposition. A nauseating stench hung permanently over whole neighbourhoods. Domestic smoke was added to the palls of industrial smoke; air pollution was early recognised as a danger to health.

Water was obtained from a pump or standpipe serving dozens, and sometimes hundreds of people. The supply was available for only a few hours a day and not infrequently was drawn from rivers into which sewers emptied, or from wells where the surface water was contaminated. For rich and poor, lack of adequate and efficient sanitation was a serious danger awaiting not only local and central government action but also technological innovations. Indoor privies of the wealthy drained into cesspits, often in their own cellar, and emptied rarely. Outdoor privies or a 'necessary' (a tub) were shared by many families of poor. Besides the filth, stench, contaminated water and insalubrious homes, the health of the labouring classes was undermined by the poor quality and quantity of food. Malnutrition was a by-product of low wages, casual labour and unemployment. Food adulteration was common, extending even to poisonous additives.

Closely allied to the degradation of domestic life in the first half of the nineteenth century were the conditions of work. Factories subjected operatives to an intensity, speed and depersonalisation of work to which the labour force had been unaccustomed. The psychological ill-effects were matched by the physical degeneration. Long, unbroken hours of work in humid, ill-ventilated and dust-laden environment (a worker could be fined if he opened a window or was caught wasting time washing himself) impaired the health of the 'Hands' and also affected succeeding generations. Outbreaks of 'fevers' and debilitating complaints were common. In addition there was much maiming and mutilation through the dangerous and unfenced machinery. Many masters were very brutal especially with their child workers.

Conditions in the coalmines were equally inhuman. In 1840, 3,000 women and girls were still working underground, hauling tubs of hewn coal by means of belts and chains attached to their bodies. Mills and mines received the greatest notoriety, but for the longest part of the nineteenth century the largest number of work people were employed in small workshops or in their own homes. In the mid-sixties three quarters of a million were engaged in the clothing, laundry and carpet industries alone. Confined twelve to sixteen hours in overcrowded, overheated rooms with their vitiated atmosphere, workers were prone to contracting lung diseases and fevers. In the sweated trades a whole family might live and work in a single room. Health and lives were gravely wasted. Government interference did not come until late, and once again, improvement was aided by technological advances in industry. It was similar with the unhealthy trades, where occupational diseases such as lead poisoning and lung affections were common almost until the end of the century.

The expectation of life is a good index of the health of the people. In industrial areas in mid-century it was 18 to 25, and 40 for the country as a whole. The general mortality rate was 22 per 1,000; this did not begin to fall until the last quarter of the century to reach 16 per 1,000 in 1900. But such statistics do not give the complete picture. A large proportion of people suffered permanently from subnormal health or some form of physical disability as a result of environmental and working conditions or undernourishment. Succeeding generations were born weakly. The 'submerged masses' of the politician had a far deeper and wider connotation. Closely interrelated with immediate health problems were the causes and the consequences of widespread promiscuity, a high illegitimacy rate, early childbearing, infanticide, orphanage, crime, brutality and alcoholism.

Obviously a great deal of medical care was required. But little was available for the underprivileged. Quacks flourished well into the second half of the nineteenth century. Countless poor could not afford treatment or medicines of any kind. After the new Poor Law of 1834 the destitute sick came under the Poor Law medical service, and this grew to great dimensions by the end of the century. But how effective was personal medical care or curative medicine? Modern medical science was still in its infancy. Medical training, practice and organization had to undergo radical improvement before the profession could cope with the increasing demands upon it. Institutional medical treatment was unpopular. It was also inadequate. Hospital hygiene, amenities and nursing were generally scandalous during the first half of the nineteenth century. This held for the workhouse sick wards, and the voluntary hospital founded to cater for the poorer classes.

Although there was dire necessity for improving curative medicine this was less vital at the time than preventing the infectious crowd diseases and epidemics. 'Environmental' disease had to be tackled by 'sanitary' measures. Preventive medicine had to combat smallpox, the fevers, cholera and tuberculosis, the greatest killer of the time, before there could be an effective scientific medical revolution in the twentieth century. The public health movement was continuous but it was fear of epidemics, particularly cholera, that immediately roused the apathetic or shook the government into legislation. The first outbreak of asiatic cholera occurred in 1831–2 and took over 50,000 lives. A Central Board of Health and ineffectual local health boards were formed. All were disbanded when the scare was over. The second epidemic came in 1848, and again there were 50,000 deaths. Between 1848 and 1854 cholera claimed a quarter of a million victims, and the third epidemic in 1854, 20,000. The fourth and last epidemic broke out in 1866 when there were 14,000 deaths.

By the 1860s there had also been four epidemics of typhoid, but the disease was endemic and accounted for about 20,000 deaths a year. Typhus, confused so long with typhoid, took 4,000 lives a year. The epidemic of scarlet fever in 1840 saw 20,000 deaths. Smallpox was one of the most dreaded diseases. It was endemic in urban areas, and throughout the nineteenth century there was an average of 6,000 deaths a year. During the epidemic of the late thirties 31,000 people succumbed, and 44,000 in that of 1871–3.

All the problems which beset Britain as she emerged as an industrial country were accentuated by the depression which followed the long Napoleonic War. Inevitably an increase in disease correlated with an increase in poverty. Large-scale government measures were imperative. But effective reforms were long delayed for many reasons. The British had no experience of state paternalism. Public action for public welfare had few champions. Neither did the people feel that the state had any obligation for improving health and welfare. Parliament, composed of a landed aristocracy, was ill-tuned to the needs of a new age. The fear of revolution, which lasted for decades, restrained many purposeful philanthropists who would have been concerned with ameliorating the lot of the labouring classes. The chaos of local administration militated against local improvement. Local authorities and private utility companies jealously guarded their rights from central interference. Vested interests were powerful opponents for generations to public health or welfare measures. The Treasury kept a tight rein on civil expenditure, and two-thirds of the national budget was allocated to military departments.

So improvement came only after much controversy and many heated battles. Local Improvement Commissioners existed in the eighteenth century but these could not cope with rapid urbanisation. Overlapping of functions and inefficiency could only be met by government intervention on a national scale. Gradually the prevailing philosophy of *laissez-faire* was undermined from many sides, for industrial expansion depended on a healthy labour force. The nineteenth century also witnessed a powerful re-surgence of humanitarianism. It also spawned whole new classes of men: doctors who became familiar with the lives of the poor, educationalists, and administrators in new public services, such as the Poor Law, Public Health and Factory. There arose many new professions directly or indirectly connected with improving health and welfare. And regularly, the outbreak of an epidemic, especially of cholera, was the catalyst in getting action out of a recalcitrant or procrastinating administration.

Everything depended on central and local government reform. Improvement in the lives of the working classes only began after the Parliamentary Reform Act of 1832, and the Municipal Corporations Act of 1835. Civil Service reform started after the middle of the century, as did the increasing use of inspectors and special bodies for implementing legislation. Also by this time it was recognised that self-interest and self-help could not cope with the ever increasing problems of health and working conditions. So the ruling upper and middle classes, long before the lower classes, became aware of the need for government responsibility and obligation in matters affecting the public health.

Most of our welfare services stem from measures for combating poverty. The architect of the new Poor Law of 1834 was Edwin Chadwick. He early recognised the close connection between poverty and sickness, and his transference in 1848 from Poor Law to Public Health is significant. In 1838–39 he instigated Poor Law investigations into the worst slums of London, following these with a monumental inquiry covering huge sections of Great Britain. The lesson still being learned from Chadwick's Sanitary Report of 1842 is that the prevention of sickness is not only a question of humanity but also of economy. This was a forceful weapon in his long struggle to convert public opinion. Chadwick was also responsible for the organisation of the Royal Commission on the Health of Towns, and although not a member, drafted almost the entire first report of 1844.

But few giants have succeeded alone or begun *de novo*. Chadwick had a few able allies and dedicated lieutenants. The progenitors of the nineteenth century public health movement were a small group of doctors in Manchester who voluntarily formed a short-lived local Board of Health in 1795 headed by Dr. Percival and his 'Resolutions'. By the time Chadwick came to power Dr. J. P. Kay (later Sir James Kay-Shuttleworth) had produced a survey on *The Moral and Physical Conditions of the Working Classes employed in the Cotton manufacture of Manchester* (1833) and Dr. Southwood Smith, had in 1825, launched the Sanitary Idea in its new nineteenth century concept with his long essay on Fevers. This was extended into a book in 1830.

As with other areas of welfare the success of the public health movement depended on the growing number of societies. Most effective were the Health of Towns Association founded in 1844, and the Epidemiological Society in 1850. The Literary and Philosophical, and the Statistical Societies of large towns, such as Liverpool, Manchester and Leeds contained large numbers of doctors and reformers who could enlighten business men and local dignitaries. The published Transactions of all societies contributed to informing public opinion and pressurising the government. And essential to every aspect of health improvement was Dr. William Farr, Compiler of Abstracts at the Registrar General's Office. For forty years, from 1840 to 1880, he appended long detailed essays to the statistical reports, not only analysing facts and figures, but also including his many ideas on reforms.

The first really effective Public Health measure was introduced in 1848. The General Board of Health was instituted for a trial period of five years and local Boards of Health could be formed as single health authorities and appoint medical officers. But the Act was only mandatory where the death rate exceeded 22 per 1,000, or if one tenth of the ratepayers petitioned. There was great delay in implementing every section of the statute, but some drainage and sanitation schemes got underway. There was unusual procrastination in the appointment of Medical Officers of Health, and these like the Poor Law Medical Officers worked only part-time. The special qualification of the Diploma in Public Health was not introduced until 1875.

The General Board of Health came to an end in 1854. It was renewed on an annual basis until 1858 when it was replaced by the Medical Office of the Privy Council. Personal opposition to Chadwick was the primary reason for the fall of the Board, and his public career ended prematurely in 1854. Chadwick's unpopularity and his genius lay in his unflinching determination to introduce strong central control and to drive an unwilling government and country into efficient rationalised administration. Further, he insisted on rigid conformity to a principle.

Chadwick's mantle fell on John Simon, the second giant in the public health movement. He instituted inquiries into every aspect of health, hygiene and living and working conditions, employing special investigators and inspectors. For a generation he published massive annual reports on the health of the country. Although he felt his work frustrated, public health interest and activity moved on a larger plane. They also gradually amended the purely Sanitary Idea and became more medically orientated. And from the fifties, whilst medical science and practice were still largely ineffective, government activity was accelerated to improve health and living standards. There were many Nuisances Removal and Diseases Prevention Acts, Lodging Houses Acts, Factory Acts. Food adulteration began to be investigated, and measures for better water supplies and sanitation were implemented, if slowly. Personal medical care was being steadily improved for the destitute by the many Orders of the Poor Law Board. The effects were cumulative and interrelated. After mid-century, the rise in the standard of living and acceleration in technological advances in many directions contributed to slow improvement in national health and welfare.

The Sanitary Idea lingered on, but the new science of bacteriology was emerging. This was to usher in additional concepts for public health. The miasmatic theory which predominated during the first half of the nineteenth century was old. Disease was regarded as originating directly from filth and excrement. The effluvia or miasma in the air had to be removed or prevented by sanitary improvement. This was linked with the battle between contagionists who believed in infection, and the anti-contagionists who doubted whether any disease could be transmitted by direct infection (The demarcation was not as strict as has been supposed; this will become evident from the reviews). Just before mid-century, John Snow with his scientific inquiries into cholera, and William Budd into typhoid, produced evidence that the cause of infection was some specific organism which was passed by intestinal discharges into sewage, and then through defective sanitation into water supplies. Although the annihilation of the organism was their primary target, they regarded the cleanliness, pure water supply and efficient sewage disposal advocated by the sanitarians as very important.

In 1849 another significant development in the medical aspect of public health occurred. Typhoid and typhus fever were differentiated. Other infectious diseases were also being described.

It was just a generation after Southwood Smith, in *The Edinburgh Review* of 1825, had published his monumental paper which marked the turning point in the theory and practice of preventive medicine from simple quarantine measures to 'sanitary science'. He had helped to launch modern public health concepts. Yet within a few decades the miasmatic theory was proved wrong and his sanitary reform ideas insufficient.

It is in the context of current medical theories, and not only the practical manifestations of the public health movement, that the texts of the journals which follow must be viewed.

The press at any time is an index of what is uppermost in the public mind. The fear of epidemics, particularly of cholera, was in the forefront in non-medical as well as medical circles. So was smallpox and vaccination. Jenner had won great acclaim at the end of the eighteenth century, but until the mid-nineteenth century his discovery aroused serious controversy. The many and very long articles in numerous journals are therefore a good indication of how much thought was devoted to the theories and practice of combating infectious diseases, either by the old quarantine regulations or by more comprehensive sanitary improvement. Further, reformers are dependent first on the public being made aware of problems and, second, on creating interest in their amelioration. The periodicals of the nineteenth century played a leading part in enlightening the middle and upper classes, those sections of the community which controlled the destiny of the whole. They must take their place alongside the Transactions and Reports of specialist and learned societies as aiding the public health movement and indirectly bringing pressure to bear on the government.

The Journals*

The nineteenth century was the great age of journals. They were generally quarterlies of prodigious size. For us they provide an index of the issues which predominated at any particular moment. Current thoughts, particular theories, and the arguments in the major controversies are made available in great detail. We can trace the evolution of ideas in politics, economics and medicine and in social reform. We learn not only more of the men known to us, but also of the lesser known who were involved in important issues. The generalisations with which we are familiar are elucidated and substantiated.

The journals were published with a dual purpose: education and entertainment. The author of *Cholera Gossip*, Dr. W. A. Guy (*Fraser's*, vol. 40, 1849), pointed out that he was writing for readers who would open the pages of the magazine for relaxation, not mere amusement. He therefore wished to speak with seriousness, but not weary the reader with formidable tables and sustained discussion. That so many authors produced both, gives us an insight into the demand, standards and stamina of the nineteenth-century reading public. It is also an indication of the earnest desire for enlightenment in every field.

As those who governed the journals held particular principles on politics or social and economic policies, contributors were chosen carefully. But articles were frequently published presenting opposing points of view, of service to contemporaries, and researchers now. *The Edinburgh Review* claimed that its reviewers were free to speak their minds, and did so in no uncertain terms. Editors and authors kept a close watch on each others' publications. In 1853 (vol. 47) *Fraser's* pointed out that the fifth and sixth numbers of *The Westminster Review* of 1825, on contagion and quarantine, had attracted a great deal of attention, but accused the writer (Southwood Smith) of bias. He had 'ignored facts propounded by experienced men who held opposite opinions'. The reviewer (unidentified) had done his homework, for he quoted the *Quarterly* (vol. 33, 1825) which came out in direct refutation of the *Westminster*, and the *Edinburgh* of September 1826 'which closed

* I am greatly indebted to the *Wellesley Index to Victorian Periodicals, 1824–1900*, vols. 1 & 2, ed. Walter E. Houghton. This gives the identity of most contributors, short general notes on the journals and a bibliography of articles. Vol. 3 of the *Wellesley Index* has not yet been published, so we have to await information regarding *The Westminster Review*.

the contest'. He concluded with a recapitulation on quarantine from the 1852 October issue of the *Edinburgh*.

It was often politic for authors to remain anonymous. But it was also the policy of the journals until the mid-sixties for their articles to remain unsigned. Ninety per cent remained so for the century as a whole, and always in the *Edinburgh* and *Quarterly*. The writers were all men of erudition and of high standing in a particular profession. Many wrote with great knowledge about a remarkable variety of subjects. All showed literary ability. One author maintained that the general reading public 'derive knowledge and form opinions exclusively from the laudatory articles'. (*Fraser's*, vol. 47, 1853)

The Edinburgh Review was founded in 1802 by Francis Jeffrey, later Lord Jeffrey, Sydney Smith and Francis Horner. Jeffrey was a celebrated Scottish judge and staunch Whig politician. He was editor from 1803 to 1829. His own contributions to the journal were collected into four volumes in the 1840s. Smith was a divine and a reformer, but also a well-known author and wit. Horner, a barrister and politician, was the brother of Leonard, the geologist and educationalist who became chief factory inspector. Lord Brougham, the radical reformer, was closely connected with these three, and was responsible for many outspoken reviews. Although the *Edinburgh* stood out for social and political reform, it tried to steer a moderate course.

The Quarterly Review was launched in 1809 by the High Tories to counter the *Edinburgh*'s opposition to the government. The founders: Lord Canning, the statesman, John Murray, the publisher, and Sir Walter Scott were, however, not reactionaries, but believed in a 'humane paternalism'. They were not apathetic to social reform, for they included essays by Lord Shaftesbury for example, on factories, child labour and ragged schools. *The Quarterly* like *The Edinburgh Review* enlisted a small group of regular contributors who wrote on an extraordinary wide range of topics.

Fraser's Magazine for Town and Country appeared in London monthly. For over fifty years it represented 'progressive thought', chiefly on politics, but also on religion and social conditions. It was the brainchild of William Maginn who was the first editor, from 1830 to 1847. He was an extremely versatile Irish wit whose work had been too outspoken for *Blackwood's*. Four of the six articles reproduced from *Fraser's* are by Dr. W. A. Guy, a pioneer nineteenth-century medical statistician and a leading sanitary reformer. Altogether Guy wrote thirteen lengthy essays on public health questions for *Fraser's*.

Probably the greatest influence of any journal on social and health issues was that of *The Westminster Review*. It came into being in 1825 and it is significant that Southwood Smith, the outstanding public health reformer, was one of the founders. He used it as his airing ground, and in it Chadwick also published many of his ideas.

In the public health field all these journals followed a similar pattern presenting much the same subjects. Thereby they illustrated which were the predominant issues at any particular time. Foremost in the early nineteenth century were the conflicting theories on the etiology of infectious diseases, contagion, quarantine and isolation, and vaccination. The 'fevers' and cholera were rightly an obsession. From the 1840s interest in public health measures was demonstrated by the emphasis being shifted to an analysis of books and reports on the health of towns, and to scientific studies on water supplies and the need for state action on a national scale. Further, it is of interest to note how many reviews gave extensive coverage to overseas experiences and developments. The international aspect was very strong.

We must remember that these were not medical journals, nor were many writers on medical subjects doctors. But as was said in *The Edinburgh Review* (vol. 6, 1806) on smallpox and vaccination, medical questions ought in general to be left to medical journals, but the topics were of such importance that they were of great interest to everyone. All the reviews were written with great knowledge and skill. To be able to amass so many facts and statistics, and to sustain arguments to such a degree was an amazing tribute to the learning and capacity for hard work of the authors. It was no less to the readers. Rarely were the articles restricted to analysing the books before them. They were generally full-scale essays embodying the reviewer's own research and opinions.

The early public health movement owed a debt to Edinburgh. Its medical school was alone in Great Britain in interesting its students in public health problems. In 1807 it appointed the first Professor of Medical Jurisprudence and Medical Police, Andrew Duncan. From 1820 to 1856 William Alison, a great public health reform enthusiast, was Professor of Medicine. Owing to the restrictions placed on medical education in England up to the 1830s, many Englishmen went for their training to western Europe or Scotland. Southwood Smith, Kay and Percival were only three of many, who returned home influenced by what they had learned in Edinburgh on the importance of viewing medicine in a broader social context.

It is therefore significant that the first volume of *The Edinburgh Review* published a study on the prevention of infectious fevers. The author of the book discussed was John Haygarth, who had pioneered the treatment of fever by isolation in 1783, and had also written on smallpox and inoculation. Haygarth addressed his work to Dr. Percival, founder of the voluntary Manchester Board of Health and one of the pioneer public health reformers. The study was first presented to the Bath Literary and Philosophical Society. (We have noted the importance of learned societies as providing a meeting place for doctors.) John Thomson, the reviewer, was one of the early influential writers of *The Edinburgh Review* group. He was a surgeon and expert on military medicine. He agreed with Haygarth's ideas on fever being contagious and that victims should be isolated to prevent its spread. Isolation wards were to be well-ventilated and cleanliness was stressed. (Such improvements were very necessary in institutions at the time.) In 1818 the *Edinburgh* published another review on fevers. It was written by either Thomson or

Dr. A. J. G. Marcet of Guy's Hospital. As all reviews, it was not only an analysis of eight publications, but a prodigious work embracing the history of fevers, and the ideas on their causes and cure in the light of medical knowledge of the time. The prevention of fevers should no longer be left to physicians but should be taken up by the politicians and philanthropists. Typhus, it was pointed out, was of several varieties (typhus and typhoid had not yet been differentiated) ' but all arise from specific contagion' and fatigue and subnormal health made people susceptible to the disease. Again, isolation, fumigation and cleanliness were prescribed, and the setting up of fever hospitals.

In 1825 Dr. Southwood Smith countered in *The Westminster Review*. As physician to the only special fever hospital in London, he spoke with wide experience of fevers. With his two long essays he has been attributed with founding the whole new concept of sanitary science which had hitherto meant quarantine regulations only. Ostensibly he was reviewing thirteen works including two books by Charles MacLean, the much travelled medical and political writer, who utterly repudiated the idea of contagion and was regarded as leader of the anti-contagionists. Southwood Smith gave a clear definition of contagious disease and the theories. With detailed accounts of yellow fever and other fevers abroad he tried to prove that fevers were non-contagious. He elaborated his own thesis of the miasmatic theory of the etiology of disease and championed the anti-contagionists. By stressing the connection between sanitary conditions and disease, he became one of the pioneers of the sanitary reform movement. He came out strongly against the absurd and ineffective quarantine regulations: he did not, as others, demand total abolition, but rather that they should form part of a sanitary code. This, he concluded, deserved the serious attention of the physician, the merchant, the statesman and the philanthropist. He succeeded.

Five years later he published an extension of these reviews in his book *A Treatise on Fever* and emphasised preventive measures. This book in turn received an exciting review in the *Westminster* (vol. 12, 1830). Apart from giving an excellent synopsis of Smith's Treatise, Smith's tenets on the pathology of fevers were compared with William Stoker's *Pathological Observations on Continued Fever*. The author presented the conflicting arguments to the general public, as well as the medical profession, for the ' controversy which now agitates this country upon the subject of Fever, is of equal importance to every class of society'. Because of the ' great national distress ', it was of the utmost urgency to find means of prevention and treatment.

By this time the threat of an invasion of asiatic cholera loomed large. *The Westminster*, true to its altered title, *The Westminster and Foreign Quarterly Review*, published a long work on the incidence of cholera overseas (vol. 15, 1831). The panic was beginning and measures for prevention were sought desperately. New and old disinfectants were among the suggestions. The author deplored the dissension in the medical profession regarding the many forms of treatment, which included bleeding and opium.

Fraser's published a review on John Webster's *Essay on Epidemic Cholera* (vol. 6, 1832). Webster repudiated the contagious character of the disease and the asiatic origin of the epidemic. He believed the new form was only a more severe strain of the bilious cholera which was always present. Dr. D. M. Moir, an authority on cholera, attacked these assertions in his survey, but proposed that the truth probably lay between the contagionist and anti-contagionist theories.

The Quarterly (vol. 27, 1822) had produced a long article analysing the controversy over contagion and epidemic diseases. As on so many occasions the plague entered into the discussion. Quarantine was also rarely omitted, and here again the restrictive, expensive system was criticised. Economic reasons were always included. In 1825 Robert Gooch, an Edinburgh physician, continued on the same theme, and in 1831 Robert Ferguson published a review on cholera. The versatility of medical men at this time is noteworthy. Ferguson was an obstetrician, later becoming accoucheur to Queen Victoria, but he wrote many well-informed papers for the *Quarterly* on a wide variety of subjects, including prisons and public health. In volume 46 he reviewed seven works on cholera, devoting forty pages to discussing the disease abroad. He then criticised the regulations of the Privy Council for combating the epidemics: 'the government of this country neither has done, nor are doing, nor even as yet contemplate doing, what we conceive to be their duty in relation to that pestilence which hovers at our doors'. After attacking the government's inertia he gave suggestions adding 'notes' for private families.

The second cholera epidemic of 1848 brought panic once again. From the journals we learn that public health-wise, little had been achieved since 1831–32. Medical ideas had also altered little. But John Snow, through the observations he made of the incidence of cholera, was enabled to present his new theories in 1849. In the same year, the *Westminster* published a review which focussed first on the great early epidemics such as the Black Death and the Great Plague. Then the startling observation followed: that asiatic cholera was not a new disease in 1817 in India, but already existed in the seventeenth and eighteenth centuries. Turning to the General Board of Health reports on quarantine, the author pointed out that this proved conclusively that quarantine establishments were useless as a means of prevention and that isolating the sick was inhuman, a relic of medieval superstition.

A new aid was by this time beginning to make significant contributions to combating disease. This was the official collection and publication of statistics. *Fraser's* (vol. 40, 1849) printed an excellent article entitled 'Cholera Gossip' in which W. A. Guy praised the facts and figures offered by the Registrar General. Well qualified to do so as a medical statistician, Guy analysed the information on the incidence and deaths from cholera. He insisted that as the places and classes of people attacked were known, something could be done by sanitary measures to prevent further epidemics.

With a third outbreak of cholera threatening in 1853, the Board of Health reports on quarantine and on the 1848–49 epidemic were closely scrutinised.

The Board was attacked in *Fraser's* (vol. 47) for its non-contagionist attitude and for relying solely on sanitary measures for the prevention of disease. The quarantine issue was still open, so was the contagionist theory. *The Edinburgh Review* (vol. 96, 1852) also published a paper on the Board's reports. James Howell, possibly an army medical officer, praised the sanitary movement, and in recapitulating public health progress, drew attention particularly to the reports made to the Poor Law Commission in 1838–39 by Doctors Southwood Smith, Arnott and Kay, as being the first to attract the attention of Parliament to the causes of sickness among the poor.

Smallpox, another scourge of the nineteenth century, was not involved in contagion theories. It had always been recognised as contagious, but controversy was aroused by vaccination. It must be remembered that Jenner lived until 1823, so probably read the tremendous amount written for and against his discovery. *The Edinburgh Review* (vol. 9, 1806) published an article exceedingly informative at the time, and interesting to the historian. On the dispute over vaccination and inoculation, it purported to survey a tract of Robert Willan, an Edinburgh graduate and well known physician and dermatologist. In fact it was the reviewer's own thesis, normal procedure in the journals. Frequently, books or reports for review were not even mentioned. The article is attributed to Andrew Duncan, the younger. He was an eminent physician of Edinburgh who had several professorships at the medical school and there held the first chair in Medical Jurisprudence and Medical Police in Britain, 1807 to 1819. He presented all arguments, including the original quotations which reveal the strength of feeling aroused. The vituperate language, not uncommon in the nineteenth century, would scarcely be regarded as ethical today!

Much of the controversy arose because vaccination was still new. The vaccine was sometimes impure, despite the National Vaccine Establishment. Re-vaccination was not known and the dosage was unsure. When vaccination became compulsory in 1853 conscientious objectors joined the medically orientated anti-vaccinationists.

In 1810 *The Edinburgh Review* (vol. 15) produced a long list of material published on vaccination, with comments by Frances Jeffrey. This, he said, was just a small portion of the literature on 'acrimonious controversy'. We learn that 'this disgraceful warfare' had, until 1809 been confined to the Metropolis and had only just crossed the Tweed. Eight years later, the *Quarterly* (vol. 19) produced a good history of smallpox in antiquity, and in other countries with their ideas for prevention and treatment. In 1825 (vol. 33) Robert Gooch, the Edinburgh physician, discussed the pamphlet of Robert Ferguson in which he lamented that in the native country of Jenner's incalculable discovery, crowds of poor went unvaccinated. In many other European countries vaccination was compulsory and mortality from the disease had greatly decreased. Gooch gave statistics and compared records with those of towns in Britain. He believed immunity was for life, but drew attention to the conjecture that the influence of vaccination might wear off.

For mitigating the severity of the disease Ferguson proposed first vaccinate, and a few days later inoculate with smallpox.

In addition to covering the medical aspects of public health, the theories and controversies and the terrible incidence of infectious disease, the journals were alive to the activity and practical aspirations of reformers. Evidence that sanitary reform was arousing wide attention in the country from the 1840s is provided by the reviews. The subject now predominated over those which we have noted. A public health policy had been established.

In 1840 Ferguson had deplored that ' England is the only country devoid of a medical police (state health policy and administration) and into which the public health has been allowed to shift for itself' (*Quarterly* vol. 66). Chadwick was just beginning. His monumental Sanitary Report was admirably summarised and discussed in the *Quarterly* (vol. 71, 1842) by Sir Francis B. Head, an author and colonial governor. He emphasised Chadwick's point: that the health of the nation was nearly synonymous with its wealth. It was the duty as well as the interest of the state to protect its 'labouring power'. The public health movement was furthered by the reports of the Health of Towns, and the Metropolitan Sanitary Commissions. W. A. Guy not only analysed these in *Fraser's* (vol. 36, 1847) but compared London with other European capitals, once again making use of his statistical knowledge. He eulogised on the sanitary reform movement and re-iterated its objectives very clearly.

The first real success of the reformers came with the Public Health Act of 1848, which understandably raised tremendous interest – and concern – in the country. The Bill had been emaciated and many very necessary improvements omitted. Whilst deploring the shortcomings of the statute, Guy called it 'An Act which, in honest, firm and willing hands, is capable of working a complete physical revolution in the disease-smitten towns of England' (*Fraser's*, vol. 38, 1848). He praised Chadwick but warned him that England ' will not suffer even an enlightened and benevolent despotism'. He was right. In 1854 Chadwick was sacked. Guy, once again in *Fraser's* (vol. 50, 1854), eulogised on the achievements of the Board of Health but outlined all the work which still remained to be done. He condemned the House of Commons for murdering eight or nine public health measures which had recently been launched and also the local opposition. As a portent for the distant future he mentiond John Simon's suggestion of a Ministry of Health.

A characteristic of Chadwick's administration was his dependence on civil engineers. For his sanitary science they were more important to him than doctors. It is therefore significant to remember the development of the engineering profession and how several branches aided public health. This was reflected in the choice of contributors to the journals by mid-century, and their subjects. The *Edinburgh* published one of its best reviews in vol. 91, 1850; the author was William O'Brien, an engineer. He was also an excellent historian of public health progress. As a disciple of Chadwick he pointed out the high cost of medical care for the poor, an expense to the parish which was to a great extent preventable. True to his training, he gave a critical account of London water supplies. A more technical study on water supply was provided in *The Westminster Review* in 1856. The ideas of Josiah Parks, the civil engineer and inventor of deep drainage, were discussed, and the experiments of Dr. Arthur Hassall, one of the pioneers of purer food and water, were criticised. Hassall was the most important figure in the *Lancet* inquiries of the early fifties into food adulteration, and again in similar subsequent government investigations. *The Quarterly Review* (vol. 88, 1850) also printed a paper by a sanitary engineer. F. O. Ward had earlier published an article on London water supplies, but in 1850 he produced 58 pages which included not only a survey of public health statutes and government reports, but in the main, advocated very emphatically the need for strong administrative centralisation and consolidation of responsible local bodies, in the interest of efficiency and economy. He was a true follower of Chadwick, but the principles were not realised until the closing decades of the century.

However necessary, the sanitary movement was too narrowly conceived for some reformers, who desired a more comprehensive approach. The *prevention* of disease was not enough. The promotion of the health of the people as a more complete policy was envisaged under a system of *medical police* – in the German connotation. The term was anathema in England and rarely used. In 1846 *The Westminster Review* dared to entitle an extensive essay: *The Medical Police of the United Kingdom*. This advocated the reorganisation of the medical profession and medical education, the appointment of full-time medical officers, public provision of medical care, and the closer relation of medicine to political economy. The *Westminster* was always a pioneer in social and health reforms.

The reviews chosen from these journals are but a selection. There are many more on closely related subjects. And there are many more journals. The mine of information presented in periodicals was essential to creating an awareness of problems and for soliciting sympathy and action. In this they succeeded. They were intended for a wider spectrum of society, and if they aimed at entertainment and relaxation, we must today marvel at the intelligence of the reader and wonder at his seriousness. It is hard for us to imagine anyone save the dedicated reformer, or reactionary opponent, appreciating the length and depth of the articles.

These reprints are not for the casually interested. They are for the researcher or for scholars who wish to fill in the gaps left in conventional histories. They must come with a sound knowledge of public health history, and their lengthy study will be amply rewarded by exciting new discoveries. They will be able to survey the domestic scene more closely and also make valuable comparisons with other countries. (It is for researchers that I have given names and a little information on authors, but the *Wellesley Index* should be consulted in conjunction with these periodicals. This would provide fuller perspective.)

For the historian, for whom it is essential that he view his special interest in broad context, the nineteenth-century journals are also a must. From the writings of the time we can recapture events, character and ideas. They are not only valuable source material but help us to live in that period and feel and think as people did then.

We must be grateful for these reproductions for making these records readily available. Even more so, when we are told that 'Victorian periodicals are doomed to rapid destruction due to chemical reactions in the pulp paper on which they are printed'.†

Ruth G. Hodgkinson
February 1973

† George W. Cook, The Victorian Periodicals Newsletter, 10, 1970, p. 37.

ART. VII. 1. *Results of an Investigation respecting Epidemic and Pestilential Diseases, including Researches in the Levant concerning the Plague.* By Charles Maclean, M. D. 2nd Edition, 2 vols. 8vo.

2. *Report of a Select Committee of the House of Commons, appointed to inquire into the Validity of the Doctrine of Contagion in the Plague, in* 1819.

3. *A Treatise on the Plague, designed to prove it Contagious, &c.* By Sir A. B. Faulkner, M. D. 1 vol. 8vo.

4. *The History of the Plague, as it has lately appeared in the Islands of Malta, Gozo, Corfu, Cephalonia, &c.* By T. D. Tully, Esq. Surgeon to the Forces, and late Inspector of Quarantine, &c. in the Ionian Islands. 1 vol. 8vo.

5. *Evils of Quarantine Laws, and Non-existence of Pestilential Contagion, deduced from the Phenomena of the Plague of the Levant, the Yellow Fever of Spain, and the Cholera Morbus of Asia.* By Charles Maclean, M. D. 1 vol. 8vo. 2nd. Edition.

6. *Report on Quarantine of the Select Committee of the House of Commons on the Foreign Trade,* 1824.

A CONTAGIOUS disease, is a disease which is capable of being communicated from person to person. An Epidemic disease, is a disease which at certain periods prevails generally over the whole, or over a large portion of a community. A Sporadic disease, is a disease which arises either in a single instance only, or of which the cases at one time are few and scattered. The cause of a contagious disease is a specific animal poison. The cause of an epidemic disease is, or rather is supposed to be, a certain condition of the air. A contagious disease prevails by the communication from person to person of that specific animal poison from which the malady derives its existence. An epidemic disease prevails through the influence of the atmosphere. The specific animal poison which gives origin to a contagious disease must have existed in some person, and have been communicated from that person to another, by actual contact, before such a disease can be propagated. The application by contact of its own specific virus is indispensable, as a first step, to the progress of a contagious disease : it is essential to every subsequent step. For the extension of an epidemic disease, on the contrary, it is only necessary that a person (provided he be predisposed to receive the malady) be surrounded by the noxious air from which the epidemic arises. A distinction has, indeed, been made between a contagious disease which is communicable by palpable matter, and one which is communicable by invisible effluvia : the distinction is truly unphilosophical. Whether the contagious matter be visible or not, it must still be matter : whether its application to any part of the body of the individual who receives it, can be distinctly traced or not, it must come in contact with some part of his body. The small-pox is communicable by the application to a healthy person of the matter contained in its pustules ; it is also communicable by placing a healthy person within a certain distance of the diseased ; in the former case, the application of the morbid matter is palpable ; in the latter case, it is not palpable, it is too subtle to be appreciated by the senses, it is conveyed through the medium of the air ; but its application is as real, and as really by contact, as when it is applied by the lancet of the inoculator.

In the whole range of politics, nay, even in that of theology itself, there is no subject on which such vague notions have prevailed ; none respecting which men's minds have been so completely and so generally mystified, as that of contagion. The subject of contagion certainly opposes to its investigation no peculiar difficulties ; but by the aid of one enormous assumption, and by neglecting to distinguish between one or two circumstances, which it is essential to discriminate, the extent to which both medical and unprofessional men, of the greatest intelligence, have allowed their understanding to be abused, is perfectly astonishing. For several centuries the subject of contagion has had the singular property of depriving the physician, the philosopher, and the statesman, of the power of applying to its investigation the commonest rules of reasoning ;

and men have argued on this topic, apparently to their own satisfaction and to that of others, in a manner which would have covered them with shame, and overwhelmed them with contempt, had they so done with reference to any other subject of human inquiry. And yet it is a subject on which it is of great importance that the ideas should be clear and the judgment sound. It is intimately connected with the life or death of millions of the human race ; it is interwoven with the commercial welfare of nations, and with the interests of this country in particular ; and the whole system of quarantine laws is entirely dependent upon it. To this subject the anxious attention of the legislature has already been directed more than once. The Committee of the House of Commons, of 1824, have thus recorded their opinion on the matter :—" The influence which this law (that of quarantine) is supposed to have in the protection of public health ; its bearing on some of our strongest prejudices ; and its containing the various precautions which have been long deemed our safeguards against the introduction of contagious diseases, from whatever part of the world the danger may be apprehended, renders every recommendation that may affect it, a matter, at once, of general interest and peculiar delicacy. On the one hand, care is to be taken, that in the attempt to relieve commerce from burthens and inconveniences which press upon it, and to afford it the greatest freedom of which it is susceptible, we do not expose the country to the most formidable risk. On the other hand, that neither ancient prejudices, nor an excess of anxiety to avert possible danger, should induce the continuance of restrictions inessential to their object ; and should thus deny to the trade any of those facilities, which, consistently with every prudential regard to considerations of protection and safety, it may be permitted to enjoy."* This subject is again to undergo the investigation of parliament early in the ensuing session. It is of the utmost importance, that those who are to engage in this inquiry should come to it with some real and correct information, and with unprejudiced minds. When the investigation was first instituted, ignorance was not blameable ; prejudice was unavoidable ; at present the case is different: there are facts which it is now criminal not to know ; there are prejudices which it is disgraceful any longer to entertain. We own that we take a deep interest in the subject : we have devoted to it much time and labour ; we have pursued the inquiry with all the calmness and caution which it

---

* Second Report of the Select Committee, &c. of 1824.

was in our power to exercise; we have succeeded, at least, to the satisfaction of our own minds, in clearing away the vagueness and mystery in which it once seemed to us to be involved; and we earnestly request the patient attention of the reader to the doctrine and the facts about to be adduced. We shall first state what appears to us to be the true doctrine of contagion; we shall next adduce the evidence on which that doctrine is founded; we shall then examine the arguments which have been urged in support of opposite opinions; and lastly, we shall enter into a full consideration of the sanitary code.

Before proceeding to investigate the subject of contagion, it may be proper to observe, that it is by no means exclusively a medical question; it is really a question of science, to be decided by facts which every one can understand; a question of testimony, to be determined by evidence which every one can appreciate. There are circumstances which render medical men peculiarly unfit to investigate the subject. Few members of a profession are capable of taking any thing but a professional view of any professional subject. In medicine, the authority of the master has, at least, as much influence over the mind of the student, as it has in any other science. On this subject, in particular, pupils, before they are capable of forming an opinion for themselves, are taught, in the schools, certain dogmas which are inculcated upon them with extraordinary earnestness; their minds are trained to take only one view of the subject, and to consider all doubt on the matter as leading to the most terrible consequences. It is therefore only now and then that a man arises, endowed with extraordinary power, or placed in circumstances peculiarly favourable to the discovery of the truth, who is found capable of making that mental effort, which it is necessary to exert, in order to unlearn; to disregard the undue authority of the master; to look into nature as an original and independent observer; to see what is passing around him with his own eyes, and to judge with his own understanding. Among the members of the Spanish Cortes, in October 1822, there were nine medical men. The subject of contagion was brought before the consideration of that body by Dr. Maclean. It was a subject in which the Spanish Cortes could not but feel a deep interest, in consequence of the fever which had so recently depopulated numerous cities of the Peninsula. So overwhelming did the evidence adduced by Dr. Maclean, to prove that neither the fever which had lately raged in Spain, nor any of those fevers which are the objects of sanitary laws, are contagious, appear to that assembly, that, in opposition to the unanimous opinion of the nine medical members of their own body, as well as to that of an immense majority of all the physicians of Spain, they rejected altogether, after a solemn debate, and by a majority of sixty-five to forty-eight votes, the project of a code of sanitary laws which had been for years in careful preparation, successively, by a commission of the Government, and two Committees of Public Health of the Cortes. Here evidence in support of an undoubted truth, relating to a question which might have been deemed exclusively professional, sufficient to satisfy a majority of sixty-five to forty-eight unprofessional members, was not sufficient to satisfy a single individual out of nine professional men !

It has been stated that a contagious disease is a disease capable of being communicated from person to person. It is produced by an animal poison, and it has no other known cause. This animal poison is the product of a peculiar secretion of the animal economy. The character which is essential to it is, the power of producing when applied to a healthy person, a similar disease.

All the diseases to which the human body is subject, are divided into acute and chronic. Contagious diseases, in like manner, are either of an acute or chronic character. Examples of acute contagious diseases are, the small-pox and measles : of the chronic the venereal disease, the itch, the scaled head, the yaws, and a few others.

That species of contagion by which certain chronic diseases are prepagated, is so obvious as to require no discussion. The morbid secretion upon which it depends is palpable; the application of it is direct; the effects are visible, and can be observed and marked through every stage, from their commencement to their termination. With the single exception already adverted to, the same is true of that species of contagion upon which acute diseases depend. The small-pox secretes a contagious matter which is contained in its pustules ; the measles secretes a contagious matter which is contained in its vesicles. Apply a portion of the fluid contained in the pustules of the one, and the vesicles of the other, to a healthy person : it will excite in the latter the same train of symptoms as existed in the individual in whom the contagious matter was secreted. Moreover, persons who approach within a short distance of the affected, and who do not come into actual contact with them, are often attacked by these maladies ; but this is never the case with chronic contagious diseases, in all of which, the contact must be direct. It has been already shown, however, that even in the former, the contact is no less real, though it is not visible, and that the contagious matter, in a form too subtle to be appreciated by the senses, is conveyed from one body to another.

The origin of contagious matter, like the origin of every natural production, is concealed from the scrutiny of man. We
know nothing of it; but of the nature of the diseases it produces, thus much, at least, is certain, that they depend upon a
peculiar animal poison, and that they are propagated by the
communication of that poison from person to person.

It would have been reasonable to suppose *a priori* that diseases arising from causes thus specific, would observe peculiar
laws : they are found to do so; and a knowledge of these laws is
essential to the understanding of this subject.

1. Contagious diseases produce certain phenomena; that is,
a combination of certain symptoms : these symptoms are determinate and uniform; they are always the same; they never vary
except in degree. In every individual, under every variety of
age, sex, constitution, and mode of living; in every country; in
every season of the year, and in all possible states of the atmosphere, these symptoms are precisely the same. The operation
of any one, or of any combination of these agents, so powerful
in modifying disease in general, is only to render the symptoms
of a contagious disease more or less mild or malignant. The
symptoms themselves are uniformly the same : the small-pox is
never without its pustules ; the measles is never without its
vesicles ; the virus of the small-pox never produces the symptoms of measles ; that of measles never produces the symptoms
of small-pox. Each disease preserves, under every variety of
circumstance, the same specific character.

2. The phenomena produced by contagious diseases are not
only determinate in themselves, but they are uniform in their
accession, in their progress, and in their termination. Beyond
certain limits, which are narrow and fixed, they never vary in
either of these respects. The small-pox produces its appropriate symptoms in a certain time after the contagious matter has
been received : first, certain symptoms arise ; these are succeeded by others ; this succession takes place in a certain
order ; the symptoms come to their height in a certain period ;
they decline in a certain manner; they terminate in a certain
time. The period also when the disease has run its course and
ceases to be contagious, that is, ceases to exist, is determinate.
All these things are regular as the course of the planets. In
small-pox the law of the disease is, that no contagion takes place
until the eruption appears ; and that it remains as long as there
is any scab on the skin. The period which elapses between the
reception of the contagious matter and the first appearance of
the disease in small-pox from inoculation is 8 or 9 days. Thus,
of 810 inoculated cases, in 519 fever commenced before the

ninth, in 219 on the ninth day. The exceptions are extremely rare in which it either anticipates or exceeds this period. In the casual, or what is termed the natural small-pox, the latent period is somewhat longer than in the inoculated; but the utmost range is only from ten to sixteen days. The latent period of the contagion of measles is from ten to fourteen days. The other phenomena of these diseases succeed each other with a like regularity.

3. The morbid matter producing a contagious disease being once secreted, that disease can be propagated at any time and amongst any number of persons. So long as it retains its energy this specific virus never ceases to produce its specific effects; these effects can be produced by no other cause. From this law it follows, that no disease which is not contagious at its commencement can become contagious in its progress. The spontaneous generation of a contagious disease is as great an absurdity as the spontaneous generation of an animal. Nor, on the other hand, can a disease which is contagious in its commencement, cease to be contagious in its progress. The notion that a fever may arise from cold, from wet, from a peculiar constitution of the atmosphere, or from any of the common causes of fever, and become contagious in its progress, originated in an ignorance of the laws of the animal economy, and has been perpetuated in consequence of inattention to those laws. No man of sense can consider what a contagious disease really is, and what the ascertained laws of the animal economy are, without perceiving that this notion of the generation of a contagious disease must be false. To suppose, indeed, that a disease non-contagious in its commencement may become contagious in its progress, or the converse, is to imagine in the animal economy, precisely the same absurdity as it would be in the vegetable, were an acorn by a change of soil or climate to cease to produce an oak, and to generate a bramble.

4. Acute contagious diseases are capable of affecting the same person once only: chronic contagious diseases are capable of affecting the same person more than once. On what this peculiarity depends we do not know; it is an ultimate fact; but the fact itself is certain. If there be an ascertained fact in medicine, it is, that the small-pox and measles attack the same person once only. Cases, indeed, are on record, of the occurrence of these diseases more than once in the same individual: allowing the perfect accuracy of the observations on which these statements are made, it must still be conceded that it is an event so seldom witnessed, that it can be ranked only with the most singular of the exceptions which are known to exist to any general rule

5. Strictly connected with this law, and as a consequence of it, there follows one negative character of an acute contagious disease ; namely, when it has once gone through its course there can be no relapse. It is impossible either in that weakened state of the body which immediately succeeds an acute disease, or in any other condition of the constitution, whether by exposure to the common causes of fever, or by an application of the specific virus in any degree of intensity, to re-excite the original train of symptoms.

It might reasonably have been thought impossible that diseases so precise, so uniform, so specific, could be confounded with any other maladies. Yet there is an important class of diseases with which they have been generally confounded, and with which they not only have nothing in common, but to which they afford a perfect contrast, namely, Epidemic diseases. Epidemic diseases are governed by laws as precise and uniform as contagious diseases ; but, as has just been said, these laws are not only not the same, but the very opposite.

The term epidemic, considered etymologically, merely signifies *generally prevailing ;* but, in medicine, it is universally appropriated to designate a certain class of fevers. These fevers are highly malignant ; they occur frequently ; they spread extensively ; they prove more mortal than all other diseases together. Supposing mankind to consist of one thousand millions ; it is computed that thirty millions die annually from all diseases, and that of this number fifteen millions, that is one half, die of epidemic maladies. These diseases, therefore, possess an extraordinary interest and importance.

It has been stated that epidemic diseases are fevers. These fevers appear to derive their origin from one cause, namely, the state of the air ; a certain condition of the air is supposed to produce epidemic diseases, because this hypothesis affords the best solution of all the phenomena which they exhibit. What that constitution of the atmosphere is which gives rise, in any case, to an epidemic disease, we do not know ; therefore we cannot know what the peculiar constitution of the atmosphere is, which gives rise to peculiar epidemics. Of both these points we are in total ignorance. It is reasonable to believe that there are certain qualities of the atmosphere which have a considerable influence in the generation of these diseases ; namely, its heat, cold, moisture, dryness, and electrical state ; but what degrees and combinations of these qualities are connected with the production of epidemic diseases, we do not know. We have derived, from experience, the certain knowledge of one fact only ; namely, that these maladies are generated most frequently, and in the most malignant form, by a moist and warm atmosphere. It has, moreover, been supposed, that certain changes may take place in the constitution of the air which are not perceptible by our senses, and that these changes may have the most important influence on human health and life. Of this conjecture it is impossible to affirm or deny any thing : the changes it supposes, even if they really take place, must for ever remain unknown to us. Yet the supposed properties of the atmosphere, which result from these supposed changes, have received a distinct appellation, and have been called its occult properties. To give a non-entity a name, is at once to convert it, in most men's imagination, into a substance. Accordingly, these occult properties have been assigned and reasoned upon, as the causes of epidemic diseases, by some of the most distinguished physicians, with no more hesitation or scruple than they would speak of oxygen and nitrogen as component principles of the atmosphere.

In assigning certain conditions of the air as the cause of epidemic diseases, we are able to advance one step. The air, it is certain, is often charged with noxious exhalations arising from the putrefaction of animal and vegetable matter. These exhalations are generated in marshy situations, or where stagnant water contains dead vegetable matter ; and their production is greatly promoted by heat. Their precise nature is not known, for they have never been obtained in a separate state ; but it is ascertained that they are suspended in the air ; that, naturally, they do not extend far beyond the place where they are generated ; that, by currents of wind, they are capable of being conveyed to a great distance ; that they exert a powerful agency in producing some of the most malignant fevers ; and that a long-continued exposure to them, wonderfully shortens the duration of human life. Thus there is said to be a place in America where, from this cause, the inhabitants do not attain more than twenty years of age. It is certain that these exhalations exert a most important agency in the production of epidemic diseases ; it is equally true, that often-times their influence cannot be traced, and that in the most terrible pestilences which, there is reason to believe, depend entirely on the condition of the air, it is impossible to attribute to such exhalations any share in producing its morbid state.

Epidemic diseases observe certain laws : these laws, it will be seen, are the complete contrast of those which regulate contagious diseases.

1. The phenomena of epidemic diseases are not determinate and uniform ; they are diversified in the highest degree ; not

only in different countries and different seasons, but in the same country and the same season These symptoms observe no regular concourse ; they do not succeed each other in any determinate order ; there is no discernible connexion between the application of their cause and the appearance of its effects ; their duration is variable. The phenomena of contagious diseases, on the contrary, as has been shown, is determinate ; the order of their succession is regular ; the period which elapses between the application of their cause and the appearance of its effects is fixed ; their duration is uniform.

2. Though there is the greatest possible diversity in the phenomena of epidemic diseases, yet in all countries, the periods at which they commence, decline, and cease, are determinate and exact. These periods correspond with certain states of the seasons. They differ in different countries according to their geographical position, and they may be anticipated or postponed by circumstances, but in general they are remarkably uniform. In Asia Minor, Egypt, and Syria they commence in March or April, and cease in June or July : in most parts of Europe, and in North America, they begin in July or August, and end in November or December. The epidemics which prevailed at Gibraltar and in Spain in 1800, 1804, 1810, and 1814 prevailed in these autumnal months. Not only in Gibraltar and Spain, but in Italy also, and in all the places which they attacked, they uniformly commenced at one period ; they terminated at one period. The yellow fever is stated, by Dr. Rush, to have appeared in America six times successively : it always commenced from the first to the middle of August ; it always terminated about the middle of October. It is remarkable, that all the epidemics in Great Britain, of which we have any certain record, prevailed in Autumn, and committed the greatest ravages in August, September, and October. The history of epidemics in every part of the world confirms these observations. Now, that diseases which depend upon the state of the air should be thus influenced by season, should commence, come to their height, and cease, at determinate periods of the year is what might be expected ; contagious diseases, on the contrary, from the very nature of contagion, could not possibly be subject to such a law. Diversity in the phenomena which they exhibit ; uniformity in the periods they observe, might be expected to characterize epidemic diseases, from the nature of their cause : uniformity in their phenomena, diversity in their periods, might be expected to characterize contagious diseases, from the nature of their cause ; accordingly, these circumstances are actually found alike to characterize and to contrast both.

3. Epidemic diseases prevail most in certain countries, in certain districts, in certain towns, and in certain parts of the same town. The reason can often be distinctly ascertained. They prevail most in those countries which are the least cultivated ; in those districts which are the most woody, the most exposed to particular winds, and to inundation ; in those towns which are placed in a low and damp situation, and which are unprotected from certain winds ; in those streets and houses, and even in those apartments of the same house, which are the most low and damp, the worst built and the least sheltered.

Winds, whether assuming the form of gales, hurricanes, tornadoes, or tempests, often produce the most important effects in the most opposite direction. " Let us suppose," says Dr. Maclean, " two local currents of wind to meet in the neighbourhood of a long morass, dividing it into two equal parts ; the persons to leeward, that is, on the opposite sides of the opposite ends would be affected with disease, whilst those to windward, that is at the reverse opposite sides of the opposite ends, would remain exempt. The effects of an interchange of visits, would in such case, be very different. The sick to leeward, by visiting their friends to windward, or laterally, would recover, and none of the persons to windward would be affected by the presence or contact of their sick neighbours. But if the windward or lateral inhabitants were to visit their friends to leeward, they would become affected with disease, through the means of the air, whilst it would be supposed under the existing belief (of contagion) to be communicated to them by contact with the persons of their sick neighbours."

In all towns there are some places more insalubrious than others : of course these are inhabited by persons who can least afford to pay for situation; that is, by the poor. The habitations of the poor are likewise generally crowded, and always ill ventilated and dirty. Accordingly, it is in these situations that epidemic diseases most frequently arise, and prove most mortal. The most certain and the first victims of epidemic diseases are those who, from their poverty or their occupations, are most exposed to the air ; and those who being strangers to the climate are least accustomed to it. The liability of persons to the epidemic of the East and West Indies, on their first arrival in those countries, is proverbial. " The yellow fever," says Dr. Mac Arthur, " is almost universally confined to men recently arrived in the country." During the plague of London in 1665, of 3,000 that fell sick in the first week, the greatest number were new comers. These facts clearly point to the influence of the atmosphere : they are incompatible with the

nature of contagion, and they discriminate the diseases which
arise from these different causes. Contagious matter being
applied to the unaffected, the disease it produces would as
readily arise in the rich as in the poor; in the well-fed as in the
ill-fed; in the well-clothed as in the ill-clothed; in the well-
lodged as in the ill-lodged; in the idle as in the laborious; in
those who dwell in a pure, as in those who dwell in an impure
atmosphere, and in the natives of a country, as in strangers.
¶ 4. Epidemic diseases commence, spread, and cease, in a
manner perfectly peculiar. They arise, for example, in some
particular quarter of a town, or in some district. They do not
proceed to attack other places in regular succession, according
to their proximity to the quarter first affected; but they break
out, at once, in the most distant, and the most opposite
directions. They prevail, suppose in a certain district, suddenly they diminish or cease there, and appear in another
quarter, it may be, the most remote from the first; then they
may again return to the place first attacked, or they may suddenly appear in a spot near to it, or in one in an opposite
direction. People are attacked, not in proportion as the inhabitants of the affected mix with those of the unaffected places;
but in proportion as the inhabitants of unaffected, expose
themselves to the *air* of affected places. The visits of the sick
to unaffected places is followed by no increase of disease; the
visits of the inhabitants of an unaffected, to an affected place,
is attended with a certain increase of sickness. On their removal from a noxious to a pure air, the sick often rapidly
recover; but they do not communicate the disease to the inhabitants of a pure atmosphere; in the history of all the
epidemics which have ever prevailed, in all parts of the earth,
there is not on record a single example of the communication of
the disease from the sick to the healthy in a pure atmosphere.
Again, the manner in which epidemic diseases terminate is most
peculiar and characteristic. It is precisely at the period when
the greatest number of persons are affected, and when the
greatest mortality prevails, that these maladies rapidly decline
and suddenly cease. There is scarcely an exception to this
law in the history of epidemic diseases. It perfectly accords
with the nature of the cause upon which epidemics are here supposed to depend; it is totally inexplicable upon the hypothesis
that they are produced by contagion. To suppose that a disease
which is propagated by contagion, can rapidly decline and
even suddenly cease, at the very period when the greatest
number of persons are affected, and when the greatest mortality
prevails, that is, when the contagious matter is proved to be in

its most active and malignant state, is utterly absurd. So true is this, that the most intelligent and candid contagionists acknowledge, in so many terms, that this important fact is perfectly inexplicable upon their system. " It is a very curious fact," says one of the most distinguished and able advocates of the common doctrine of contagion, " *and perhaps wholly unaccountable upon any theory of the propagation of contagion,* that pestilential diseases, after running an indefinite course, notwithstanding all the measures adopted to restrain their progress, frequently cease spontaneously, at a time when the walls of the houses, furniture, &c. must still be supposed to be highly impregnated with the contagion. The fact is authenticated by Dr. Russell, Dr. Lind, and several other physicians of equal respectability." The fact is indeed certain ; it is most distinctive of these two classes of diseases ; it is alone sufficient to prove that they are essentially different.

5. Epidemic diseases are capable of affecting the same person repeatedly ; in every epidemic some cases occur of successive attacks in the same individual ; in general, relapses are so frequent and so fatal, that they may be ranked among the chief causes of the excessive mortality of these diseases.

Such, then, are the laws which characterize and discriminate contagious and epidemic diseases. That these maladies are not only distinct from, but incompatible with each other, no one who considers what has been stated can doubt ; but they have been so completely confounded, not only by unprofessional observers, but also by great authorities in physic, that it may be proper to establish their incompatibility by some separate proofs.

Were the common use of the term epidemic confined to its strict etymological signification *(generally prevailing)* it would be correct to say of the small-pox, for example, when generally prevailing, that it was epidemic. But this term has been appropriated to the designation of a class of diseases observant of the laws which have been stated. To call any disease epidemic, therefore, merely because it is generally prevailing, unless it be also obedient to all the other laws which characterize epidemic diseases, must lead (and the history of this subject affords abundant proof that it has led) to the most pernicious confusion of ideas.

1. It is certain that epidemic diseases are not contagious, because there is no proof that they are. The absence of evidence completely irresistible, on this subject, is itself sufficient proof that there is no evidence whatever. For, were epidemic diseases really propagated by contagion, it could not possibly

be a matter of controversy: the facts establishing the truth would be so clear, so numerous, so overwhelming, as to place it beyond all question. No one can doubt, no one ever did doubt, that the small-pox is contagious; the proof of it is simple, precise, complete; it must necessarily be so with every disease which depends upon a specific cause, and which produces specific effects; it is not so with a single epidemic; this alone must be sufficient to decide the matter in the judgment of every philosophical mind.

2. Epidemic diseases are not contagious, not only because there is no evidence that they are, but because the evidence that they are not, is as complete as the proof of a negative can be. It has been shown that the causes, the phenomena, and the laws of epidemic, are dissimilar and opposite to those of contagious diseases. But diseases which are dissimilar and opposite in their causes, in their phenomena and in their laws, must necessarily be inconvertible and incompatible.

3. Epidemic diseases are not contagious, because if they were so there must be a spontaneous generation of a specific animal poison in the progress of every epidemic. This, it has been shown, is contrary to the ascertained laws of the animal economy. We repeat, that no man of sound understanding can consider what a contagious disease really is, and what the ascertained laws of the animal economy are, and believe, for one moment, that a disease non-contagious in its commencement, can become contagious in its progress; or that a disease contagious in its origin, can cease to be so in its course; we repeat, that such an event in the animal economy would be as contrary to the laws of nature, as it would be in the vegetable, were an acorn, by a change of soil, or of climate, to cease to produce an oak and to generate a bramble.

4. Epidemic diseases are not contagious because the human race continues to exist. Were these maladies really capable of spreading by contagion, mankind must long since have been exterminated. To the devastation of acute contagious diseases, nature has set limits by rendering them capable of affecting the same person once only; but epidemic diseases are capable of affecting the same person repeatedly; and, in point of fact, the same person is often attacked, several times successively, by the same disease during the prevalence of the same epidemic. Were such a disease capable of propagation by contagion, it is obvious that it would be impossible to set any bounds to its ravages. Every person in health who came within a certain distance of the diseased would become affected; these would communicate it to others; as the disease spread, no person in

society could long continue beyond the sphere of its influence; the separation of the healthy from the sick would be impossible; no one could remain healthy, because even those who had had the disease would be again and again seized by it. Whilst a single individual of the community remained alive, it could never cease. Had the contagion of the small-pox been capable of affecting the same person repeatedly, no precautions could possibly have prevented it from being in a state of constant circulation; wherever it once broke out it would never disappear so long as there was a healthy person to be seized. Fortunately for the human race epidemic diseases do not thus spread; do not thus perpetuate their devastation. Even in the places and the seasons in which they exert their most powerful and malignant influence, the number of individuals is always small compared with the bulk of the community which remains unaffected; and, as has been already stated, it is precisely at the period when the greatest number are attacked, and when the greatest number perish, that is, when the contagious influence, if it really existed, must be most extensive and most active, that these maladies rapidly decline and suddenly cease. This fact, as has been already shown, is utterly incompatible, and is acknowledged to be so, with the property of contagion : it is alone decisive of the question.

But it will be asked, how could diseases so dissimilar and so opposite, have been confounded? How can medical men in particular have fallen into the delusion, and why do they continue to be misled by it? It is not difficult to assign the true cause; we particularly request the attention of the reader to this point, because if he will take the trouble to understand it, we are satisfied that the whole of this subject, so obscure and so mystified, will at once appear intelligible.

It has been shown that fever is capable of being produced by two causes; by a specific contagion, and by a peculiar constitution of the air, which, for the sake of distinguishing it from its other states, and of expressing the fact that it is the cause of epidemic diseases, may be termed its epidemic constitution; it is commonly called a pestilential constitution; but fever is capable of being produced by another, and a totally different condition of the air, namely, by the corruption of it. This corruption may take place in various ways, and exist in various degrees of intensity, and its effects will vary accordingly from the head-ache, produced by a crowded theatre, to the mortal fever occasioned by such a corruption of it as occurred in the black-hole of Calcutta, or such a state of it as exists naturally in the Grotto del Cane. There is this evident difference between an epidemic constitution of the air, and a corruption of it. We know nothing whatever of the change of properties of the air which renders it capable of producing pestilential fever : often we are able to ascertain completely both the nature and the source of that corruption of the air which produces common fever. The effects of an epidemic constitution of the air extend over a whole country, or over a large portion of it ; the effects of a corruption of the air are confined to that particular spot in which the deterioration takes place.

The modes are various in which the air may be so corrupted as to produce fever; the subject of contagion cannot be understood without attending to the causes which are capable of producing this corruption of the air ; yet these have hitherto not been noticed. It is ascertained that this corruption may be produced by three causes : 1. By the confinement of the healthy exhalations of the human body. 2. By the confinement of the morbid exhalations of the human body. 3. By exhalations arising from the putrefaction of dead animal and vegetable matter. In point of fact these causes are among the most common and powerful agents in producing fever, and their operation can often be accurately traced.

1. Fever may be produced by the confinement of the healthy exhalations of the body; as in crowded and ill-ventilated apartments. The facts which establish this point are numerous and decisive. Allusion has already been made to the deterioration of the air which took place in the black-hole of Calcutta. Mr. Howell and others who escaped from that horrible situation were seized with typhus fever. Typhus fever may at any time be produced on board a ship simply by shutting down the hatches and keeping the persons on board confined between decks for a few days. Dr. Lind states, that in a frigate which sailed from North America with a healthy crew, a malignant fever broke out before her arrival in England during very bad weather ; this fever affected a considerable number of the men ; and the surgeon's mate, boatswain, and some others died of it : in this case a seasoned crew was attacked with a malignant fever in consequence of the hatchway being shut down. Sir James Fellows states, that towards the latter end of January, 1811, two English transports (Metcalf and Phyllerea) arrived in the bay of Cadiz from Gibraltar, having between 4 and 500 German recruits on board. They had been kept on board under quarantine for upwards of a month in Gibraltar-bay; and unfortunately, on the arrival of the transports in Cadiz, the weather became so tempestuous that the crews of these vessels and the soldiers were obliged to be kept below. During *the few days* that the hatches were

covered over, in consequence of the heavy rains, a complete typhus fever had been formed. In his examination by the Committee of the House of Commons, Dr. William Gladstone states, that men of war were formerly ballasted with shingles; that this ballast was often not shifted for many years; that when it was turned it produced fever in several of the ships, and that this fever assumed the character of the prevailing fever of the station (whatever it might be) at which the vessel happened to be at the time. Sir John Pringle states, that he has observed a mortal fever to arise in the hospital of an army, not only when crowded with sick, but at any time when the air is confined, and especially in hot weather. " I have observed the same sort to arise," he adds, " in full and crowded barracks, and in transport ships when filled beyond a due number and detained by contrary winds; or when the men have been long kept at sea under close hatches in stormy weather." For this reason hospital ships for distant expeditions have been generally destructive both to the sick and their attendants. Of course, fever is more readily produced and becomes more malignant when uncleanness is added to confinement. For both these reasons it most commonly arises, and is most malignant, amongst the poor.

2. Fever is capable of being produced by the confinement of morbid exhalations from the human body. Wherever people labouring under any diseases are crowded together, more especially if the apartments are imperfectly ventilated, malignant fever is sure to be generated. Sir John Pringle remarks, that it is incidental to every place ill-aired and dirty; that is filled with animal steams from foul and diseased bodies; and on this account, jails and military hospitals are most exposed to this kind of pestilential infection; as the first are in a constant state of impurity, and the latter are so much filled with the poisonous effluvia of sores, mortifications, dysenteric, and other fetid excrements; nay, there is reason to apprehend, that when a single person is taken ill of any fetid disease, such as the small-pox, dysentery, or the like, and lies in a small close apartment, he may fall into this malignant fever. A remarkable fact, stated to us as occurring under his own observation, by a distinguished surgeon attached to one of the large hospitals in London, is alone decisive of this point. He mentions, that, in a particular ward of his hospital, whenever the number of patients contained in it, that is, surgical patients (for it was a surgical ward), amounted to twenty, typhus-fever was sure to be generated; and that whenever the number did not exceed fifteen, the fever never appeared. This event was observed to happen so constantly, that, at length, it was made a rule not to

place more than fifteen patients in this ward, from which period fever never occurred.

3. Fever is often produced by the exhalations arising from the putrefaction of animal and vegetable matter. Typhus fever often spreads over the adjacent country when the dead are left unburied on the field of battle. Forestus mentions a malignant fever which raged at Egmont in North Holland, occasioned by the putrefaction of a whale which had been left on the shore. Senac gives an account of a malignant fever which was excited by the accumulation of the offal of a city without the walls. It was received into a ditch filled with water; while covered by the water no bad consequences resulted; but when the quantity increased so that it rose above the surface, a dreadful fever spread through the city and its neighbourhood, so that where four hundred used to die yearly, the deaths were increased to two thousand. The malignant fevers which prevail in low marshy situations, particularly in warm weather, are examples of the effect of the putrefaction of vegetable matter in producing these diseases.

Now, contagion has hitherto been universally confounded with this corruption of the air. The fevers produced by this corrupted atmosphere, have universally been stated to be produced by contagion. Every author, with scarcely a single exception, who has observed and recorded facts similar to those which have been mentioned, has represented them, not as proving the power of a corrupted atmosphere to excite malignant fever, but as establishing its power to generate contagious fever. But it is obvious that they do not afford the slightest evidence of the existence of a contagious influence; that the supposition of contagion is entirely gratuitous; that the exact, and the only point they prove is, the power of a corrupted air to produce malignant fever; that other evidence is necessary to prove that the fever so produced is contagious, namely, evidence that when once generated, it re-produces itself, by contact of the sick with the healthy in a pure atmosphere, and that it observes all the other laws of contagious diseases. So far is this from being proved, that every fact is in direct contradiction to it; it is certain that these fevers do not, in a pure atmosphere, re-produce themselves by contact; it is certain that they do not observe a single law of contagious diseases. The single error of thus confounding the influence of a corrupted atmosphere with the generation and communication of a specific animal poison, has produced the most extraordinary and universal confusion of ideas on this subject; we are satisfied that the removal of this source of misconception is all that is now needful to render it perfectly luminous ; we hope, and believe, it will be felt to be so by every intelligent and unprejudiced mind.

There are two fevers, for the especial purpose of elucidating the nature of which, we have entered into this discussion ; namely, the yellow fever and the plague. The point to be ascertained is, whether or not these fevers are contagious ; and in order to arrive at the truth, it is only necessary to examine whether they conform to the laws of contagious or of epidemic diseases. Let us, then, attend to the history of these fevers with a special reference to this matter ; and first, of the yellow fever. This fever frequently prevails in various parts of Spain, and in Gibraltar, and proves extremely fatal. In 1821, whilst Dr. Maclean was in Spain, it attacked Barcelona, and with his wonted zeal he hastened to the spot in order that he might fully investigate its nature. Dr. Maclean is one of those extraordinary men who is capable of concentrating all the faculties of his mind, and of devoting the best years of his life, to the accomplishment of one great and benevolent object. In order to demonstrate what epidemic diseases really are, and what they are not, and to put an end to the errors which have so long, and so universally prevailed on this subject, errors which he believes to be the source of incalculable misery, and of certain death to millions of the human race, Dr. Maclean, with an energy scarcely to be paralleled, has devoted thirty years—a large portion of the active life of man. In this cause he has repeatedly risked that life ; and for its sake he has encountered all sorts of suspicion and abuse ; but the demonstrations of respect and gratitude which he has received from private individuals, and from public bodies, in all the countries which he has visited, have proved that the benevolence of his intentions has been recognized, and the value of his labours appreciated ; and he may enjoy the further satisfaction of knowing, that his opinions are making a steady progress, not only in his own profession, but among well-informed men in every station ; and that at no distant period they will universally prevail. Of the fever of Barcelona, in 1821, he has given so complete and masterly an account, that in order clearly to exhibit its nature (and it may stand as a paradigm of yellow fever), it is only necessary to select from the facts with which he has supplied us. In conjunction with ten native and four foreign physicians, who agreed regularly to assemble two evenings in the week, Dr. Maclean in the city which it was devastating, entered upon a minute and patient investigation of the nature of this disease. The names of the persons forming this association are recorded ; they consisted of physicians of four different nations : they were volunteers in the cause of science and humanity, serving at their own expense; they were actuated neither by the hope of reward, nor the dread of displeasure from any government or sect, or corporation, or individual; they acted in direct and obvious opposition to their minor personal interests; the resident physicians of Barcelona, especially, exposed their reputation and their fortune to great hazard; the investigation was continued regularly for the space of two months, and it is from the facts which were established in the course of it, the statement of which completely turned the current of opinion in Spain, that we derive the information we are about to offer.

1. In the first place, then, it appears that this disease was singularly diversified in the forms it assumed; that the combination, the succession, and the degree of its symptoms were so different in different cases, that it was difficult to assign to it any fixed and invariable progress, and that it was exceedingly irregular in the slowness or the quickness of its course. In all these respects it conformed to the first law of epidemic diseases, and was in contrast with that of a contagious disease.

2. This fever commenced in August, that is, precisely at that period of the year in which epidemics have always been known to manifest themselves in Spain and similar latitudes. Thus, in the epidemic which prevailed in Andalusia, in 1804, out of the twenty-three towns which it attacked that year, it commenced in the month of August in ten, and in September in eight. The fever of Barcelona continued to increase till the middle of October: the greatest mortality took place on the 19th of that month. This, also, is in strict conformity to the regular course of epidemics. In the epidemic of 1804, in sixteen towns in Spain, the greatest mortality took place in the month of October; in Cadiz, in Alicante, and at Gibraltar, by a singular coincidence, it took place on the same day, namely, the 9th of that month. From the 19th of October, the fever of Barcelona gradually declined, and subsequently it continued to diminish, in a regular and progressive manner, until its total disappearance. Thus this fever conformed to the second law of epidemic diseases.

3. It appears, that in Barcelona, from the neglect of the public police for many years, the sewers, drains, canals, and other channels for carrying away the impurities of the city, had been choked up, and become foul to such a degree, that towards the end of June it was impossible to pass by the sea wall, where they were discharged into the harbour, without being incommoded by the stench of accumulated and putrefying animal and vegetable substances. A committee which was charged with

the office of cleansing the port, discovered that the water-course was obstructed at its mouth by a bank of sand, which prevented its discharge, and, consequently, that a large quantity of stinking water was collected, the product of various manufactures, slaughter-houses, wash-houses, and other establishments situated on its banks, exhaling an insufferable stench. The foul water which stagnated around this sand bank was one foot higher than the level of the sea. Now, in the houses of Barcelona which faced the port, in the streets de los Encantes, de la Merced, Mencado, and others adjoining the focus of infection, the mortality was horrible, and nearly general; whilst in the streets of Santa Ana, Tallers, San Pedro, which are higher, and in others which are exposed to the north, and which are more distant from the focus of infection, there were very few sick. At a certain elevation, and at a certain distance from the south-east wind, which was the conductor of the noxious exhalations, as is proved by the course of the epidemic, not an individual sickened who had not been exposed to the causes affecting the lower part of the city. Indeed, the higher parts of Barcelona enjoyed a total exemption from the disease. These facts prove that the disease was a true epidemic ; they are inexplicable on the supposition that it was propagated by contagion.

4. Certain facts connected with the origin, progress, and termination of this disease, afford irresistible evidence that it was an epidemic fever, and could not possibly be propagated by contagion. Thus it was common to see four, six, or even eight individuals of the same family simultaneously affected ; that is in the same day, the same hour, the same instant. This might have arisen from an exposure to a pestilential air, it could not have arisen from contagion. It broke out in numerous points at once ; it committed the most dreadful ravages in certain spots, while places in the closest proximity were entirely exempt from its attack. In a narrow street of Barcelona called Calle de la Daguizea, 130 persons died ; in a place within ten yards of it not one perished. This difference appears to have depended upon the different position of the streets and houses in respect to the south-east wind. In Barcelonetta there were two families which resided close to each other—they both lived about the middle of the south side of Calla Santa Barbara—the houses were of the same size, plan, and structure. The easternmost family, that of Andrea Gallup, consisted of six persons, they kept a grocer's shop, and were in constant communication with the public—here not one was sick. The westernmost family consisted of ten members, they kept a wine and liquor

shop, and were also in constant communication with the public — here every one sickened and nine died. The grocer whose family did not suffer at all, was sheltered from the south-east wind; the spirit merchant's family, every member of which suffered, was directly exposed to it.

These facts are in perfect harmony with the usual cause of fever in this country. Of the fever at Gibraltar, in 1813, Mr. Gardiner, surgeon to the naval hospital, observes, that the disease did not spread from any focus, but broke out in fifty different places at once. " The rise and progress of our epidemics," says Mr. Amiel, "have never been traced in a satisfactory manner from a single point of contagion to a gradual number of individuals or families ; and instead of creeping slowly from one district to another, cases have made their appearance unconnected and scattered at different points ; and in some instances it has spread with the rapidity of the electric fluid, attacking persons who had never approached the sick or any assignable cause of contagion."

Like other epidemics, it was when the fever of Barcelona had acquired its greatest degree of extension, and produced its greatest mortality, that it began notably to decline. That day, as has been stated, was the 19th of October : on that day there died 246 persons, on the 2nd of November there died only 98 ; subsequently it diminished in a regular and progressive manner until its total disappearance.

This disease was never, in a single instance, communicated from person to person. When those who had contracted it in the city, removed into the country, whether they died or recovered, not a single case occurred of the communication of the malady, even to their nearest relative, *if the latter had not been in Barcelona.* Great numbers of persons passed the whole day in the capital, who retired at night to their families, either in country houses or in the nearest villages ; in no case did they communicate the disease to any individual. There was a daily traffic of carriages, sick persons, mattresses, linen, clothes, and other furniture from that part of the city in which the disease was most prevalent and mortal, to unaffected places; these never conveyed the malady beyond the ditch which surrounds the city·; nor was the disease transplanted, neither could it by any means be transplanted beyond that ditch.

The danger, so far from being in the direct ratio of intercourse with the sick, was, in many instances, in the inverse ratio. Whenever the hospitals were placed in healthy situations, the attendants on the sick, in these establishments, enjoyed even a greater exemption from disease than the inhabitants of the town generally. The average proportion of persons who were seized, estimated upon the whole community, was about one in seven. In the General Hospital, the proportion of those who sickened among the attendants, was also one in seven; in the Lazaretto of the Vice Queen of Peru, it was one in eight; in the Hospital of the Seminario, it did not exceed one in thirty; in the Lazaretto of Nazareth, which was considered the foul Lazaretto, or the receptacle of the worst cases, there were thirty attendants on the sick : of these not one was seized. Surely this is evidence which no mind can resist, that this disease was not contagious.

Several families isolated themselves in their houses, and employed the most exact precautions for avoiding communication with the sick ; but they did not by such means preserve themselves from the malady. Those who shut themselves up in good air, and who possessed the means of surrounding themselves with the conveniences and comforts of life, were uniformly exempt from disease ; those who shut themselves up in the pestilential atmosphere, and who had not the means of rendering their condition comfortable, were sooner affected than those who mingled in indiscriminate intercourse.

We shall only advert to one circumstance more in proof that this disease is not propagated by contagion; but that is decisive ; we refer to the effect of emigration. Those persons who left Barcelonetta, and who retired to a healthy situation, invariably remained unaffected, with the exception of a small number who were seized soon after they left the town, and who had evidently contracted the disease there. But neither those who, having come from the place where the disease was most prevalent, remained in health, nor those who fell sick, communicated the malady in a single instance, to the healthy inhabitants of the healthy places to which they removed. Mark the contrast. A barrier having been established between Barcelona and Barcelonetta so as to place the latter town in a state of isolation—what was the consequence ? The barrier was established on the third of September ; on that day there were in Barcelonetta nine sick persons ; by the tenth the number increased to one hundred and sixty-two. Thus, in seven days from the isolation of the town, the daily mortality had increased eighteen-fold. Precisely the same effects followed a removal of the troops in the same fever which prevailed at Gibraltar. Mr. Martindale, in his official reply respecting this fever, states that in Dillon's regiment, which was quartered in the blue barracks, near the Moorish castle, a great number of the men took the fever ; that several died ; that, in consequence of this, the regiment was sent to the neutral ground and encamped, and that *immediately* the fever stopped ; that the 8th battalion of the 66th regiment arrived from Cadiz in a healthy state ; that they were encamped in the governor's meadow ; that shortly afterwards they went into town and were quartered in the cooperage range ; that the fever *instantly* raged amongst them ; that both officers and men suffered severely ; that they were then sent back to the encampment, and that the disease, as in Dillon's, immediately ceased as if by magic. Further, Mr. Playfair, surgeon of Dillon's, records the following very important and illustrative fact :—That even after removal to the camp, in the governor's meadow, while the men of Dillon's regiment were allowed to enter the town, on fatigue duty, the fever still continued to prevail ; but that from the day of their confinement to the neutral ground, they were quite free from it, *although they had equal intercourse with the inhabitants coming from town in which the disease was at that time very destructive.* And Mr. Amiel states that, no individual labouring under epidemic fever, on being removed to a pure and ventilated place, such as the neutral ground or Europa point, ever communicated the disease to those in the closest contact with him.

These facts afford the most irresistible evidence that this fever is a true epidemic. It conformed in every respect to the laws of epidemic diseases ; it was without a single character of a contagious disease. So complete is this evidence, that it produced the fullest conviction in fifteen physicians, who assembled from all parts of Spain and of Europe to investigate the disease, and it produced a practical conviction in the Spanish Cortes, contrary to all their ancient, and deep-rooted prejudices ; and, notwithstanding, that they had so recently witnessed the appalling extension and the horrible mortality of the disease. In America, also, Dr. Rush, who had been a warm advocate for the doctrine of the contagious nature of this malady, on a more patient and strict examination of its phenomena and history, became convinced that he was in error, and with a magnanimity, which has but few parallels, proclaimed to the world that he had thought and written on this very important subject in a manner calculated to mislead. " In the fourth volume" (Med. Enquiries and Observations), says this celebrated physician, " the reader will find a retraction of the author's former opinion of the yellow fever spreading by contagion. He begs forgiveness of the friends of science and humanity, if the publication of that opinion has had any influence in increasing the misery and mortality attendant upon that disease. Indeed, such is the pain he feels in recollecting that he ever entertained or propagated it, that it will long, and perhaps always deprive him of the pleasure he might othei vise have derived from a review of his attempts to fulfil the public duties of his situation."

It is then impossible to resist the evidence that the yellow fever is an epidemic and not a contagious disease ; let us in the same manner examine what the facts are with reference to the plague.

1. The phenomena of the plague are so exceedingly diversified that they embrace almost every symptom of disease which the human body is capable of exhibiting. Among these there is not one which may be considered pathognomonic, " It is as various," says Fra Louigi di Pavia, who attended a plague hospital thirty years, " as the complexions and constitutions of those unfortunate persons whom it attacks." Every where it has obtained the name of the proteiform disease. In Smyrna they reckon fifteen kinds of it. In the plague of Marseilles in 1720, the French physicians state that they could distinguish five distinct species. Every author gives a different account of the period which is necessary for the development of the disease, after the supposed application of the contagious matter. Demoullins says, " it is two or three days ;" Giovanelli, " there is no certainty, as it depends on the constitution of the patient ;" Theny, " the interval from the infection to the seizure is various ; sometimes it acts slowly, sometimes like a stroke of lightning ;" Verdoni, " generally the disease shows itself at the instant of the touch ; sometimes it does not appear for several days ;" Fra Louigi, " the infection shows itself in twenty-four hours, more or less, according to the difference of temperament ;" Julius Cæsar Kelli, " it does not appear till after the second or third day ;" Samoilowitz, " the interval between the infection and the appearance of the disease extends from ten to fifteen days inclusively." This malady, then, conforms to the first law of Epidemic diseases ; its symptoms are various ; their concourse and succession are indeterminate ; their duration is uncertain ; there is the utmost discrepancy of opinion as to the period which is necessary for the supposed contagious matter to produce the disease ; were it really contagious, all these phenomena would be the exact reverse.

2. Like other epidemics, the plague begins and ceases at periods surprisingly regular ; these periods correspond exactly to the usual epidemic seasons ; thus, in Asia Minor, it prevails from April to July ; at Smyrna, from February to June ; at Constantinople, from July to December ; in Europe, in the same Autumnal months.

3. The places in which it first appears are those in which epidemics invariably arise; namely, in the unhealthy situations occupied by the poor. In Smyrna, it originates and prevails most in particular low narrow streets, in which the houses are close, and which are inhabited by the lowest classes of the people. The plague which affected London in 1626 and 1636, first broke out in Whitechapel. In 1665 it made its first appearance, and produced its principal mortality, in St. Giles's. That of Marseilles, in 1720, appeared first, continued longest, and proved most fatal, in the *Rue de Lescalle*. In this respect it corresponded exactly with the late epidemics of Cadiz, which appeared first in the Santa Maria quarter, as those of Gibraltar broke out in Boyd's buildings. It has been shown, that a disease depending upon a specific contagion must prevail alike in all seasons, in a pure, as well as in an impure atmosphere, amongst the rich as readily as amongst the poor; and that the only influence of these adventitious circumstances would be to render the disease more or less severe.

4. The plague, in its commencement and progress, disappears and re-appears, and leaps from point to point, in a manner which is wholly incompatible with the nature of a contagious disease. In the great plague of London, which commenced in November 1664, between the first two deaths and the third, there intervened the period of a month: between the third and fourth, six weeks : the fourth did not happen until the 12th of February 1665; from that period, none took place until the 25th of April, an interval of upwards of nine weeks, or nearly twice as long as the utmost assigned duration of the supposed capability of communicating contagion. Three several times it ceased, and re-commenced in less than five months before it was fully established. But this faculty of subsiding and resuscitating, is wholly incompatible with the nature of a contagious malady. In the western parishes, as St. Giles's in the Fields, St. Andrew's Holborn, &c., it came to its height about the middle, and declined towards the end of July. In the north-western suburbs, as Cripplegate, &c., it came to its height towards the middle, and declined towards the end of August. In the eastern suburbs, in the city, and on the Southwark side, it did not come to its height till towards the middle, nor decline till towards the end of September. Whilst the disease was raging in the west, and there died of it in the two parishes of St. Martin's and St. Giles's, 421, there died in the city but 28, in Southwark 19, in Aldgate but 4, in Whitechapel but 3, and in Stepney but 1. Had the disease been contagious, this geographical progress would have been utterly

impossible. In the manner in which it terminated, it equally conformed to the law of epidemic diseases. It was exactly at the period when it raged with its utmost virulence, when the shutting up of houses and all other precautions had been abandoned in despair, and when from thirty to forty thousand persons were still labouring under the disease, that its further propagation, at the usual termination of the epidemic season, suddenly declined and ceased. No contagious disease could possibly have thus spread; could possibly have thus terminated : but supposing it to have depended upon the noxious qualities of the air, which may be so partial and so fluctuating, and which may increase, or diminish so slowly, or so instantaneously, all the phenomena which attended this, and which invariably attends similar diseases, are explained in the most satisfactory manner.

5. The plague, like other epidemics, is capable of attacking the same person repeatedly. Mr. Green, in his examination by the Committee of the House of Commons, states, that this is an ascertained fact : that it is the universal belief in Turkey, and that the Abbé who had the care of the Frank Hospital at Constantinople, was afflicted with it ten or twelve times. Mr. Edward Hayes, who was born at Smyrna, and resided there upwards of forty years, states to the same Committee, that he has known persons to be attacked by the plague ten times. When persons are convalescent from plague, the greatest anxiety is always entertained by their friends lest they should relapse.

But, besides this proof, derived from its strict conformity to all the laws of epidemics, there are numerous and most decisive facts, which demonstrate, that this disease is not contagious. It is the custom in Turkey for the relations of those who die of plague, to wear the clothes of the deceased, or to sell them in the public Bazaar ; they are never destroyed : they are, invariably, either worn by the relatives, or sold at the public market; there is no instance on record of the communication of the disease by this means; the persons who deal in the clothes are not infected ; the persons who wear them remain free from disease. The bedding of the dead is also sold. If a stranger die of plague, the Pacha takes possession of his property; the clothes form a part of that property; they are his perquisites : he orders them to be sold for his own benefit, and people dare not destroy them. The just inference from these facts, is stated by Mr. Green to the Committee of the House of Commons. " The plague," he observes, " frequently ceases suddenly, and does not recur for two, three, four or five years ;

now the clothes of those who die of the disease, not being destroyed, but generally distributed and worn, as well as the
bedding, I conceive that, if they were contagious, it would be
impossible that we could be without the plague during that
period."

The plague is not communicated by the contact of the
affected with the unaffected. In Constantinople, persons with
the plague upon them, mix daily with the rest of the people,
visit the coffee-houses, and other places of public resort, without communicating the disease. Dr. Maclean states, that the
servants of the Pest hospital, after having held the patients in
their arms, and dressed their sores, went daily to the market
without the smallest restraint, and without any communication
of the disease. During his residence in the Greek Pest House,
beyond the walls of Constantinople, near the Seven Towers, in
1815, in which he took up his abode while the plague was
raging, for the sole purpose of investigating the nature of the
disease, this enterprising physician states, that there were
about twenty persons, who were in the most close and constant
intercourse with the sick; that out of all this number, there
was but one individual, and that was himself, who was attacked
by the malady; that the persons who remained exempt, lived
in the wing of the building which was occupied by the sick;
that, for the most part, they inhabited the same rooms with the
affected; that he, on the contrary, occupied the wing on the
opposite side of the hospital; that he visited the patients every
two hours through the day; that, consequently, the intercourse
with the sick was more constant on the part of those who
remained exempt from the malady, than on that of the person
who was seized by it: that, on the other hand, the part of the
building which he occupied, was directly exposed to the influence of a north-east wind, which was the noxious blast at that
time of the year (August); and that, in its course it blew over
the adjacent marshy ground, while the opposite side of the
square, which faced the south-west, and which was occupied
by the principal servants of the establishment, was sheltered
from this pestiferous blast. It is the more necessary to state
these circumstances, because the advocates of contagion have
triumphed exceedingly at the trick which the plague wickedly
played the doctor, as if in revenge of his unceasing endeavours
to strip it of one of its most noble and appalling attributes.
But, notwithstanding this partial victory of the disease over
its arch enemy, and notwithstanding the joy testified by the
believers in contagion, at its triumph, the fact will remain a
standing proof, that the darling attribute of the former does

not exist, and that the cause of the latter is without hope :—
the fact, that in the Pest hospital, to which the worst cases of
plague that occurred in Constantinople were sent, in which
circumstances peculiarly favoured the accumulation, and tended
to exalt the malignity of the contagious matter, if it had really
existed, out of twenty persons in the most close and constant
intercourse with the sick, dressing their wounds, ministering
to their necessities, performing all the offices which persons
thus desperately afflicted require—only one individual was
attacked by the malady, and that, the very person whose intercourse with the diseased was the least intimate and the least
frequent. Instead of being an argument in favour of the
existence of contagion in the plague, this fact is a proof arith-
metically as nineteen to one against it.

But that persons may maintain, for any length of time, the
closest possible intercourse with those who are affected with
the plague, and who ultimately die of it, without being attacked
by the disease, there is the most abundant evidence. Mr. Green
states to the Committee of the House of Commons, that at
Smyrna, in the year 1778, when the plague first broke out in
that city, the son of an Armenian merchant was taken ill; that
an intimate friend was sent with this young man to a place called
Ortaquey, a village about four miles from Constantinople, on
the banks of the Bosphorus ; that the patient remained there
nine days ; that at the end of that time he died ; that his malady
proved to be the plague ; that his friend attended him day and
night, during the whole of his illness ; that he slept in the same
room, probably on the same sofa (for the sofas go all round the
room), and yet was not affected by the disease ; that afterwards
the family removed to another village, where two of the servants
were attacked with the plague, one of whom died ; yet that
neither his friend, nor the master nor mistress of the house,
nor any other person was afflicted with the malady. Men
who have perished by the plague, have lived with their
wives, and women with their husbands, without communicating it. The Rev. Mr. Dawes, in his account of the
plague of Aleppo, among many particulars, which he says are
no less extraordinary than well attested, states, that a woman who
suckled her own child of five months, was seized with a most
severe plague, and died after a week's illness ; that the child,
though it suckled her, and lay in the same bed with her, during
her whole disease, escaped the infection ; that while the plague
was making terrible ravages in the island of Cyprus, in the
spring of 1760, a woman, after losing her husband and two children, who died in her arms of the plague, made it her daily em-

ployment to attend her sick neighbours, and yet escaped infection; that a Greek lad made it his business for many weeks
to attend on the sick, to wash, dress, and bury the dead, and
remained unhurt: that a blacksmith, who worked at Cartha-
gena, but whose residence was at some distance without the
walls, contracted the disease, and died in the same bed with his
wife, yet neither herself nor their children were infected. Mr.
Green states to the Committee of the House of Commons, that
he has himself known instances of persons who have slept with
others affected with the plague without taking the malady;
that, for example, Mr. Staars, a Dutch merchant at Smyrna,
had two daughters who slept together, that one was taken ill;
that her sister continued to sleep with her; that at last the
former died; that upon examination it was found she had died
of the plague; that they found the buboes on her; that, nevertheless, her sister did not take the malady, nor did any of the
family. He further states, that Mr. Parkins, an English merchant at Smyrna, had two daughters who also slept together;
that one of them was seized with the plague; that she got
well; that her sister continued to sleep with her during her
illness; yet that she did not take the disease, nor did any of
the family.

But it may be said that these are isolated facts; that, in this
argument, individual cases, however striking, however calculated
to impose on the imagination, ought to be reckoned as nothing;
and that no events but such as are on a very large scale can
warrant any general conclusion. Be it so. There are proofs
of the same thing on as large a scale as can be desired. Mr.
Green states in the Committee of the House of Commons, that
if the plague exist at Constantinople and not at Smyrna, and
persons affected with the plague go down from Constantinople
to Smyrna, although they die there, the plague does not spread
at Smyrna; and *vice versa;* that whenever it is carried into a
place in which it does not exist, it never spreads; that about a
year ago an English ship, the Smyrna, Captain Farmer, carried
down two Turkish passengers from Constantinople to Smyrna;
that one of these men died on board, of the plague, and that the
other was landed at the port, about seven or eight miles off
Smyrna; that the ship on her arrival performed forty days quarantine; that neither the captain nor his crew were affected
with the disease; and that there is no instance on record of any
English sailor dying on board the British merchantmen in
Turkey. Dr. Russell has recorded a fact in confirmation of
the non-contagious nature of this malady, which, for the singular completeness of the proof it affords, is one of extraordinary

value. In the month of April, 1759, a Turkish vessel from Alexandria was wrecked on the island of Cyprus; a great part of the crew who were saved happened to be infected with the plague; the contagion spread with great rapidity to the towns and villages. Mark the singular exception :—The town of Larnica, he says, at this time was remarkable. It had received a part of the infected crew; it had maintained a constant inter- course with the infected quarters of the island; peasants and mule-drivers from these parts with the pestilential sores on their bodies were daily in the streets and markets. Some of them died in the houses of Larnica; two vessels also arrived which landed infected passengers and sailors. Notwithstanding this new importation, none of the inhabitants of Larnica were known to have contracted the plague; *and yet the very year following it suffered most severely from plague,* in the months of February and March, when few or none of the affected recovered. The daily funerals were from twenty-five to thirty, and many of the inhabitants fled to the mountains. Here men affected with the plague, enter a town and have communication with its inha- bitants; the disease spreads rapidly. Parts of the same crew, affected with the same disease, disembark in another town, and have the like communication with its inhabitants; the malady does not attack a single individual. What is the in- ference? what must every intelligent and unprejudiced man admit to be the only rational explanation? That in the towns and villages in which the plague appeared, there was that year a pestilential atmosphere, which would have produced the dis- ease whether the crew of the ship from Alexandria had landed or not; that at Larnica, on the contrary, the atmosphere not being pestilential, the disease was not produced, notwithstand- ing the importation from Alexandria : that, however, on the fol- lowing year the atmosphere in this place was pestilential, con- sequently the malady was produced, and would have been equally produced whether there were importation from a fo- reign region, whether there were intercourse with an affected place, or not.

We shall adduce but one fact, or rather one class of facts more in confirmation of the opinion which the preceding state- ments are more than sufficient to establish; it cannot, at least, be objected to these, that they are not on a scale sufficiently large. Sir Robert Wilson, in the Committee in the House of Commons, states, that while in Egypt he saw many cases of plague; that that part of the army, Turkish and British, which moved against Cairo, passed through the country where numerous villages were infected with the plague; that during

the march the soldiers had constant communication with those
infected villages; that at Menoef, where the plague had raged
with the greatest violence, it was found necessary to establish
a bakery for the use of the army; that, however, none of the
persons who attended that bakery became affected; that at
Rahmanick there was a lazaretto or plague hospital; that it
contained several men who were lying infected with the plague,
and that many were brought out of it already dead; that others
were dying in the environs of the town of the same disorder;
that the Turks stript the bodies of all, indiscriminately, of their
clothing; that there was no restraint whatsoever in the communication of the army with the inhabitants; that the inhabitants had also free access to the camps; yet that no plague
was communicated to the troops; that the city of Cairo had
lost a great many of inhabitants the same year by the plague;
that when the army arrived at Cairo, and united with the Grand
Vizier's army, many of the graves in which the inhabitants had
been buried who had died of the plague were opened, and the
bodies stripped of their clothing with which the Turks covered
themselves; and yet that no soldier of either the British or
Turkish armies became infected with the plague : that the disorder ceased between the 17th and 24th of June, at the precise
time when its cessation had been anticipated.   Moreover, that it
was affirmed by the French officers that, although the plague
raged in Cairo that year with very great violence and carried off
some of the French army, yet that notwithstanding a constant
communication was held between the garrison stationed in the
citadel, and the inhabitants of the town, *the soldiers in the citadel
were not affected with the disease.*   That many thousands of the
inhabitants of Lower Egypt had died that year of the plague;
that the Indian army passing through Upper Egypt had traversed
a country in which about sixty thousand inhabitants were said
to have perished; that whole villages were destroyed ; yet that
the troops of that army brought no infection with them; nor
were any precautions adopted to prevent contagion on their
junction with the British and European army.   "To these circumstances," he adds, " I was myself an eye witness.   I
would wish also to state, that as we moved through the country the inhabitants pointed out to us particular villages that
were infected with the plague, *and which plague did not
extend out of those particular villages to any of the contiguous
villages, although there was no precaution whatever used as
to the communication with the inhabitants of the infected villages.*   Conversing with Dr. Desaguettes, the chief physician
of the French army, and M. Assilini, the head surgeon of the

French army, they assured me that, whenever a battalion, infected with the plague, had been marched out of the infected place, the soldiers recovered, AND NEVER CONVEYED THE INFECTION TO OTHER GARRISONS; and that troops marching into that infected garrison which had been vacated, did not become themselves affected, *unless they remained there longer than eight or ten days.*" What makes the phenomena of this disorder more remarkable, continues this witness, " is, that the villages are insulated, and built on parallel lines, not more than 500 yards asunder ; and though six or seven of those villages in one district may be affected with the plague, and though the inhabitants of those infected villages constantly pass through villages not infected, on their route to the Nile, yet though there is such a daily traverse and communication, the infection will remain in the villages where it broke out, and not extend infection through the district."

Now we do affirm, that if a man were to set himself to invent proof, that any given disease is not contagious, he could, by no effort of the imagination, suggest proof more precise, more complete, more overwhelming than that which is afforded by this narrative. It cannot be necessary to multiply testimonies : many others are on record, and might easily be cited ; but without advancing another argument of any kind on this subject, we would merely put to any man of candour the following question : Suppose what we contend for to be true ; suppose that the plague is really not contagious ; suppose that this were a truth fully ascertained, and universally admitted, what proof could there be of it ; what evidence is it possible to conceive which we do not possess ? The disease obeys every law of an epidemic ; it does not obey a single law of a contagious disease ; it is not communicated by wearing clothes impregnated with the sweat, pus, and ichorous matter from the bodies of those who have died of the malady ; it is not communicated by sleeping in the uncleansed beds of those who have perished of it ; it is not communicated by coming into the closest possible contact with their living body ; it is not communicated by sleeping in the same bed with them ; the husband who dies in the arms of his wife communicates it not to her ; sister communicates it not to sister ; the child deriving sustenance from the breast of its mother, who is perishing, and who does perish by it, receives it not ; the sick who fly for succour to a purer air, impart it not to the inhabitants of these more favoured places ; whole armies continue in unrestrained and constant intercourse, with affected towns and villages, without receiving it in a single instance ; again, then, we demand what proof is it possible to imagine, that this malady is not contagious, which we do not actually possess? The Committee of the House of Commons, in their report on the doctrine of contagion in the plague, intimate, that this evidence is insufficient. That they should have so thought at that time is not surprising; the subject was new; it was not possible that such facts, brought before their view for the first time, should be comprehended in all their important bearings, or produce their full impression; these facts are now better understood; the argument is much simplified; the evidence is more complete; the mystery in which the subject was enveloped is removed; ancient prejudice is shaken; reason and science have put to silence the clamour of medical authority, more ignorant than it fancied itself learned, and still more illogical than ignorant; that voice has forced itself to be heard; it will continue to be heard, and the truths it announces will prevail: we trust we shall find, in the result of the investigation about to be instituted in the British Parliament, that the period of their triumph is at hand.

We are obliged, reluctantly, to postpone the investigation of the facts (as they are called) which are alleged to prove the contagious nature of the plague; we shall embrace an early opportunity of considering these " facts;" we shall weigh in the balance of justice the medical authority, and examine with some strictness the medical reasoning on which they are founded; we shall then enter into a full consideration of the Sanitary Code.

Art. X.   1. *Remarks on the Yellow Fever of the South and East Coasts of Spain ; comprehending Observations made on the spot, by actual Survey of the Localities and Rigorous Examination of Facts, at Original Sources of Information.* By Thomas O'Halloran. M. D. &c. &c. London. 1823.

2. *A Treatise on the Plague, designed to prove it Contagious, &c.* By Sir A. B Faulkner, M.D. 1 Vol. 8vo.

3. *The History of the Plague, as it has lately appeared in the Islands of Malta, Gozo, Corfu, Cephalonia, &c.* By T. D. Tully, Esq. Surgeon to the Forces, and Inspector of Quarantine, &c. in the Ionian Islands, 1 Vol. 8vo.

4. *Report from the Select Committee of the House of Commons, on Contagious Fever in London,* 1818.

5. *First Report from the Select Committee of the House of Commons, on the State of Disease and Condition of the Labouring Poor in Ireland,* 1819.

6. *Observations on Quarantine ; being the Substance of a Lecture, delivered at the Liverpool Lyceum, in October,* 1824. By Charles Maclean, M. D.

7. *Report on Quarantine of the Select Committee of the House of Commons, on the Foreign Trade,* 1824.

IN considering the subject of contagion in our last number, we stated in detail the laws which regulate contagious and epidemic diseases ; we pointed out the source of error which has led both medical and unprofessional men to confound maladies so opposite and so incompatible ; we adduced the evidence, that Yellow Fever and Plague belong to the class, not

of Contagious but of Epidemic diseases ; and we proved, that
neither of these affections is capable of being communicated
by one person to another. We were obliged to postpone the
consideration of the evidence, on which the advocates for the
contagious nature of these diseases ground their faith. As it
is our wish to exhibit to the reader a complete view of this important subject, we proceed with the statement of that evidence,
after which he will have the whole case before him, and will be
competent to form an opinion of it for himself.

We hoped we should have been saved the trouble of going
over the facts alleged to prove the contagious nature of the
Yellow Fever. That disease has lately been so strictly investigated, and so great a proportion of those who have had an
opportunity of observing it, have been satisfied that it is not
contagious (and we refer for proof of this to Dr. O'Halloran's
interesting work), that most professional men are now ashamed
to avow themselves the advocates of a prejudice which is nearly
obsolete. There are circumstances of recent occurrence, however, which appear to have revived the expiring faith of some
devout believers in the common doctrine ; and to these it may
be proper to advert, especially as it will afford a specimen of
the kind of evidence which satisfies the minds of these persons,
and which they represent as irresistible.

In 1823, the yellow fever prevailed at Sierra Leone, in the
Bann sloop of war, and at the Island of Ascension. In all
these places the disease is supposed to have had a common
origin, and Sir Gilbert Blane believes, and has endeavoured to
prove, that it arose on board a merchant timber vessel called
the Caroline, and was propagated thence by contagion. The
facts are as follow. The Caroline arrived at Sierra Leone, from
Europe, with a crew perfectly healthy ; she landed her cargo at
Tomboo Island : during this time, which was considerable, she
lay in a low, swampy situation, surrounded with mangroves ;
in about a month after she had been on this station, her crew
became sickly ; but it was not until *three months* after her
arrival on the coast, that any of her men became decidedly
affected with yellow fever. Almost simultaneously with, yet
somewhat previously to, her sending to the hospital on shore
the first man affected with this disease, it had appeared in the
colony. " *At this time,* says Dr. Barry, the physician of the
hospital, the fever had begun its ravages on shore ;" and consequently, as this gentleman observes, the disease could not
possibly have been communicated to the colony by the Caroline. While the crew of the Caroline were in a sickly state,
she was visited by the master of the Bann, by the master of

the Snapper, and by the carpenter and carpenter's mate, of the Owen Glendower frigate; these persons remained on board several hours; one of the officers, namely, the master of the Bann was afterwards taken ill of fever, and he continued ill two days; in the mean time, the crew of the Caroline had constant communication with the boats' crews of the different men of war, at the watering place, without communicating the disease to a single individual. She sailed for England on the 5th of May; she arrived there on the 29th of June; during her passage, all her invalids recovered, and not one of her passengers, of whom there were several, became affected with disease. From this narrative, it is plain, that this vessel could have had no influence in communicating yellow fever, either to the shore, or to the vessels near it.

The Bann sailed from Sierra Leone, on the 27th of March; four days afterwards three of her men became affected with fever; in three days more, four others were added to the list, and from this period the disease spread amongst the crew very rapidly, and proved extremely fatal. She reached the island of Ascension on the 25th of April; her sick, forty-five in number, were immediately landed: tents were pitched at the distance of five hundred yards from the garrison, and all intercourse was interdicted. At this period the garrison was in good health; two days after the sick had been landed, one case of fever occurred in the garrison; twenty days afterwards, another person belonging to the garrison was taken ill, and subsequently the disease attacked twenty-eight persons. While the Bann was at Ascension, the Driver sloop of war arrived from Sierra Leone with her crew in perfect health; two clerks were sent from her on board the Bann; they were both taken ill; two other officers visited the Bann, neither of whom became affected. The Bann sailed from Ascension on the 2nd of June; she arrived at Bahia on the coast of Brazil on the 10th of the same month; among other vessels she found there the Tartar frigate; a boat from the frigate came alongside her *during a heavy rain;* the boat's crew sheltered themselves on board; in a few days afterwards some of this crew were attacked with fever.

Such are the facts, and so clearly do they prove, in the opinion of Sir Gilbert Blane, that yellow fever is a contagious disease, that he conceives he has settled the controversy by the statement of them; and a writer in the Medico Chirurgical Review for January last says—" We think that few men, not completely blinded by prejudice, or wedded to some favourite doctrine will reject, or doubt the evidence which has been brought forward respecting the contagious character which this fever evinced in the Bann, both at Ascension and Bahia. *If this evidence be questioned, it is in vain to look for further testimony in human affairs."*

Now, in reference to the fever of Sierra Leone, it is sufficient to observe, that it was the usual fever of the climate, and the usual Epidemic season. In reference to the fever on board the Bann, it is obvious, that the crew were exposed to the same epidemic constitution of the air as the people on shore ; and the surgeon of the vessel states, that they were, moreover, subjected to severe labour in re-fitting the Bann, and the San Raphael, a Spanish schooner, which the Bann had captured, and to great exposure to the heat of the sun, while they at the same time indulged in " irregularities." The continuance of the disease after the vessel left Sierra Leone is attributed by the same gentleman " to vicissitudes of the weather," which he states were great, and observes in his Report, that " *the men were generally taken ill in the night, when exposed to chills on their watch."* It appears, also, that relapses were so frequent (events which we have shown to be of most rare occurrence in a contagious disease) that out of the number seized by the malady, twenty-two had *two* attacks, two had *three* attacks, and one had *four* attacks. With reference to the alleged communication of the disease from the Bann to the Island of Ascension, it appears certain from the facts adduced by Dr. Burnett, that this island is subject to the visitation of fever " exactly similar " to that which prevailed on board the Bann; it is probable, that its epidemic season is precisely that at which the events of which we are treating took place ; it will be observed, that the first case of fever in the garrison occurred two days after the landing of the sick, which is too short a period for the operation of contagion : while the next case did not happen until twenty days after, which is too long a period for the contagion to have remained quiescent, if, as is affirmed, notwithstanding " nominal restrictions," the communication between the garrison and the sick was, in point of fact, immediate and direct. The disease, it appears, prevailed at the springs, that is, at the lower posts on the island, which is precisely the situation in which epidemics always prevail; while at the higher post, namely, that at the Green Mountain, 2,500 feet above the level of the sea, *there was not a single individual attacked, although the communication between the persons at this post, and those at the others, was kept open for eighteen days, and one of the soldiers stationed at it had actually been on board the Bann, and remained there some time.* With reference to the

alleged communication of the disease from the Bann to the
Tartar frigate, at Bahia, we suppose no one will expect us to
reply to an argument, in favour of the doctrine of contagion,
founded upon the circumstance, that part of a boat's crew, who
had taken shelter in a vessel during a heavy rain became some
days afterwards affected with fever; and with reference to all
these events, we fear the reader will scarcely forgive us for
detaining him with things so frivolous, although in a Medical
Journal, published not three months ago, it is affirmed, that
they establish the contagious nature of yellow fever in so clear
a manner, that if this opinion be " henceforward questioned, it
is in vain to look for further testimony in human affairs."

The facts alleged to prove, that the Plague is contagious,
may be arranged under those of ancient (not ancient, indeed,
in the common acceptation of the term) and of modern date.
The earliest fact of this kind on record is that stated by
Fracastorius in 1547, who affirms, that " out of one leather
coat, there died five-and-twenty Germans, who put it on one
after another." This " fact" is said to have happened thirty
years before, during a plague at Vienna; the narrator does not
pretend to have witnessed it; he gives no testimony, on the
authority of others; the scene is laid in Italy; the victims are
Germans. Alexander Benedictus [Lib. de Peste, cap. 3.]
informs us, that there was a feather bed which was thrown
aside into a remote corner of the house, because it was " suspected to hold the plague in it, and that it raised the plague,
by being shook up, seven years after, of which 5,900 people
died in twelve weeks in Wratislaw." And in another place, we
are told by the same author, that " the pestilent contagion was
shut up in a rag for *fourteen years!*" Forestus affirms, that a
young man was seized with the plague, only " by thrusting his
hand into an old trunk wherein there was a cobweb, which in
that instant made a plague sore." The plague of London in
1665 is attributed to a Frenchman, who is said to have died of
the disease in Drury-lane, and to have had in his possession
some Turkish silk, which had been imported the preceding
year from Holland, and in which the contagion resided, although
there is no proof even of the existence of this Frenchman,
much less that he died of the plague with silk in his possession,
and that this silk came not from Lyons, but from Constantinople. During the epidemic in 1698, says Noah Webster,
" a flock of quails flew over the chimney of a house, in which
several diseased persons were, and five of them fell dead upon
the spot!" Such are the facts on which the elder contagionists
relied : the three first are the principal circumstances adduced

by Sennertus, to prove that the plague is a contagious disease, and they appear to have been the main, if not the only foundations, on which Sanitary laws were first established.*

Most of the facts adduced by the later contagionists are of a similar character. Dr. Wittman informs us that the brother of the French general Julien, who died of the plague in Egypt, had " received the infection by taking a pinch of snuff from a box, out of which a person who had the plague on him at the time had also taken snuff." It has been affirmed that a man dropped down dead of the plague by standing on a Turkey carpet, and that a lady by only smelling at a Turkey handkerchief died of the plague on the spot. Yet Dr. Russell declares that amongst the many thousands whom he saw ill of plague he never met with an instance where the person was sensible of the stroke of contagion at the time ; and Assalini observes—" It has often been said that, in breaking open a letter, or on opening a bale of cotton, containing the germ of the plague, men have been struck down and killed by the pestilential vapours. I have never been able to meet with a single eye-witness of this fact, notwithstanding the inquiries which I have made in the Lazarettos of Marseilles, of Toulon, of Genoa, Spezia, Livournia, Malta, and in the Levant ; all agree in repeating that they have heard of such an occurrence, but that they have never seen it . happen." Nevertheless, Dr. Augustus Bozzi Granville relates to the Committee of the House of Commons that in Corfu in 1815 a priest who went into the church and touched the cloth of the great altar so as to shake it, in order to purify it, was seized with the plague; that he instantly fell down on the steps of the altar, and that in three hours, even before he could be carried to the Lazzaretto, he expired, with buboes under the arms and livid spots over the body. Dr. William Pym, " Confidential Adviser of the Privy Council on matters of Quarantine," states to the same Committee, that although he is not acquainted with the plague by personal observation, yet that he *knows* one instance of its communication at sea by direct contact : namely, on board his Majesty's ship the Theseus, which, according to his account, having captured some French gun-boats that were ordered alongside, the person who went " on board to issue provisions, &c. received the infection of the plague." Dr. Robert Tainsh, however, was subsequently examined, who states that he was surgeon of the Theseus ; that five persons affected with plague were, indeed, taken on board this vessel, but that

* See Sir Richard Manningham's Discourse concerning the Plague, &c. 1758, p. 25.

the disease was not communicated to any individual in the ship; not to a single man, although there was both direct and indirect communication between the ship's crew and the sick.

Abundance of stories of the like kind respecting equally the yellow fever and the plague are related by many medical men, and with a strange credulity are believed by others; but to enumerate no more of such absurd fictions, let us attend to the alleged facts which are deemed by grave authority as irrefragable and decisive.

Sir Arthur Brooke Faulkner, M. D., who was at Malta during the prevalence of the plague in that island, in the year 1813, considers himself, and appears to be esteemed by others, as the great modern authority on this subject. This gentleman was examined by the Contagion Committee of the House of Commons, and his evidence is given at considerable length in their Report: since that period he has "deemed it necessary" to publish a book, expressly, as he tells the College of Physicians, in the dedication of his work to that learned body, "in consideration of the weight attached to his evidence:" and certainly the college have given some indications that they rely upon him as their main prop. He informs us that he has had peculiar and excellent advantages for ascertaining the nature of the plague: that he has availed himself of his opportunities with the utmost diligence, and that whenever he has related any circumstance which did not fall under his own personal observation, he has employed the greatest caution in investigating the truth. The result of his labour he details in the following order:—" I propose to comprise the arguments and facts collected during my services in Malta, in support of the contagious property of the plague, under the following divisions: 1. The extension of the disease to Valetta from the infected vessel, San Nicolo. 2. Its extension to the individuals who were infected by communicating with the first case in Valetta, and to the Augustin Convent. 3. And its extension to certain of the Casals, and to the island of Gozo." The propositions, then, are, that the plague extended by direct communication from the San Nicolo to the city of Valetta; that the person first affected in Valetta communicated the disease to other individuals; and that thus extending through the city, it was communicated to the Casals or villages in its neighbourhood. The whole argument depends, it is obvious, upon the clearness with which it is made out, that the first infected person in Valetta had communicated with the infected vessel : the evidence to establish this fact must, to use our author's own term, be "direct," because upon that fact every other rests; it is the first link upon which every other that composes the chain hangs. What then must be the astonishment of every one, to read in immediate succession to the propositions just quoted, the following words: —" The evidence will in each of these instances of communication be made out by *direct* proofs, *excepting in the first*, which, for want of facts derived from satisfactory authority to establish fully an actual communication between the San Nicolo and the city, &c," In the outset, then, he admits that he is destitute precisely of that very evidence which, according to his own showing, is essential to his argument. " The evidence of communication will be made out by direct proofs excepting in the first instance :" but the first instance is precisely that in which it is essential to make out the fact of communication by the most clear and irresistible evidence : yet he admits, in so many terms, that there is " a want of facts derived from satisfactory authority to establish fully an actual communication between the San Nicolo and the city." His argument is, that the plague is contagious, because the disease was conveyed by direct communication from the San Nicolo to the city of Valetta : that the San Nicolo was the *fons et origo malorum*, and that there was direct communication between this vessel and the city ; yet he himself states that there is no direct evidence of this communication : that there is a want of facts to establish any communication whatever. By this single admission he has himself proved that his whole argument is baseless and his entire evidence nugatory. But he maintains that although there is no direct evidence to establish the alleged fact of communication between the San Nicolo and the city of Valetta, yet that the indirect evidence is sufficient to substantiate it. Were this really the case, it would follow, that the evidence he has adduced is wholly inferential : that with all his opportunities and all his experience he has been unable to find a single positive proof of the proposition he maintains, and that the utmost he has achieved is the collection of certain rumours, and the narration of certain stories which, IF true, afford a presumption of that which no man of sense ought, or can believe, without the most direct and irresistible evidence. This " indirect" evidence, however, which is to supersede the necessity of all positive proof, is—what may the reader suppose? A letter addressed by himself to the commander of the forces a few days after the arrival of the San Nicolo at Malta. This letter consists of an expression of the violent panic into which he was thrown by the arrival of this vessel in the harbour, and of a suggestion that it should be removed to a greater distance from the city. The letter was written on the 10th of April; on the 16th, that is, six days after it was presented to his Excellency, the first case of plague is rumoured to have occurred in the town of Valetta, and this Sir Arthur Brooke Faulkner considers as an absolute and perfect demonstration that the plague is a contagious disease. The argument is—A vessel arrives in the harbour of Valetta; throws the doctor into a panic; he writes to the governor on the 10th of April: on the 16th a person is taken ill of the plague in Valetta; therefore this person was affected with plague, in consequence of direct communication with this vessel; whence it follows that the plague is a contagious disease. On stating this argument to the Committee of the House of Commons, and on being requested to trace the connection between the vessel and the family first affected, he says—" I hold it as hardly requiring proof that the disease should have found its way from an infected ship in the harbour, when I consider the *apparent* connection between the cause and effect arising out of the arrival of the vessel; and the almost immediate verification of my prediction to the governor. I consider these circumstances as conclusive." Here the very thing to be proved, is stated to require no proof, and accordingly is taken for granted. " I think it an event not improbable," he continues, " that some of the family might have got goods from this vessel." And in another place, when asked if he had no better proof to advance, he says—" I think when the whole evidence I have given is well weighed and considered, the proof is made out as far as presumptive evidence can well render it." Then, were all his evidence valid, and all his induction just, the utmost he would have effected, even according to his own statement, would be the establishment of " an apparent connection:" the rendering an event " not improbable;" the making out a " presumptive" proof; and on this it is that we are asked to rest our faith in the tremendous doctrine of pestilential contagion!

Such is Sir A. B. Faulkner's language before the Committee of the House of Commons. Mark the difference when he sits down in his study to compose his book in order " to guard against the least appearance of inconsistency or mis-statement : to do justice to the information he can afford, and to convey his opinions in all the force of which they are susceptible." Then so complete, so " intuitively obvious " does the evidence of the contagious nature of the plague, afforded by his letter to the governor, appear in his estimation, that he doubts whether any attempt to render it more so, would not " as in the case of axiomatical truth rather tend to tarnish its clearness :" that no one can hesitate a moment to conclude that it establishes the fact " that the presence of the San Nicolo, and the plague which manifested itself in Valetta do stand to each other in the relation of cause and effect." " This, I confess," he continues, " appears to me, as a learned authority observes, one of those consecutions which are so intimately and evidently connected to, or founded in, the premises, that the conclusion is attained, *quasi per saltum*, and without any thing of ratiocinative process, even as the eye sees its object immediately and without any previous discourse."—" To allege in the face of the above letter," he adds, " that the breaking out of the plague in Malta on the arrival of the San Nicolo, was a fortuitous coincidence, would be not less rational than to maintain that an explosion taking place at the time of applying fire to gunpowder was a mere contingency; that the *only* difference in the two cases is, that, in respect to the fire, the effect is more constant and immediate than with reference to the plague ship;" but he considers this " want of constancy in the succession of causes and effects" as trifling, and of no consequence in this argument.

But further—Sir A. B. Faulkner states that the manner in which the plague was introduced into Valetta from the San Nicolo, was by a piece of linen, part of her cargo, which was purchased by one Salvatore Borg, a shoemaker, whose family was the first infected. When strictly questioned as to this fact by the Committee of the House of Commons, he acknowledges that he does not know any thing which could have conveyed the disease from this vessel to this family, excepting this linen; yet immediately afterwards he admits that he cannot speak with confidence as to the linen being found in Borg's house, much less is he sure that, if it were there, it came from the vessel. " I beg to be understood in giving this evidence that I was not present myself, and therefore I cannot speak with confidence as to the linen being found in Borg's house. I did not see the linen myself. It was confidently rumoured to have been brought from the infected vessel. I am not aware of any thing which could have conveyed the disease from the ship to the city except the linen. I rest my whole evidence upon what I before specifically stated, namely, the circumstance of my prediction," &c. &c.

Having accounted in this very satisfactory manner for the introduction of the plague into Valetta, in the first instance, he proceeds to show that the disease must be contagious, because from this first point, it proceeded in the direct line of contact. From Salvatore Borg's family, he affirms, it proceeded in a direct line to that of Maria Agius; but the only reason assigned for this is that the two families of Borg and Agius were intimate, and he distinctly admits that he only had the case from report

" I *heard* that Maria Agius and others she immediately communicated with, were attacked by the disease." The malady
having thus extended " in the direct line of contact " to these
two families, it was communicated by them, according to his
account, to other individuals in Valetta; and from these to
others, until the whole city became affected; and from the city
it was extended, still in the direct line of contact to the casals
or villages in its neighbourhood. These circumstances he adduces as facts : they must be facts, and substantiated in the
clearest manner, to render his argument of the least value; yet
he produces no evidence whatever of their 'truth ; on the contrary, he admits in so many terms that he has no evidence to
produce.   " I could not trace," he says, " the progress of contagion from Agius to any other family.   I dropped the inquiry
there : it appeared to me impossible to carry the investigation
in a *direct line* farther." How then does he know that it proceeded
in a direct line from these families to others, and from the city to
the casals? In what manner he ascertained the former he does
not inform us, but that it proceeded in a direct line from Valetta
to the neighbouring casals, he endeavours to substantiate by the
testimony of one of the captains of the Lazaretto.   " I am in
possession of documents furnished to me by one of the captains
of the Lazaretto, showing that the contagion made its way in a
direct line from Valetta into the affected casals and villages."
This account, together with his acknowledgment that even the
cases of Borg and Agius which he had so positively stated to be
cases of plague, were not known to himself to be so, but were
only rumoured to be plague, appears to have excited the scepticism of the Committee, for they immediately put to him the
following question :—" Then not-one of these cases in which you
state, &c. &c. *was from your own personal observation?"* Answer.
" *Not one.*"   And yet there were cases which did come under his
own personal observation, and they afford an excellent contrast
to those which did not.   A few of the soldiers became affected
with the plague : *the disease did not spread, however, amongst the
troops, although the soldiers lived, as all soldiers do, in the most
gregarious manner.*   This was one fact.   Moreover, he states
that he was in attendance on the military hospital, which was
the pest hospital; that he was personally and constantly close
to the sick ; that he is not certain whether he himself caught
the disease; that he is, however, quite sure, that the other
medical attendants did not ; that the orderlies, also, who were
employed under him in the care of the sick, and who were
necessarily in contact with those who had the plague, escaped
to a man,   Thus, in the only two instances in which he had an

opportunity personally of observing the disease, it is certain that it did not spread in a direct line, or in any other manner. Not to a single medical attendant—not to a single man out of all the orderlies, the nurses of the sick, who were in the closest possible contact with them, was the malady communicated. Every case of communication recorded by him was derived from rumour : the Committee of the House of Commons remark this : they represent to him that not one of the alleged cases of communication was from his personal knowledge, while of the numerous cases which fell under his own observation, the disease did not in a single instance communicate to persons, and he admits the truth of the observation.

Such is the evidence adduced by Sir Arthur Brooke Faulkner of the contagious nature of the plague as it manifested itself at Malta. To what does it amount ? A vessel reported to have the plague on board arrives in the harbour of Valetta ; Sir A. B. Faulkner is dreadfully frightened on seeing " its yellow flag with the black ball in its centre :" forthwith he writes to the commander of the forces : six days afterwards the first case of plague is reputed to have occurred, but there is no proof that this was really a case of plague : the medical man who saw it, and who is stated to be a physician of high respectability, declares that it was not plague, but typhus fever ; whatever were its nature, however, there is not the shadow of evidence to prove that it arose from communication with this vessel ; no connection whatever can be traced between them ; several individuals of the same family became successively affected with fever of a similar character : at length a person, in another family, is taken ill, it is rumoured, with the plague; this case is connected with the first only by the circumstance that the two families were intimate ; there is the same doubt whether it was really a case of plague : further than these two families, the extension of the disease by contact to other families in Valetta is not pretended to have been ascertained ; it is said, but it is a mere report, an entire assumption, that from Valetta it was communicated by direct contact with the nearest villages ; not the slightest evidence is advanced to prove that this was the case ; the soldiers who were taken ill with the malady did not communicate it to their companions ; the medical officers who attended the sick did not become affected ; the orderlies, who were the nurses of the sick, escaped in every instance. And yet this is the proof, this is the " series of decisive facts and concatenated evidence," by which Sir A. B. Faulkner states that he has " no doubt of being able to substantiate that the plague is produced by a specific contagion, and communicable only by contact or close approximation with infected persons or materials," and of which there is too much reason to believe that the College of Physicians, in their official report, declare that it " fully ascertained the contagious nature of the plague !"

As Sir A. B. Faulkner may be considered the representative of the college of physicians, so Mr. Tully is understood to be the defender of the faith of the Army Medical Board. He also has written a book on the Plague at Malta, which is valuable not for the additional facts which he has supplied, but for the reasoning which he has advanced. We have had a specimen of the facts which satisfy the contagionists ; it is right to attend to the reasoning with which they " exhort, rebuke, and confirm." After stating with as much confidence as though it were an undoubted and indisputable truth, that the original source of the plague was Egypt; and informing us, amongst many other things respecting its early history and progress, that it was first introduced into Europe at the period of the Crusades, in consequence of the intercourse which took place at that time, between the European nations and the inhabitants of the East, Mr. Tully says—

' The contagion of the plague is THUS *proved* by the general history of its progress, and medical *science* has been for centuries past accustomed to speak of it, and to treat it as a contagious disease. Fanciful theorists have sometimes hazarded a contrary doctrine ; but *experience* has always proved its fallacy. Thus, of the plague of Marseilles in 1720, the physicians of Paris believed that it was not contagious ; the fatal consequences are too well known : 60,000 persons fell victims to the disease in the short space of seven months. The faculty of Sicily declared the distemper which ravaged the city of Messina in 1743 not to be of a contagious nature, and in the short space of three months 43,000 individuals were sacrificed. The *theoretical* doctrine of non-contagion is *in these instances refuted* by the plain *demonstration* of *facts*.'

Thus, because the physicians of Paris believed the plague of Marseilles not to be contagious, *therefore* 60,000 persons died in seven months; because the faculty of Sicily declared the distemper which ravaged Messina not to be contagious, therefore 43,000 persons died in three months ; and because these events happened, the doctrine of non-contagion is proved to be " theoretical, and is refuted by the plain demonstration of facts." Whatever may be thought of the logic of this argument, it undoubtedly shows that Mr. Tully is as well acquainted as Sir A. B. Faulkner with the meaning, and as severe in the application of the terms " proof, science, experience, demonstration," &c.

Of the argument of Dr. Maclean and others, that if " the

plague depended entirely upon contact with persons and things, its ravages would never cease, in those countries where no precautionary measures are taken to prevent communication between the affected and the healthy, Mr. Tully complains, that it is urged too triumphantly; yet he admits, that to a certain extent the inference is correct, " inasmuch as we rarely hear of the total cessation of plague in Turkey : there are only temporary intervals of calm, in which the disease slumbers for a time, breaking out perhaps with increased violence in the succeeding year." But if there be rarely a total cessation of the plague in Turkey, there is sometimes a total cessation of it; -and if there be ever, no matter for how short, or how distant a period, a total cessation of it, the argument of Dr. Maclean, notwithstanding Mr. Tully's objection to the term, is triumphant! Mr. Tully's metaphor is not happy. A specific virus cannot enjoy " a temporary interval of calm;" an animal poison cannot " slumber ;" so long as it exists and continues in contact with an animal body, it must work its work of destruction without sleeping night or day. We may not allow Mr. Tully to get out of a bad argument by the most graceful figure ; much less can we permit him to escape from a bad argument, by a worse metaphor. But our author, animated by this imagery, waxes bold to such a pass, that he at length absolutely declares, that this very argument of the non-contagionists, " is equally calculated to establish the doctrine of contagion, as to prove the contrary :"—how ? " inasmuch as the plague may be said to be constantly prevalent in Turkey, from the circumstance of its continually recurring after its occasional disappearance." The argument is—the plague sometimes, though rarely, ceases in Turkey ; the plague constantly recurs after its disappearance ; therefore the plague constantly prevails. Mr. Tully, however, admits that this syllogism does not satisfactorily explain why contagion has not entirely depopulated the countries in which no precautions are taken. He assigns, as a farther reason, that upon some individuals diseases, undoubtedly contagious, have no effect at all, and that there are persons who are unsusceptible to the virus of small-pox itself. In order to render this reason good, it must be shown, that every person in Turkey who, on coming in contact with the plague, remains unaffected, possesses a peculiarity of constitution similar to that which renders some individuals incapable of receiving the contagion of the small-pox. It is calculated, that the exemption from the contagion of the small-pox is as one in twenty ; it is probable, that the proportion of those who escape the contagion of the plague in

Turkey, even when the epidemic is very prevalent, is six-sevenths of the whole population; were these six-sevenths therefore to possess a constitution similar to that which is now possessed by one in twenty, that constitution would no longer remain peculiar; it would be the prevailing constitution, it would form the rule, not the exception; the plague, how contagious soever, would become sporadic and never epidemic; the multitude of mankind must always be free.

Mr. Tully proceeds—

' What has been already said will be considered, by all those whose minds have not been strongly pre-occupied by the contrary opinion, as a complete refutation of the principal and favourite argument of the advocates of the non-contagion of the plague. But, lest our reasonings on this subject should be deemed inconclusive, we shall proceed to *prove,* that this objection which has been brought against the doctrine of contagion, is equally applicable when opposed to the system of non-contagion. Let us, then, for the sake of argument, suppose, that the plague is propagated by a diseased state of the atmosphere. This is a cause equally general in its operation with contagion: it might even be said to be more universal in its influence; but thousands of human beings have breathed the same air with those victims of pestilential distemper, who were hourly dying around them, and have yet remained unaffected; therefore, the plague is not disseminated by any atmospheric cause.'

Admitted: grant that the plague is not disseminated by any atmospheric cause; does it therefore follow, that it is propagated by contagion? The hypothesis, that the plague is produced by a morbid constitution of the atmosphere is adopted, because it appears best to connect and explain phenomena; if it be shown that this hypothesis is ill-founded, it must be abandoned; but what follows? that the doctrine of contagion is established? Certainly, according to Mr. Tully's argument. " I shall prove, says he, that this objection is equally applicable when opposed to the doctrine of non-contagion;" and his proof consists of an attempt to show, that the plague is not dependant upon the atmosphere, in which attempt, for reasons that we cannot now stop to assign, he has entirely failed; but, in which, had his success been complete, he would have left his cause just where he found it. Mr. Tully should have foreseen this fatal blow to his " proud argument." This gentleman may be a very excellent surgeon, but he certainly does not succeed as a logician.

Thus have we selected for the edification of the reader, the strongest facts, and the best arguments we could find in favour of the contagious nature of the plague; we had noted, for his information, several others of a similar character, but, besides that our space will not admit of further detail, we fear it would neither interest, nor instruct, and we are quite sure that we deserve, if we do not receive, the gratitude of every sober believer in contagion, for not scrutinizing the evidence and the reasoning, for example, of Dr. Augustus Bozzi Granville, for we do not remember ever to have seen any thing so contemptible, advanced with so much effrontery—witness his story of the priest of Corfu, to which we have already adverted, and his ignorant attempt to reconcile the occurrence with the laws of physiology. Dr. William Pym, and Dr. Frank may also be thankful for our silence. We make our appeal on this question to the judgment of the reader ; we seriously and earnestly ask him if he can give credence to such tales, or place confidence in such reasonings, as have been adduced, and above all, whether he can believe, that they are sufficient to set aside the evidence detailed in our last number, to prove that contagious and epidemic diseases are opposite and incompatible—evidence derived from the nature of those diseases, and from the laws which they are found invariably to observe.

We must, in conclusion, advert a moment to the common epidemic of our own country, namely, Typhus Fever. Typhus fever is plague modified by the climate, &c. of Great Britain : plague is typhus fever modified by the climate &c. of the Levant. The two diseases are identical, and present as strict an identity of symptoms as the same disease existing in such different climates can do. The physicians of the London Fever Hospital, and all other physicians who are extensively acquainted with the typhus fever of the metropolis, know that the plague constantly exists in London ; that is, they know that cases constantly occur in this city with symptoms *exactly similar* to those of plague : namely, with bubo, with swelling, and suppuration of the glands of the axilla, and with carbuncle superadded to all the other symptoms of malignant fever. There cannot be a doubt that typhus fever is a true epidemic ; it obeys every law of an epidemic ; it is without a single character of a contagious disease. Into the evidence of this we have not at present space to go, nor is it essential to the argument ; it will be sufficient to state briefly a few facts which decisively prove that it is not contagious.

1. The seat of typhus fever is strictly local. Around the places in which it prevails, a line can be drawn with as much precision, as that which divides one geographical district from another. In London, for example, from the first inquiry into this subject, up to the present hour, it has been found to pre-

vail with invariable regularity, in its eastern and north-eastern
parts : namely, Shadwell, Whitechapel, Bethnal-green, the
neighbourhood of Shoreditch, the parish of St. Luke's ; Old-
street and Golden-lane ; Cow-cross and Saffron-hill ; Holborn
and Gray's-inn-lane ; the neighbourhood of Clare-market and
Drury-lane, St. Giles's ; the parish of St. George's, Kent-
street and the Borough.   From these places it is scarcely ever
absent; beyond them it very rarely extends, though it does
occasionally occur in other situations.   Were it really contagious this confinement of it to particular spots would be
utterly impossible ; it would certainly spread in the " direct
line of contact" to the nearest persons, houses, streets, parishes,
and districts ; it would be impossible by any human means to
prevent its extension.   The causes which really perpetuate it in
these places are ascertained ; they are the narrowness of the
streets and lanes in these districts ; the closeness, the want of
ventilation and the filth of the houses, and the great number of
persons who are invariably crowded into these wretched habitations.

2. Typhus fever is dependant on the state of the weather.
There is a state of weather in which after it has prevailed for
some time there is scarcely a case of fever to be found ; there is
a state of weather in which fever immediately arises and extends
with great rapidity ; for example, whenever the atmosphere is
loaded with moisture and the temperature is at the same time
mild.   Immediately that this is the case the wards of the London
Fever Hospital become crowded ; this is an event as certain and
uniform as the succession of the seasons ; the prevalence of
the epidemic during the last Autumn and Winter affords an
illustration of this fact ; in consequence of the continued rains,
and unusual mildness of the season, this institution has been
so crowded with patients, that several times admission has been
refused to applicants for want of room ; a circumstance of very
rare occurrence ; and much oftener, it has been necessary to
postpone admission for many days.

3. Typhus fever is sure to be generated, to prevail extensively
and to prove highly mortal wherever there is a scarcity of provisions, or wherever the food is of a bad quality.   Dr. Bateman
in his examination by the Committee of the House of Commons
states, that the extensive prevalence of the epidemics which
originally led to the establishment of the London Fever Hospital,
was preceded by two years of great scarcity. The account which
Dr. Cheyne lays before the Committee, of the state of Ireland,
preceding and during the epidemic which ravaged that unhappy
country in the years 1816, 1817, 1818, and part of 1819, is
truly horrible.

' Two unproductive seasons in succession,' he observes, ' had reduced the labouring class to the greatest poverty. Little or no employment could be had for labourers. The clothes of the poor were nearly worn out, and many of them slept in their body clothes for want of blankets ; from the wetness of the weather, turf for fuel could not be saved ; potatoes were wet, scarce, and dear ; wheat was every where malty,.so that when the fever began, the poor were in many places living on weeds. In the neighbourhood of Kilkenny, they were feeding on hips, on nettle-tops and other weeds. Near Strathbally, many families had fed on the tops of the wild turnip (brassica napus) ; and at Castledermot this weed called brasha bwee, and a little malty flower, formed the chief article of nourishment. There were in Castledermot, I was told, at least 200 willing labourers without employment out of 500, the wages of the labourer being only 4*d.* a day with food, potatoes being $3\frac{1}{2}d.$ a stone, and it being computed that a labourer at his three meals will consume a stone daily.'

Under such circumstances the usual fever of the county, of course, became epidemic ; and proved dreadfully mortal. There is no parallel to the folly of attributing to contagion the extension of fever in a community thus reduced to a state of famine.

4. Typhus fever never spreads in the neighbourhood of institutions established solely for the reception of cases of fever. When the House of Recovery, now the London Fever Hospital, was first opened in Gray's-inn-lane, Sir Walter Farquhar and nine other eminent physicians of the metropolis, with a view of quieting the fears of the public, signed a declaration that " there was no reasonable ground of apprehension on the part of the neighbouring inhabitants ;" nevertheless the neighbours made two applications to the Sessions for the removal of the establishment as a nuisance, and so great was the terror of the people that they would not approach the building, but walked on the opposite side of the street ; yet long experience of such institutions in London, Chester, Manchester, Waterford, &c., has proved that all such apprehensions are perfectly idle ; and the Committee of the House of Commons in their report state, " that not only no hazard of spreading infection has been incurred by these establishments, but that, in point of fact, the number of contagious diseases has been greatly diminished not only in the town, but in the very district and neighbourhood where houses of recovery have been instituted."

5. In the wards of large hospitals typhus fever is never communicated by persons labouring under this disease to patients affected with other maladies. In almost every hospital in London it is the practice to mix indiscriminately the fever patients with those labouring under other diseases ; yet fever never

spreads in these wards.   Dr. Edward Roberts, of St. Bartholomew's, in his examination by the Committee of the House of
Commons states, that " in that hospital they have no fever
wards ; that fever patients are intermixed with others ; that he
never knew an instance of the communication of the disease
from one patient to another; that the medical officers have all
been of opinion that to separate the fever patients from the rest
would not be so good a practice as that which now prevails, *because they have not perceived that the fever has been communicated : that he has been physician to the hospital twenty-four
years, and has never seen the complaint communicated from bed-
side to bed-side.*" When asked if it be his opinion that fever is not
generally communicated, he replies, " I think not. We sometimes
have patients brought in upon deal boards, and in some instances they come in and die in a very short time, in a state of the
highest putridity ; we should expect if a patient of that description were put into a ward for forty-eight hours, that ward would
be affected ; but I never have been able to trace fever from such
a cause, I never saw such a thing happen.   If, therefore, there
be free ventilation, I should think typhus fever not communicated." Dr. Thomas Young, of St. George's Hospital states, that
fever patients are mixed with others, and that no inconvenience
has been found to arise from that practice.   Dr. Nevinson, also
physician to St. George's Hospital states, that he never knew
an instance of the communication of fever for nearly twenty years,
during which he has acted as physician to that charity, nor during
nearly six years that he was in attendance as a pupil there
before, though he has certainly seen some of the worst states of
typhus in that hospital.   Sir J. L. Tuthill, physician to the
Westminster Hospital states, that in that institution there is no
fever ward ; that fever patients are mixed with others ; that no
inconvenience to his knowledge has arisen from this practice, and
that no fever has ever been generated.   Dr. H. H. Southey, of the
Middlesex Hospital states, that they have no fever ward ; that
fever patients are mixed with the others ; that no inconvenience
has arisen from this practice ; that no fever has ever been generated in the hospital since he has been connected with it, nor
before as he has been informed." Were persons labouring under
small-pox mixed indiscriminately in a ward with other patients,
or were only a single case of small-pox placed in each ward, the
disease would certainly spread, and so would typhus fever were
it really contagious.

6. The medical officers of fever institutions are in general not
attacked by the disease. " During four years attendance in
the hospitals of Edinburgh and London, and afterwards during

thirty-one years in private practice in Chester, and fourteen years and a half in the Chester Infirmary, and three years at Bath, I have been," says Dr. Haygarth, " in the habit of breathing air strongly impregnated with the infectious miasms of fever. In many, very many instances, I have visited patients ill of infectious fevers, in small close and dirty rooms ; yet never but once about thirty years ago had a fever. The physicians of the Manchester Infirmary, for many years, and particularly during the late widely-spreading epidemics in that large and populous town, have, with great fortitude and humanity, constantly visited the home patients ; that is, they have in innumerable instances breathed the most pestilential air in the most concentrated state with perfect impunity." Dr. John Mitchell in his evidence before the Committee of the House of Commons observes—

' I lived about three years in the Royal Infirmary of Edinburgh. It was my regular duty to visit the sick three times a day ; in the forenoon before the physician's visit, at mid-day in company with the physician, and in the evening alone. This evening visit generally occupied a considerable time : since at the bedsides of the patients admitted through the day, I had to make memoranda in writing of every fact and circumstance connected with the case, for the purpose of being recorded in the journals of the house. Frequently the evening duty was exceedingly severe, it was particularly so during the time the Russian sick were received into the Infirmary, when it was not unusual to receive on the same day, ten or a dozen fresh cases ; most of these were bad fevers and the subjects of them so exhausted, some even *in articulo mortis*, and withal so filthy and dirty, that I could not refrain from lending my assistance to strip off their clothes and get them comfortably laid in bed. Notwithstanding all this exposure in my own person to every way by which it is conjectured febrile contagion is received, by breath, contiguity, and contact ; notwithstanding, that I was called for successive nights out of bed to the fever-ward, where I have remained administering in cases of necessity, wine and cordials, and occasionally obliged to draw off the water of the patient by means of the catheter, an operation necessarily exposing me to the effluvia arising whilst the bed clothes were turned down, yet I never caught fever.'

He then states other facts, such as that he never saw fever patients communicate fever to other patients in the same ward, that he never saw fever communicated to the nurses and other attendants on the sick, and adds,

' In short I will state, that I never saw one instance of contagious fever in the Royal Infirmary of Edinburgh ; and if it be allowable, I may add the testimony of Dr. Rutherford, the able physician under whom I acted, to the same effect. He had been physician to the house, for many years ; and a man more accurate in observation or more gifted with ability in his profession, and enlightened by general science, is not, as the many who know his modesty will acknowledge, to be met with.'

Dr. Roget, who had been physician to the Fever Institution at Manchester from 1804 to 1808, states to the Committee of the House of Commons that no officer of the establishment has at any time been affectéd with fever generated within its walls. Dr. Holme, physician to the same hospital from its first establishment to the present period, confirms this statement in its full extent. Dr. G. G. Currey, physician of St. Thomas's Hospital states that fever has never been communicated to any of the medical attendants of that institution. The same and other physicians bear uniform and decided testimony to the fact that even the nurses in these institutions are not more subject to fever than other individuals of the community ; on the contrary, that they are in general remarkably exempt ; that, sometimes, however, for example, during the prevalence of an epidemic, when the wards become unusually crowded, and they are exposed to unusual fatigues they are now and then attacked ; but that it is a circumstance of extremely rare occurrence.

Now each of these facts taken separately, is a proof that typhus fever is not a contagious disease ; the evidence arising from the whole taken together is irresistible. And yet *there is no doubt that typhus fever is capable, under certain circumstances, of generating fever.* It is a fact established by frequent observation, that if the apartment of a person labouring under typhus fever be small, close and dirty ; if it be unventilated, and if the effluvia from the body be allowed to accumulate in it, the air will become so contaminated as to produce fever in those who breathe it, or who remain in it for any length of time. For example.—Some time ago there was a poor family consisting of four persons who were attacked with malignant fever ; they all lay in the same bed in an exceedingly close and dirty apartment ; they were visited daily by a physician who always took the precaution when he entered the room to throw open the window, to station himself between the window and the bed while he examined the sick and to remain with them but a short time ; he had repeated his visits daily during a week with impunity when he was accompanied by another physician ; the latter took no precaution, but examined the skin of the patients minutely and closely, standing on that side of the bed towards which the air from the window impelled the effluvia and so near as to receive both the effluvia and the breath in the most concentrated state ; he is said to have felt a sudden disagreeable sensation at the moment of exposure and he immediately became affected with fever which proved fatal. In the hospital of Hockenhearn after the battle of Det-tingen there were at one time 1,500 men all affected with ma-lignant or jail fever, accompanied with what was termed dysen-tery. Of course the hospital was excessively crowded, and the air of it speedily became contaminated in the highest degree; under these circumstances almost all the apothecaries, nurses and other attendants on the sick were attacked with fever. At the same time some persons affected with the same disease were placed in the large church of Maestricht where there was abun-dance of room ; *here no disease whatever took place among any of the attendants on the sick.* These two cases afford an excellent illustration, the one on a small, the other on a large scale, of the fact on which we wish to fix the attention of the reader. The physician who relates the first case adduces it as a decisive proof of the contagious nature of typhus fever, and it is certainly one of the most precise and complete facts in favour, apparently, of that doctrine which we remember ever to have met with. Sir John Pringle, who gives a full detail of the circumstances which occurred after the battle of Dettingen, was not only a be-liever in, but a champion of the doctrine of contagion, and con-siders the events to which we have adverted as establishing his opinion. And such, in truth, are all the cases on record alleged to prove the contagious nature of typhus fever ; we venture to affirm that it is not possible to adduce a single example of the communication of typhus fever from person to person which is not of this description. The fact is, as we have already stated, that fever produced by this contamination of the air, has hitherto been universally confounded with fever produced by a specific contagion ; but all that we have written on this subject, has indeed been a vain labour, if it be not at once obvious, that fever arising from this cause is as distinct from fever produced by a specific contagion, as common fever is distinct from small-pox ; *no fever produced by contamination of the air can be communi-cated to others in a pure air ;* there never was an instance of such communication ; that alone is sufficient to distinguish every fever of this kind from a contagious disease, which is communicable, and equally communicable in every possible state of the atmosphere ; and yet cases of this kind are con-stantly adduced, nay cases of this kind *alone can be adduced* to show that typhus, or that any epidemic fever, is contagious. Nothing tends so much to render and to keep ideas clear as the designation by appropriate names of things that differ ; it is therefore highly desirable that this class of cases should be dis-criminated by a distinct term ; for this reason we would denominate them CONTAMINATIVE. Thus in the enumeration of the causes capable of producing fever, so far as that disease is connected with the subject of contagion, we would say that fever may be produced 1st, by a specific contagion, 2ndly, by an epidemic constitution of the air, 3rdly, by a contamination of the air. According to this nomenclature there will be contagious fever, epidemic fever, contaminative fever. A contagious fever depends upon a specific animal poison, and can produce nothing but a disease in every respect similar to itself. An epidemic disease depends upon a morbid state of the air, or upon some other cause not ascertained; it cannot, however often it be affirmed, become contagious in its progress, because every disease that is contagious must depend upon a specific poison; but it may become contaminative; that is, in its progress it may so contaminate the air of the apartment in which the patient is confined as to produce fever in those who breathe it. It must, however, never be forgotten that in the same manner, and for the same reason, common continued fever, typhus fever, the confinement of the healthy as well as the morbid exhalations of the body, in fact, not only every disease but every circumstance which is capable of producing a certain deterioration of the air, may be the cause of fever : and of this no one will hereafter doubt who will take the trouble to read the few words which were said on this subject in our last number, [pp. 149, 151]. If it be said that in thus admitting that plague, yellow fever, typhus fever, common continued fever, or any other disease, may generate a something (whatever it be termed) capable when diffused in the air, and brought into contact with a healthy body, of producing fever, the whole controversy between the contagionists and the non-contagionists is reduced to a mere dispute about words, and that no contagionist believes more than is implied in that concession, we answer —We are of opinion that no contagionist does really believe more than is implied in that concession, but so little are the contagionists themselves aware of it, that they blame their brethren exceedingly for not having a larger faith ; and with respect to the controversy being a mere dispute about words we reply in the language of Condillac "that we think only through the medium of words; that the art of reasoning is nothing more than a language well arranged ; that however certain the facts of any science may be, we can only communicate false or imperfect ideas of them to others, while we want words by which they may be properly expressed, and that the sciences in general have improved not only because philosophers have applied themselves with more attention than formerly to observe nature, but because they have communicated to their language that precision and accuracy which they have employed in their observations. By correcting their language they have reasoned better."

When the distinction which is here pointed out between a contagious and a contaminative disease shall become generally understood and adopted, which we think will be at no distant period, every difficulty connected with the subject of contagion will disappear. The fear of contagion—that fear, the physical and the moral operation of which is productive of such incalculable mischief, will be at an end. All the precautions which can be taken against the propagation of disease by causes really capable of producing disease, will continue to be adopted. The necessity of cleansing the filthy habitations of the poor, and of removing this class of persons from their confined and wretched dwellings the moment they become affected with fever; the utility of separate hospitals, for the reception and treatment of that fatal disease; the importance of securing the most free and complete ventilation wherever fever prevails, and the danger of a long-continued exposure to air contaminated by effluvia arising from the bodies and the discharges of the sick, in small and close apartments, will remain, and will appear just the same. But while the general security, not only cannot be diminished, but must be increased by the extension of sober and just views on this important subject, the gain on the part of humanity will be greater than can be estimated. We do not speak without weighing the import of the words we use, when we affirm that, in the whole range of physical and moral agencies, there is not one capable of producing in human beings, feelings and actions of such gross selfishness, and therefore capable of rendering human beings so utterly base, as the belief of the common doctrine of contagion. The history of every epidemic furnishes but too abundant evidence of this truth. " I have seen the fears and credulity of many so wrought on," says Dr. Mitchell, speaking even of the ordinary epidemics of our own country, " that the house where a fever patient lay sick, was deserted and shunned by the very relatives." " These opinions respecting its contagious nature," says Dr. Barker, " speaking of the late epidemics which ravaged Ireland, seem to have taken complete hold on the minds, even of the poorer classes, *as appears by the practice so generally followed by them of excluding from their families those who had sickened with fever.*" " There is good reason to believe," he continues, " that one-fourth of the inhabitants of the town of Limerick were attacked with fever; at one time the hospital was so crowded, that in many of the rooms there were four ranges of beds strewed on each floor, some containing six, many four, and few, very few, appropriated to one patient: so that in a small room of twenty-four square feet the number was not unusually forty. Such was the conviction of the contagious nature of the disease, that the ties of family affection were in some instances dissolved, and the nearest relatives when seized with the disease were forced out of the cabins into huts, generally placed by the road side to prevent infection, and to obtain charitable relief." Dr. Cheyne gives a particular account of these receptacles, which " family affection" provided for the sick. " When any individual of a family was affected with fever," he says, " the rest were so much impressed with the danger of contagion, that they had him removed to a barn, or out-house (where they had prepared a bed and broken a hole in the wall, to admit of their handing in medicine and drink) and locked the door which was not unlocked till some time after the disease was over. When a stranger, or a labourer who had no cabin of his own, took the disease, it was quite customary to prepare a shed for him by the road-side; this was done by inclining some spars or sticks against a wall or the bank of a ditch, and covering them with straw. Under these sheds which the rain penetrated, the patients lay on a little straw. All ranks and classes of the people believed in the contagion of the epidemic. In several instances cottages were burnt, in order to destroy a latent contagion, which resisted all the ordinary means of disinfection: and so convinced were the poor of the disease being infectious, that their conduct in many places towards itinerants, and, in particular, itinerant beggars, from being kind and hospitable, had become stern and repulsive; they drove all beggars from their doors, charging them with being the authors of their greatest misfortunes, by spreading disease through the country." The causes which produced mendicants in frightful numbers, are thus explained by Dr. Barker. " The better classes were disabled from giving employment to the poor : the poor unable to pay their rents, quitted their tenures, or were ejected from them, and assembled in wandering hordes." And yet these are the unhappy beings against whom there was such a cruel combination, that " constables were stationed on the highways to drive them away, and prevent them from entering the towns; finger-posts were put up in several places, warning them off; several Catholic clergymen from the altar denounced the practice of harbouring them, and in Roscommon, the magistrate, attended by a physician and the priests, went through the town and admonished the people not to harbour them." During the prevalence of epidemic fever in America, we are informed, that the instances of " the abandonment of the sick, even by parents and children, are often most horrible." Among these, we are told of the case of a person who, having sent his wife and children from a town in which fever was prevailing, to a relation's in the country, while he himself remained in town until attacked by the disease, was desirous when he found himself ill, of joining his family ; and was taken to them in a cart. But " the cart was not suffered to enter the yard, or approach the house. The poor man got out of it, and was called to, not to approach, and at last a gun was brought, and he was threatened with being shot if he did not go away. He crept into an out-house, where he expired without any one going near him." " Amongst Europeans," says Olivier in his travels in Egypt, " the tenderest ties, the closest affections constantly yield to the alarm which this fell malady inspires. The desire of self-preservation breaks in a moment through the bonds of consanguinity, and stifles the most virtuous sentiments." That is the text : Howard the philanthropist gives the commentary. " I was informed," he says, " that lately in a hamlet belonging to the Ragusian state, all the inhabitants died of the plague, with the exception of two or three, *who were shot by order of the magistrates to the surrounding guard.* The 30th of January, 1784, it was perceived, that a man, called Simon Chiapiglia, from the burg of Luzaz, belonging to Spoleto, after five days of fever had a tumor in the arm-pit, of so much the more suspicious a nature, that he had been employed as a door-keeper in a lazaretto from which he had been discharged on the 21st of the same month, after having been made to perform quarantine. He was well watched ; but on the following day, as in a fit of delirium he endeavoured to escape, he was *killed with a musket shot* by the centinel." Sir A. B. Faulkner states, that during the prevalence of the plague at Malta in 1813, it was ordained, that if any person should *conceal his illness,* he should be punished with death, and that, accordingly, " a Maltese of the name of Antonio Borg, who was detected concealing his illness, whilst labouring under pestilential symptoms, *was publicly made an example of and shot.*" Mr. Tully informs us, that during the same epidemic, the inhabitants of Casal Curmi were " declared to be out of the king's peace ;" that " a military commission was established in that casal, for the purpose of carrying martial law into execution ;" that, at length, the inhabitants were entirely " shut up within their own precincts, by the erection of double walls, and by the establish-

ment without these walls, of cordon over cordon :" and that
" so effectually was this work performed, that retreat was
rendered impossible." The consequence was, that the mortality
was truly horrible.   Well may Mr. Tully say of Malta, during
this frightful period, that self-preservation was the only
acknowledged law; that all alike dreaded their fellow creatures ; that,

> " Dependants, friends, relations, Love himself,
> Savaged by woe, forgot the tender tie,
> The sweet engagements of the feeling heart."

Well may he deprecate the accusation of giving an exaggerated
account, and if, as he further states, " scenes have been painted
to him by eye-witnesses, of a yet far deeper shade," and if he
have himself repeatedly witnessed similar occurrences, in still
more distressing forms, we can well conceive, that " the
impressions which they left upon his mind can only cease with
existence."

Of the system of sanitary laws, which it was our intention to
have examined in detail, it is necessary, after the full consideration which we have given to the subject of contagion, to
say only a few words.   If we are right in our argument, the
whole system of sanitary laws falls of course: it is equally
without a basis, and without an object.   Sanitary laws consist
of those expedients which are adopted, during the prevalence
of an epidemic, to separate the diseased, or those suspected to
be diseased, from the healthy ; all these expedients resolve
themselves into confinement of the sick, either in a house, a
lazaretto, a ship, a town, or a district : and the means adopted
to secure this confinement are, to close up the houses, to draw
lines of circumvallation around the town, or district, and to
station beyond these lines cordons of troops.   This system
must be considered first, in relation to its operation in the place
in which an epidemic prevails : and secondly, in relation to its
efficacy, as a means of preventing the extension of the disease
to other places.

1. Since it has not been found possible by any expedients
which human ingenuity has hitherto devised, to prevent the
healthy from coming into contact, either directly or indirectly,
with the sick, the first and most obvious effect of this system,
in the place in which an epidemic prevails is, to preserve so
many nuclei of infection whence the disease may be perpetually
diffused. 2. Its second effect is, to increase the mortality of the
disease to a prodigious extent.   It must necessarily be attended
with this consequence, because its operation is, to confine the

sick to the pestilential air, which is the chief cause of their malady. Dreadful proof of this is afforded by every epidemic in which the system has been adopted. Thus, on the 3rd of September, a barrier was established between Barcelona and Barcelonetta, so as to place the latter town in a state of isolation. On that day there were in Barcelonetta nine sick persons; by the 10th the number had increased to one hundred and sixty-two; that is, in seven days from the isolation of the town, the daily mortality had increased eighteen-fold. In Casal Curmi, " a populous village," which was surrounded in the manner that has been stated, by lines of circumvallation and cordons of troops, almost all the inhabitants were exterminated. Of between eighty and ninety persons that were sent to the Lazaretto, at Malta, in 1813, *only two survived.* There is not a single fact on record to prove that these measures have the slightest effect in preventing the extension of the disease, or in shortening its duration. Sir A. B. Faulkner attributes the declension of the plague at Malta to the vigorous police regulations which were at length adopted; but according to his own account, although " the inhabitants of Valetta were shut up in their houses, and other strict measures of quarantine adopted," yet there was no material diminution of the disease until August, that is, precisely the month in which the epidemics of the island regularly decline. We have seen how completely the village of Casal Curmi was isolated. What was the result? The last case of plague occurred in Valetta on the 19th of October; the whole island was declared to be free from disease on the 7th of January, *with the exception of Casal Curmi;* there the plague continued its ravages till the 7th of March. This single fact is decisive. 4. This system tends in the highest degree to excite and perpetuate terror, which is universally allowed to be one of the most powerful concurrent causes of sickness and mortality. " The main import," says Dr. Mead, speaking of the plague of London, " of the orders issued out at these times was, as soon as it was found that any house was infected, to keep it shut up, with a *large red cross, and " Lord have mercy upon us* " on the door; and watchmen attending day and night to prevent any one going in or out except physicians, surgeons, apothecaries, searchers, &c. allowed by authority; and this to continue at least a month after all the family were *dead* or *recovered.* It is not easy to conceive a more dismal scene of misery than this. Families seized with a distemper, which the most of any requires help and comfort, locked up from all their acquaintance; left, it may be, to the treatment of an inhuman nurse (for such are often found at these times about the sick), and strangers to every thing but the melancholy sight of the progress death makes ; with small hopes of life, and those mixed with anxiety, and doubt whether it be not better to die, than to survive the loss of their best friends and nearest relations." 5. The knowledge, that they are to meet with such treatment induces the sick to conceal their illness until it is no longer possible to afford them any relief. 6. Medical men themselves, under the influence of this base fear, abandon their duty. During the prevalence of the plague in London, almost all the physicians fled from the city. At Oxford, during the prevalence of the malady, which arose at what was called the Black Assize in that town, almost all the physicians fled. When the yellow fever raged in Philadelphia, in 1793, many of the physicians abandoned the city, and in the Levant it is seldom that pestiferous patients have medical aid. 7. An insuperable obstacle is thus opposed to any increase in the knowledge, or any improvement in the treatment, of this fatal disease. And 8thly, not the least of the evils consequent upon the terror produced by this system, and by that belief in contagion on which it is founded, is the interruption occasioned to the supply of provisions in times of pestilence. People in the country will not risk their lives by bringing provisions to an infected city. The effects of this were dreadfully experienced, both in the plague of London, in 1665, and in that of Marseilles in 1720. Of the former it was truly said, that those who escaped the pestilence died of famine; thousands perished in the fields from want. Such are the invariable and inevitable consequences of a belief in contagion, and an adoption of sanitary laws, in the place where an epidemic prevails.

That part of the sanitary system which relates to the expedients adopted to prevent the extension of epidemic diseases to uninfected countries is called Quarantine, which consists in subjecting persons to a seclusion, and merchandize to a purification of forty days. The reason why forty days have been fixed on as the period necessary and sufficient to exterminate contagion in all its known and unknown states, no one has ever pretended to assign. Let us look at the system in relation to merchandize. The argument against quarantine as applicable to merchandize is short ; it is perfectly unanswerable ; it is wonderful that any doubt should remain upon any mind for a single moment, which has been made acquainted with the fact upon which it is founded. It has been proved that it is the universal custom in Turkey for the relations of those who die of the plague to wear the clothes of the deceased ; that garments saturated with sweat, pus, and ichorous matter from the bodies of those

2 N 2

who have perished by the malady, are invariably either worn by the relatives, or sold at the public market; and that there is no instance on record of the communication of the disease by this means. Then, what can be the use of establishing quarantine laws to prevent the communication of plague by means of merchandize from Turkey? The only way in which it is possible for merchandize to become impregnated with the contagious matter of the plague, even allowing that matter to exist in the greatest abundance, is, by its being exposed to the pestiferous atmosphere, or by its being handled by plague patients. But little or no importance is attached by the believers in contagion to the influence of the atmosphere in contaminating merchandize; the only way, therefore, in which goods can be contagioned is by being handled, or by coming in contact by some means or other with those affected with plague. But plague patients cannot labour in the fields to gather in the raw material; they cannot labour at the various processes by which the raw material is manufactured; they cannot labour in the warehouses, at the wharfs, or on board, in order to pack and to stow these goods; it is not, then, particularly easy to see how merchandize can become impregnated with contagious matter; but allowing that it may be so, surely no one will contend that it can possibly receive a thousandth part of the quantity of that matter with which the clothes worn by plague patients are imbued. If then in the very country in which the plague rages, at the very time that it is committing its ravages, the clothes of such persons are constantly worn by the unaffected, and invariably worn with impunity: if such be the fact, we again ask, whether in the whole history of human affairs there be an instance of such stupendous folly as that of supporting, at a great expense, an establishment, and subjecting commerce to innumerable inconveniences, for the sole purpose of preventing the introduction of the plague by merchandize!

Moreover, it is a fact allowed on all hands, that goods are actually and constantly conveyed from places where the plague prevails to certain other places without ever transporting the disease. The plague frequently prevails, for example, in Aleppo. Caravans proceed regularly with goods in bales from Aleppo eastward through the continent of Asia, and have never been known to convey the plague to a single place: since this commerce has existed, there is no instance on record of the communication of the disease by these caravans or their merchandize to a single individual in the whole continent of Asia. It is useless to add other reasons or other facts. He who is not convinced by the single reason and the single fact here stated, would not be convinced by a thousand.

A great impression has already been produced upon the government of this country. They have gone so far as to release all vessels coming from the Levant with clean bills of health from the necessity of performing quarantine ; that is, they have repealed 46 out of 47 parts of the quarantine system : having done this, they must repeal the remaining part; they must in consistency do so ; for Dr. Maclean has demonstrated in the clearest manner in his Lecture at Liverpool (a careful perusal of which we would earnestly recommend to every one who is interested in this subject), that bills of health can afford no criterion whatever of the state of merchandize with respect to its freedom from a contamination by pestilential contagion, even were that phantom a real existence. Bills of health are documents from Consuls to ships sailing from places subject to their consular jurisdiction, certifying the state of the health of these places in reference to pestilential diseases at the time of the departure of the vessels. A foul bill declares the presence, and a clean bill the absence of pestilence, in the sea-port from which a vessel departs at the period of her sailing. Now suppose two ships to load with clean cargoes in a period of health ; one sails a day before the other ; in the mean time a single case of plague occurs in the port; this obliges the detained ship, although she may have had no communication whatever with the shore, to sail with a foul bill. On their arrival in England one ship is immediately released ; the other is obliged to perform quarantine. Again, two ships load with foul cargoes during pestilence : one sails thirty days after the plague has ceased ; she must carry a foul bill ; the other waits ten days more, when she is entitled to a clean bill. The ship with a foul bill will be obliged to undergo quarantine, that with a clean bill will discharge her cargo at once ; but it is obvious that the danger in each case is equal ; and were the danger real, the ship with a clean bill must of necessity convey contagion to the market in which her goods are sold. Once more, a ship loads with a foul cargo during pestilence ; she waits forty days after its termination and sails with a clean bill. Another ship loads with a clean cargo during these forty days ; she is detained a few hours, and a case of plague is reputed to have happened in the port; she has no communication with the shore, yet she is obliged to sail with a foul bill. In this case, also, a contagioned cargo is covered with a clean bill ; and a clean cargo is accompanied with a foul bill. It is certain, therefore, that were contagion capable of being conveyed by goods, the cargoes of ships with foul bills would often be without the slightest danger ; while the cargoes of ships with clean bills would frequently be extremely perilous.

From these facts it is clear that the system of quarantine can not be supported by bills of health, the last prop on which it stands.

We cannot now stop to state that no expurgator of goods in England has ever been attacked with plague; that in point of fact no person coming from the Levant, or from any other country, has ever been known to arrive in England with the plague upon him; neither can we detail, as we intended, the expense of the quarantine system, nor the operation of the sanitary code, of which it is a part, on commerce in general; nor the mischievous influence and power which it gives to despotic government. We have already dwelt upon the subject, we fear, too long for the patience of the reader. The facts we have adduced, and the reasons we have urged, will produce their proper effect only upon that mind which reflects upon and weighs them; but in proportion as they are considered, we are satisfied, that the conviction of the soundness of the deduction to which they lead will strengthen. And surely, whether we regard the extent of the benefit to be conferred, or the amount of evil to be avoided, there is no subject which better deserves the serious consideration of the physician, the merchant, the statesman, and the philanthropist.

Art. X.—1. *A Treatise on Fever, &c.* By Southwood Smith, M. D. &c. London. 1829.
2. *Pathological Observations on Continued Fever, Ague, &c. Part II.* By William Stoker, M. D. &c. Dublin. 1829.

A CARELESS manipulation in the prosecution of an analysis may adulterate a long and laborious investigation, but the disappointment occasioned by such a failure can only be measured, when we know the practical consequences of the genuine result. In studying the laws of dead matter, an ungrounded conclusion will seldom endanger life, or induce sickness; in ascertaining the weights and distances of the heavenly bodies, the discrepancy of a few grains or inches can never be a fatal error. Mind may be analyzed according to the taste of the metaphysician, and dissected into five or fifty rudimental principles; stars may be weighed by avoirdupois or apothecaries weight, as it may suit the fancy of the astronomer; and the world may stand for ever marshalled into two or more conflicting sects on any abstract question of theoretic science, without involving in their differences the welfare of a single interest, or the safety of a solitary individual. But in medicine nothing can be more desirable than unanimity; nothing more destructive than partial and opposing views. In a science, having for its objects the prevention of disease, and the preservation of health —of all desired objects the most desirable—the simplest theory cannot be indulged in without bringing into stake a thousand lives. A random step upon such sacred ground must lead to danger, may lead to death. The lives of our fellow-creatures are the *materiel* we experiment upon, their happiness or misery is the issue to which every experiment must tend. A faithless rule, or a fanciful remedy, in the hands of a loose and inaccurate practitioner, may prove the cause of more real evil than a wide and woeful pestilence. Reasoning therefore in such a science should be conducted on the most rigid principles, and the chaste prose of sober truth should never be adulterated with the meretricious poetry of drunken fancy.

o 2

An examination of the two works at the head of this Article has insensibly led to this admonitory strain. Written by talented members of the same profession, devoted to the same subject, and constructed out of distinct experiences, which from their variety and extent lay claim to equal consideration, they are, nevertheless, seldom agreed on any point, save that of taking different views of the same subject. How writers of the same standing and of the same day, cultivators of the same science within the same kingdom, and attendants upon the same disease, should observe so differently, and infer so oppositely, must appear strange to any one who has never been behind the scenes, and who is unacquainted with the sources of such discrepancy. Of all diseases fever is the most uncertain in its external character. It may appear in a thousand different aspects, and originate a thousand different sentiments. It is modified by age, by constitution, and by temperament; by internal mechanism and external form; by moral character and physical condition; by climate, latitude, and origin. It varies in solitary cases, and in sweeping epidemics; in town and country; in thinly-populated districts and crowded cities. This year it may be characterized by mental depression and corporeal debility; in the next it may be distinguished for general excitement and topical disease. To-day it may require bleeding, and to-morrow wine. In the same individual, at different periods, it may wear very different physiognomies; while, in different individuals, at the same period, it may be peculiar only by exhibiting the same symptoms.

In this capriciousness of external character may be discovered one reason why, by some, fever is regarded as a disease essentially active, by others as an affection of debility : why one maintains that it is an effort of nature to relieve the system of some noxious humour, while another holds it to be one of the most frightfully fatal maladies to which flesh is heir : why this pathologist considers it as a local inflammation, producing general symptoms; that as a constitutional disease, implicating generally and alike every texture and organ : why one physician nurses it with wine and bark, while another starves it with purging and depletion : why every province has its own theory, why every town has its own practice.

But it may be asked, can the source of all our wide and woeful differences be found in this single cause ? Do they exclusively originate in the multiformity of the disease itself; or may they not partly arise from the imperfection of our own conceptions as to what fever essentially is, and how fever should be studied, to be studied with success ? These are most important questions, involving the very essence of this important subject; and should we, during their investigation, be compelled to differ from great and grave authorities, we trust that love of truth,—the common and centre spirit of all our inquiries,—shall be to us what we regard it with relation to them, an acknowledged and sufficient passport.

' The degree in which the science of mind is neglected in our age—and country, may it not be justly added ? especially in our profession—that science upon the knowledge of which the conduct of every individual mind is so dependent—is truly deplorable. Medicine is an inductive science, the cultivator of which is peculiarly exposed to the danger of making hasty assumptions and of resting in partial views, yet it is not deemed necessary that he should be at all disciplined in the art of induction, or should be cautioned against any sources of fallacy in the practice of making inferences. All the partial and imperfect views of fever which have now been brought before the eye of the reader, originate in one or other of the following errors, obvious as they all are : either that of assuming as a fact what is merely a conjecture ; or that of assigning to the genus what belongs only to the species ; or that of characterising the disease by what appertains only to a stage ; or that of mistaking the effect for the cause. On careful examination it will appear that one or other of these errors, which are as serious as they are palpable, has vitiated in a greater or less degree every generalization of fever that has hitherto been attempted.

' Thus the believers in debility derive their notion of the whole disease from the phenomena which occur in the first and the last stages only : in these, it is true, they may find abundant evidence of debility : but then they overlook the intermediate stage in which there are generally the most unequivocal indications of increased sensibility in the nervous, and increased action in the vascular systems : in this manner they characterise the disease by what appertains only to certain stages of it. Again, when they contend that debility is not only the essence of fever in general, but is really characteristic of every type of it, they affirm what is indisputable of fevers in particular seasons, in particular climates, or in particular constitutions ; but beyond this their generalization cannot be extended : in this manner they assign to the genus what belongs only to the species. And when Cullen goes on to affirm that the proximate cause of all the morbid phenomena is a " spasm of the extreme vessels," he commits the additional and more palpable, but not less common error, of assigning as an undoubted fact, as a real and ascertained occurrence, what is only a conjecture, and for which there is not, and for which he does not even attempt to adduce, the shadow of evidence.

' Precisely similar to this is the error of those who for the most part belong to the same school, and who attribute the essence of fever to a morbid condition of the blood. The blood may be diseased in fever, but if it be so, these writers do not know it, or at least they do not adduce any evidence that they are in possession of such knowledge : they do not appear so much as to have questioned chemistry ; at all events, it is certain that they have hitherto received no satisfactory answer. There is no evidence on record that the alleged deterioration of the blood takes place in every type and every degree of fever . and if there were it would still be but one event among many, and one that occurs late in the series, and therefore could possibly be nothing more than an effect.

In like manner those who maintain that inflammation of the brain is the sole cause of fever, assume as an established and admitted fact the universal and invariable existence of inflammation of the brain in this disease. Inflammation of the brain, without doubt, is demonstrable of many individual cases, and of some whole types : but beyond this there is no proof that the generalization can be carried : the evidence indeed in regard to many cases is entirely against the assumption, and is as complete as negative evidence can well be : consequently it must be admitted that even this hypothesis, in the present state of our knowledge, is founded on the error of assigning to the whole genus what belongs only to particular species : and it would be trifling with the reader to attempt to prove, that this is still more certainly and strikingly true with regard to inflammation of the mucous membrane of the stomach and intestines—an affection which in innumerable cases in which its existence is certain, clearly appears on the slightest examination of the succession of events, to be an effect and not a cause.

‘ No comprehensive view can be taken of fever, no just conclusion can be arrived at relative to its nature and seat until it be studied with a consciousness of the liability to such errors and a vigilant endeavour to avoid them. The present investigation has been undertaken with a deep consciousness of the danger and a watchful and unremitting care to avoid it. Even if the effort prove to be without success, the example can scarcely remain without use.

‘ The frequent and formidable disease on the investigation of which we are entering, cannot be understood until clear and exact answers are obtained to the following inquiries. 1. What is the series of phenomena which constitutes fever ? 2. What are the particular phenomena which are common to all its varieties and combinations ? 3. What is the order in which these phenomena occur in the series ? 4. What are the organs, and what their states, upon which these phenomena depend ? 5. What are the external signs of these internal states, or what are the indications by which their existence may be known ? 6 What is the external noxious agent or agents, or the exciting cause or causes of the disease ? 7. What is the particular remedy, or the particular combination of remedies which is best adapted to each state of each organ ? When these questions can be clearly and perfectly answered, and not till then, we shall know the disease and its treatment. In order to make any real progress in this knowledge we must therefore prosecute these inquiries. It appears to me that we are already in possession of ascertained facts, adequate to answer with a high degree of certainty, though perhaps not with absolute certainty, several of these questions.   In keeping these inquiries steadily before our view in our investigation there will be this great advantage, that it will enable us clearly to perceive what we really know and what still remains to be ascertained.—pp. 30—34.

So writes Dr. Smith, and we heartily concur with every sentiment expressed.   A fairer opportunity than the present could be seldom found for showing how sadly regardless the generality of medical writers are of the science of reasoning, and how frequently their inferences are drawn from premises in themselves equivocal, and which, moreover, are imperfectly understood.   That specific fever is " one and indivisible" can, in our opinion, be as indisputably demonstrated as the simplest problem in Euclid's Mathematics, and that our jarring systems as to its essence, seat, and cure do not arise exclusively out of the wayward fickleness of its external signs it is easy to prove. There is no doubt but that it wears a thousand varieties of aspect; that it is modified by climate, constitution, and treatment; that during one and the same attack it may be weak and strong; that in one and the same person, at different periods of its progress, it may be marked by nothing but torpor, or be remarkable for nothing but activity.   All this is true; all this not unfrequently occurs.   But this playfulness of form is a mere matter of degree.   In all cases the seat and sort of mischief are unchangeably the same; the same internal action is going on; the same external contour of feature may be ever recognized.   A stroke more or a stroke less may impart an individual peculiarity to a portrait, which had been previously a faithful resemblance; even a hair's-breadth deviation of the pencil from the path which it ought to traverse may constitute a characteristic deformity.   And hence it is, that one and the same painting, in the hands of a skilful artist, can assume five thousand modifications of countenance, ten times five thousand varieties of likeness, without losing or receiving a single feature, without even materially altering the original outline.   Now that which may be easily done by a limner's pencil working upon canvass, is daily wrought by the hand of Nature upon the constitution.   Fever, viewed as a unique and generic disease, wears certain features which are as constant and as characteristic as are those composing the original portrait of the painter.   In the first place, the nervous system is always deranged;—the mind is dull, heavy, and confused.   In the second place, the functions of the heart and lungs are always disordered;—the pulse is altered, either in strength or frequency, or both, and the respiration is either quick and imperfect, or slow and laboured.　In the third place, the secretions are diseased ;—the stools are offensive, the urine is either limpid or turbid, the skin is dry, the saliva is viscid, the heat is irregular—sometimes low, more frequently high, the appetite is defective, the thirst is ardent.　In every pure case of fever these phenomena are as steady and as sure as are the ordinary features in the artist's portrait.　They may be variously proportioned, both in intensity and number, just as the limner's colours may be modified.　In one case the brain may be more affected than the heart ; in another the lungs may suffer more than either,　In one instance the functions of the intestines may be especially deranged ; in another the prevailing symptoms may pertain to the head.　One constitution may be weak ; another may be strong.　In one case the morbid cause may be active, in another it may be moderate ; in the self-same case we may have the nervous, sanguiferous, and digestive organs successively attacked, so that the fever which began as cerebral and acute, may terminate as abdominal and typhous. Within the precincts of a short article it is impracticable to detail every modifying cause of fever; the preceding are merely a specimen of the many which might be adduced ; but, as the present purpose is to canvass general principles rather than minute particulars, this specimen will be quite sufficient for all the ends of argument.

　　It follows, then, from the preceding observations, that there are certain general symptoms characteristic of febrile action ; that these symptoms are essential to the presence of fever ; that accidental circumstances may modify their original character to a very multifarious extent, but that they still remain substantially the same ; and that, like a well delineated portrait, which may be transformed by the introduction of a few trifling alterations into endless resemblances, fever may present a multitude of aspects, and yet possess the same rudimentally essential character.　Ignorance of or inattention to this view of the subject, we believe to be the fruitful source of all our differences respecting this disease.　The original portrait is overlooked or lost amid the confusing transformations to which it has been subjected ; and what was nothing but a mere creature of circumstance and degree is embodied with the consequence of an original and independent entity.　Modes are thus converted into substances, types into species, and epidemics into genera. An entire and indivisible disease is broken down into as many distinct maladies as there are shades in the intensity of the exciting cause, in the strength of the patient's constitution, or in the activity of the internal mischief.　To know all these

variations in the form of fever is highly important; just as im
portant to the physician as it is to the limner to know what
effects different proportions of light and shade can work upon
his original portrait. A perfect understanding of the former is
as necessary to a successful practitioner, as that of the latter is
to a successful painter; and the general eminence of either will
not be widely disproportioned from the degree of success which
has been attained in this department. But, between a knowledge of these varieties, as abstract forms of disease, and a
knowledge of them, as aberrations from one common malady,
there is an inestimable difference. Two cases of fever may be
vastly different in external sign, and yet be identified in essence;
just as two portraits may be vastly different in general expression, yet have individual features strikingly alike. The elements of both may be symptomatologically, pathologically, and
in every sense the same, and the *pathognomonia*, or individual
peculiarities of each, may be found only in the proportion
which one element bears to another; and it were surely a sad
confounding of all order to mistake such matters of degree for
essential distinctions, and because of a few shadowy differences
to discover no similarity of substance.

A man, in previously good health and spirits, is seized with
the common continued fever of this country. He shivers and
feels cold, sensations of heat succeed, his mind is dull, his
strength is impaired. Severe pain is now complained of in the
head or chest, his pulse is full and strong, his skin is warm,
his thirst is ardent. A few days are allowed to pass before he
is again seen, and the following symptoms are present; the
head-ache is now dull, and accompanied with a sense of confusion and vertigo, his mind is always torpid and occasionally
confused, his pulse is quick and easily compressed, he sleeps
badly, his thirst is less ardent, his teeth, lips, and tongue are
covered with black and putrid matter, and his strength is much
reduced. Allow this state of disease to proceed for a few days
further, and then we shall find that no complaint of any kind
is acknowledged; his pulse is fluttering and weak, his mind is
alienated and noisy, his stools and urine are passed unconsciously,
his debility is so extreme that he is unable even to turn in bed,
his muscles are much convulsed, his hand trembles, and he
lies prostrate and helpless in the bed. Now, in this case,
which is a very fair and ordinary example of continued
fever in London, there are three very distinct periods, each
characterized by symptoms peculiarly its own. In the first
there is obvious excitement, combined with considerable activity; in the last there is nothing discoverable but weakness

and want of strength ; and in the intervening period there is a confused intermixture of both. Suppose that three practitioners were called in at different periods to attend these three stages of disease, a single period being allotted to the care of each, is it likely that any two of them would agree, either as to the type of the fever, or as to the plan to be adopted in its cure ? To one it would appear principally strength, to another principally debility, and to the third a perplexing compound of strength and debility. The old fable of the Cameleon would certainly be played over again, and while each rested confident in the accuracy of his own conclusion, all would be, were they to judge exclusively of a single stage, misled by a partial view. Wine would be recommended by one party, bleeding by another, and the third might find equally strong objections to either. It is not insinuated that any one of these parties would be wrong in differing from his neighbour ; on the contrary the symptoms justify them in drawing very different conclusions, and the treatment adapted to the first stage would be as destructive to the last, as that of the last stage could be to the first. What is advocated is, that the leading error, into which most writers upon this disease are betrayed, consists not so much in drawing false conclusions from the cases which are before them, as in generalizing these conclusions so as to adapt them to any and every case which may occur. A conclusion may be logical enough in its construction, and might be useful enough in its application to practice were its application confined to that form of cases out of which it was constructed ; but, by straining it to suit fever of every country and every stage, it becomes over drawn and is of suspicious applicability to even any case.

Here then, out of a single instance of fever can we manufacture Brunonians and Clutterbuckists, Systematists and Localists, Bleeders and Stimulators, and every opposing heresy which has crept into this department of medicine ; and what this history teaches as a single case it may also teach as the prototype of entire epidemics. Fever is more active at some seasons, in some countries, and in some constitutions, than others. We have seen it where the lancet, even at its commencement, could not be employed with safety ; where mental anxiety and corporeal depression were coeval and coequal, and where the strength was materially affected by an active purge. But such cases, at least in England, pertain to the rarest form of this disease. It is more frequently observed, if the early symptoms have been witnessed, that they indicate a greater or less degree of action, and that debility of any consequence does not betray itself until after the decrease or subsidence of this activity, and that then debility appears in a tolerably direct ratio to the degree of the preceding action. The train of inferences, therefore, which may be deduced from this case as a solitary illustration of fever, will equally result from it as exemplifying in its various stages the various epidemics and constitutions of this pestilence. And we have preferred a single case, consisting of three stages, as illustrative of the principal types of fever, in preference to three or more separate cases, drawn from three or more distinct epi- demics, that we may more easily explain the causes of these varieties and thus harmonise into one view the antagonising theories of the day, and also show in the strongest manner the necessity of general premises, before general conclusions can be formed. If one and the same disease can exhibit symp- toms of strength to-day, and symptoms of debility to-morrow— if one and the same patient can be bled with profit in the morning, and require wine for support in the evening—if three practitioners shall disagree, and shall have good reason for dis- agreement, about the nature and treatment of one and the same case, merely because they have witnessed different periods of the same action; surely it cannot be denied, that it is worse than folly to judge of all epidemics by the character of a single epidemic, or of all instances of fever by the character of a single instance. In the same ward of the same hospital have we examined twenty cases upon the same day, and in no two of any of them have we recognised the same symptoms. Patients occupying neighbouring beds, and coming out of the same house; people living under the influence of the same habits, having constitutions as much alike as age, temperament, and health could render them, will exemplify the most opposite types, will require the most opposite treatment, and may betray the unguarded into the most opposite views. Yet in the midst of all this contrariety and distinction, there are always points of family likeness discoverable; there are always generic bonds of union pervading every species. One epidemic or one case may differ from another epidemic or another case, just as the first stage of one and the same case may differ from its middle, or last stage. Yet in all these—whether they be entire epidemics, or individual instances; whether they be the fevers of extensive cities, or of trifling hamlets; whether they be preying upon the young and rich, or upon the old and poor—there are common signs, reciprocal resemblances, sufficiently striking to refer them all for their origin to one general class of causes, for their nature to one general form of action, and for their treatment to one general plan of cure.

Having now endeavoured to establish three points ;—that fever may be modified into a thousand forms by age, season, climate, constitution, cause, &c.,; that the varietiesof symptom, which individual instances afford, arise not from any difference iħ the nature but in the degree of the action going on, and that all cases and kinds of fever are linked together by certain common and characteristic signs ; it follows, and we would dwell upon the importance of these inferences, that fever cannot be generally known, if it be not seen and studied in patients of every age and constitution, in countries of every climate, and in every season of the year ; that any theories formed of it, or treatment proposed for it upon the knowledge of an epidemic of a single year, or of a single province, must be partial and un-founded ;—that all types of fever are merely creatures of degree, rather modes than entities, and not the results of distinct causes ; and that whatever peculiarities may present themselves, however many or marked they be, they must originate in circumstances intimately conneçted with the intensity of the morbid cause, or the character of the patient's constitution. To maintain, then, that because the fever of 1818 was distinguished for debility, the fever of 1829 must be remarkable for the same feature ; that because the fever of one country requires wine, that of another country cannot admit of bleeding, is extravagantly pre-posterous. Yet, strange to tell, this is the very error which most of our Pyrotologists have committed—an error less subversive of logical precision, than it is of practical principle. Anxious to con-struct imposing generalizations, which would comprehend within their range every quarter of the globe and every quality of consti-tution, these authors gathered together the reasonings and results of a confined experience, and mixing them up with some feasible speculations, wove them into a smooth and specious looking texture,which they took to market, and vended as honest goods of universal currency, adapted to the use of any purchaser in any country ! Thus is it that the fever of the half-starved peasantry of Dublin, during 1818, has been made the present fever of the world ; that the Adynamia of the Borough has not only crept over London, but is groping its way into the outskirts of the British empire ;—that the Gastro-Enterite of Broussais has proved an ignis fatuus to the French pathologists ; that the Typhus of Sunderland has formed the basis of a new theory, and of a new treatment still more remarkable than the theory which precedes it ; that Inflammation of the brain is held out to be only one step removed from continued fever ; and that there is no such thing as Idiopathic or specific fever, febrile symptoms being in every case nothing but the physical indications of some o cal inflammation.

It has been said that symptoms of equivocal origin do frequently appear; that they are not always proportioned in intensity to their cause ; that the most malignant mischief may be undermining the stamina of life with a degree of silence to be equalled only by its certainty. These are facts of too great notoriety to be disputed, and of too serious interest to be lightly passed over. Ulceration of the intestines may proceed through its every stage, even to perforation of the gut, without betraying adequate, or any tokens of its very presence. The brain may be deluged with watery effusion, and yet cerebral symptoms appear moderate or mild. All this is undeniable, and it shall afterwards be our business to shew why all this may happen ; but to maintain that fever is immethodical and wild, that it is bound down by no principles, directed by no laws, is gross error, and has been the cause of much evil. If an organ be diseased, or if a function be disordered, both the disease and the disorder are under the controlling agency of vital principles ; and the symptoms announcing these conditions, as well as the conditions themselves, proceed under the guidance of certain laws, and are obedient to the authority of specific causes. Every symptom in every case of fever is indicative of some internal morbid state ; every change of symptom is a sensible manifestation of some change in this internal state. The defect lies not in the fallacy of the symptoms which are present, but in the absence of symptoms which might have been expected to be present. The symptoms which are present are true enough in their indication as to the nature of internal action, although they may fail in announcing its precise degree. And we have only to regret that cases do occur, in which internal action, and that of fatal character, may be in existence without making itself known by any appreciable sign. Speaking of abdominal cases of fever with relation to this point Dr. Smith observes :

'The uniformity of the symptoms which denote that these morbid changes are going on, is as remarkable as the regularity with which the changes themselves occur. Their great peculiarity, which it is as important to know, as it is to understand their indication itself, is their want of prominence. They are always to be discerned, or with extremely rare exceptions ; but they seldom or never force themselves upon the notice of the careless or extort the attention of the unobserving; still they are not the less constant in their occurrence because they come without noise, nor is the indication they give of their presence less significant because it is unobtrusive. They do not announce their presence by the excitement of violent paroxysms or by inducing intense pain, because the state of the system in which they take place is incompatible with acute sensation of any kind. The prominent symptoms during life are almost always in the head ; the great changes of structure found after death are always in the intestines ; and this, which the pathologist learns from observation, the physiologist might have predicted from his knowledge of function. The affection of the intestines in fever is never a simple or single affection : it never occurs alone, but always in combination with an affection of the brain ; and the cerebral affection is always antecedent, the intestinal invariably subsequent ; while the certain consequence of the cerebral affection is a diminution, and ultimately an abolition of sensation. It is therefore quite impossible, from the very nature of the derangement that takes place in the animal economy, that the intestinal affection should ever be attended with violent pain. Occasionally, indeed, when the abdominal affection is very much in excess, and the cerebral affection is unusually slight, severe pain may be felt ; but that is rare, and the total absence of pain, and even the total absence of tenderness on pressure, is more common. It is not then to the patient's own complaint of pain in the abdomen that the practitioner must trust for the discovery of abdominal affection in fever.

'But though the patient seldom complain of pain in the abdomen, yet in the great majority of cases the abdomen is tender on pressure, and it is so in all, excepting when the cerebral affection is peculiarly severe or is very far advanced. These exceptions render this symptom not absolutely constant, although at the bed-side of the sick the practitioner will find it very rarely absent. The symptom which is still more constant, as the reader must have observed in the perusal of the preceding cases, and which therefore affords a very certain guide to the detection of the disease, is a loose state of the bowels. Whenever both concur there can be no doubt of the diseased process which is going on within the intestine : but as the tenderness may be obscured or lost from the intensity or advancement of the cerebral affection, so it is very remarkable that, in the progress of the intestinal disease, the bowels sometimes become regular and even constipated. The physician who sees the patient for the first time in this stage of the disease, can ascertain the condition of the mucous membrane of the intestines only by obtaining an accurate account of the preceding symptoms. And when it is possible to procure a distinct and complete history of the disease from its commencement, it is commonly found that nausea and vomiting were among the early symptoms, while, as we have seen, the latter is not unusually present in the more advanced stages. The result of the whole is that, excepting when the cerebral affection is most intense and overwhelming, the existence of inflammation and ulceration in the mucous membrane of the intestines in fever is denoted by signs which are quite constant, and in the fidelity of the indication of which we may repose implicit confidence. The importance of the diagnosis may perhaps plead our excuse for repeating them again. They are tenderness of the abdomen on pressure ; loose stools ; redness of the tongue, especially at the tip and edges, in general preceded by nausea and vomiting, and in the most exquisitely marked cases, and in their advanced stage, followed by a mixture of blood in the stools and a swollen, hard and tympanitic state of the abdomen. All these symptoms by no means always concur in the same case : but the presence of one or two of them will be sufficient to guide the attentive observer to the knowledge of the disease.'—pp. 288—291.

Is it then not highly injurious to the interests of this inquiry to overlook these leading principles and laws ? Is it not exceedingly empirical to treat unseen disease by unknown symptoms ? Is it not derogatory to philosophy to attach the importance of a general cause to a single consequence ? To confound a naked symptom with the covert action which brought it forth, and to sweep into one confused generalization, things in themselves as distinct as light and darkness? Probably there is no case of fever in which there are not present some specific and expressive symptoms ; no symptom which does not indicate some condition of internal parts ; and that there is no chance of knowing what fever is, or requires for its management, unless we keep this etiological connexion between external signs and internal states constantly in view, treating the one as indicated by the other. By so doing nature is studied in her own way, the veil of mystery is withdrawn from the face of disease, and whether it be an important organ which is afflicted, or an important function which is attacked, a careful and experienced eye may not only ascertain the nature, but measure the extent, of morbid change, wherever, however, and whensoever, it may exist.

The next question of interest, which here deserves attention as inseparably connected with the last point, is, what is the nature of that internal condition which gives origin to these external signs ? Some assert that it is pure inflammation ; others that it is something different from pure inflammation ; and a third party maintain that it is neither pure inflammation, nor something different from pure inflammation, but that first and last it is pure debility. To enter into a critique of all these opinions, cum multis aliis, would be endless and useless. Some of them are too fanciful for serious argument, and others stand so feebly propped that they invite compassion much more than they do conflict. In a practical sense two more especially require examination, and as the works which are now before us may be fairly held as the ablest advocates which have as yet appeared in their defence, it will be more than interesting to find how well they measure in each other's company. Dr. Stoker believes that fever is essentially adynamic ; that its seat is in the blood ; that the blood is in a dissolved and diseased state ; that depletion of almost all kinds and degrees is injurious; and that tonics and restoratives are the most effectual medicines :—

' Common epidemic fever, says Dr. Stoker, especially when contagious, as I have frequently asserted when speaking of its pathology and treatment, has not appeared to me at any time to be essentially inflammatory. Adynamic fever, a denomination for typhus fever, which I shall employ, as I have hitherto done to express the putrid or malignant fever of Sydenham; the slow nervous fever of Huxham; the nervous fever of common language; the synochus, typhus mitior, and gravior of Cullen; the gaol and hospital fever; the *fièvres essentielles* of the French; the epidemic of the Irish writers; the contagious of Bateman; the typhus of Dr. Armstrong; and the proper idiopathic, or essential fever of Dr. Clutterbuck : whether it exists separately or independently; or is combined with any of the other forms of febrile disease, sporadic or symptomatic.

' Typhoid or adynamic fever I consider to be generally symptomatic of morbid changes in the physical characters of the blood, and have, as on former occasions, stated what those morbid changes are—but I have arranged inflammation under the head of symptomatic fever, merely because it is more usually connected with some change in the structure of parts, discoverable after death : on the other hand, typhus fever is connected with morbid changes, that *primarily* take place in the fluids, and produce morbid actions, and sometimes permanent changes of structure in the said parts. These changes too in the condition of the blood are distinguishable from those which we have stated to occur in inflammation ; and the morbid actions excited relatively by those changes in the blood are also distinct. In inflammatory fever on the one hand, increased action, in typhoid fevers on the other, debility, is almost the immediate consequence. On account of this debility being an essential character of typhoid fevers, I denominated them adynamic.'

In the Medico-Chirurgical Review for August, 1829, it was shown, in opposition to Dr. Stoker, that the depressed character of some of the Dublin epidemics was not the unmixed result of pure febrile disease ; that the state of the poor (out of whom a great majority, if not all, of the patients admitted into the Cork Street Fever Hospital, to which the Dr. belongs, were taken) was such as to modify and give a peculiar cast to the original affection; that this modification consisted in a preponderancy of adynamic symptoms ; and that, consequently, it only tended to mislead the public to urge upon them such a type as a fac-simile of fever. It was further argued that the blood is in no instance the primary seat of this disease ; that disorder in this fluid was a mere consequence, and probably the first consequence, but not the cause ; that in the first stage of action it presented no symptoms of disease ; that its dissolved appearance came slowly on as the fever advanced ; and that in many pure cases no such appearance has been witnessed at any period of the malady. The earliest febrile symptoms, it was maintained, were connected with the nervous system—these were languor, lassitude, mental depression, malaise, sense of cold and pallidity of the surface; the heart then sympathised more palpably, and with disorder in the circulation came on deranged function in every organ, and diseased secretion in every tissue. The unfairness of making the fever of Dublin, and more especially such a fever, the fever of the world, was strongly insisted on, and arguments were drawn from the acknowledged character of the Irish constitution, from the experience of many Irish writers, and from personal acquaintance with the disease among the resident as well as the emigrant Irish, to prove that they are in general little more remarkable, if not a little less, than their neighbours for adynamic fever. And, lastly, it was shewn that the fever of London is essentially inflammatory, that its treatment requires the lancet more than wine, and that the Irish are just that class of patients who stand most in need of full and free depletion. The work of Dr. Smith confirms these views in every point, and establishes them on the basis of a pathology which it is impossible to shake. The fever of London, we repeat, is anything but a disease of weakness. Is increased arterial action a proof of weakness, or is acute pain, or is improvement under depletion, or is the aggravation of every symptom under stimulating treatment? Are increased vascularity, change of structure, deposition of lymph, formation of pus and membranes, the ordinary and legitimate results of debility? Whoever witnessed wide and spreading ulceration from adynamia? Whoever saw the membranes of the brain thickened, adherent, and charged with blood from want of action? What have we after death from ordinary inflammation of the brain and membranes, but what we find in fever? Have we any thing beyond turgid vessels, effused lymph and serum, and altered structure? If we have, it should be pointed out. Have we any thing in Pleurisy, or Pneumonia, or Bronchitis, beyond disorganized or inflamed lungs, inflamed and thickened membranes, increased secretion, adhesion and effusion of lymph and pus? If we have, let them be pointed out. Have we any thing more indicative of action, and of strong action, in Enteritis, or Peritonitis, or any other itis that may be fixed upon, than intestines loaded with engorged vessels and matted into one adhering mass, cavities filled with phlogistic depositions, structure softened into lacerable pulp, ulcerations wide as they are deep? If we have, it were for the sake of truth to make it known. Yet these are the morbid appearances after death from adynamic fever, from fever whose essence is weakness, whose seat is relaxed and effete blood, in which we are cautioned from leeching, prohibited from bleeding, advised to try transfusion, and which we are strongly recommended to make merry with wine!

Now let Dr. Smith be heard. He, we think, has given an unanswerable summary of the pathology of fever, drawn from a multitude of dissections, which, if contrasted with any which can be brought against them, are as unequalled in their superiority as number; and, as it would form the best proof of what has been advanced, we feel sorry that its length renders its introduction impossible, while it were only to give half the required proof did we mutilate the passage. The following masterly extract may form a sufficient substitute :—

' The account of the pathology of fever is the history of inflammation, and the description of the individual changes that take place in the organs that constitute the febrile circle, is an enumeration of various products of inflammation which are formed within them. There is scarcely a fatal case of fever which does not afford, in one or other of the organs of that circle, some inflammatory product; there is no considerable number of fatal cases which does not furnish a specimen of every inflammatory product. And what are the severest cases of fever, and why are they the severest ? With the single exception immediately to be stated, the severest cases are those in which, together with a severe primary affection of the nervous system, this inflammatory action is in the greatest degree of intensity, and is seated in the greatest number of organs ; and they are the most severe, not only on account of the severity of the primary affection of the nervous system, but also because it is in them that the inflammation is the most intense, and because that inflammation attacks the system at one and the same time in the greatest number of points. From among the preceding cases, fix upon any one in which the powers of life were, from the commencement, the most completely overwhelmed, and in which they were the most rapidly exhausted, and when the last struggle for existence is over, examine the changes that have taken place in the internal organs—what is it that is found ? traces of inflammation, legible, deep, extensive; while, in almost every case, these traces are thus legible, deep, and extensive, in proportion to the apparent intensity of the fever, and to the rapidity with which it extinguished life. In this point of view, how important, how instructive, how invaluable, is the lesson which the mixed cases of fever afford ! With few and rare exceptions (and in all diseases some exceptions occasionally occur to what appear to be the best established and the most invariable laws) these are the cases in which the symptoms are the most urgent, and in which they run their course with the greatest rapidity ; these are the cases in which the debility is the most striking; in which it comes on the most early, and pro ceeds to the greatest degree of prostration ; these are the cases which are the most purely typhoid, the most truly adynamic ; these are the cases which, in general, commence with the most sudden and alarming deprivation of physical and mental power; in which all pain and uneasiness are soonest lost in stupor, in which the stupor most rapidly increases to insensibility ; in which delirium comes, perhaps, as early as the third or fourth night, accompanied with its attendant, muscular tremor, and too often with its most formidable ally, erysipelas ; in which, at this early period, the respiration is short and hurried, the skin dusky, the colour of the cheek purple, the tongue brown and dry, the lips and teeth sordid, the abdomen tender, and the stools loose ; in which, in a day or two more, the abdomen is swollen, tense, and tympanitic, the stools passed in bed, the patient prostrate on his back, completely senseless and powerless, while the pulse is 120 or 130, and so feeble that it can scarcely be distinguished. But what is this debility ? in what does this adynamic state consist ? It consists of a peculiar affection of the nervous system, followed rapidly by intense inflammation of the brain or of its membranes, or of both : by intense inflammation of the mucous membrane of the bronchi, and by intense inflammation or extensive ulceration of the mucous membrane of the intestines. And why is the patient weak or adynamic ? Because he is not only assailed by an affection of the nervous system, which deprives the organs of the stimulus necessary to enable them to perform their functions with due vigour, but, at the same moment, inflammation is set up in three of the great systems, the healthy action of which is most essential, not only to strength but to life : thus the citadel is attacked at one time at three of its capital points. It is not asserted that inflammation alone constitutes the state of fever, nor that the danger of the patient is always in exact proportion to the degree of the inflammation. How it differs from inflammation, and what is superadded to the inflammatory state, will be shewn immediately ; but it is a most important fact, that the degree of the debility is most intimately connected with the intensity and the extent of the inflammatory action. Now and then, as has been already stated, the intensity of the nervous affection is so great, and so rapidly destructive of life, that there is no time for an inflammatory process to be set up, much less for an inflammatory product to be formed. The patient is struck dead as if by lightning, or by Prussic acid, or by apoplexy. In this country, he does not actually die as instantaneously as he might be destroyed by the electric fluid or by poison, although there are countries, seasons, and particular spots, in which the concentration of the febrile poison appears to be sufficiently great to extinguish life instantaneously ; and even in this country, life is sometimes destroyed by a stroke of fever as rapidly as it is by a stroke of apoplexy, when the latter does not prove fatal in the first few hours.

Now the peculiarity in these cases is, that the internal organs, after death, exhibit no signs of inflammation, unless vascularity be inflammation. The organs which, in ordinary cases, are inflamed, are in these cases turgid with blood. Are the terms debility or adynamic appropriate expressions to designate even this condition of the organs ? Just as appropriate as they would be to express the condition of a person who is struck dead by lightning, whose muscles are incapable of contraction, and whose blood will not coagulate. Those who apply these terms even to such forms, and, à fortiori, to any other forms of fever, must be ignorant either of the nature of the disease, or of the constitution of the human mind. If they know the disease, they know that the patient appears to be weak because the primary operation of the disease is upon the nervous system—an operation which, as has just been stated, while it disturbs that due and equal distribution of nervous influence which is necessary to the healthful action of the organs, and, therefore, to the general strength of the system, is not incompatible with, but promotive of an excitement of the vascular system, which terminates in inflammation. Debility is the last, the ultimate result of the disturbance of the functions of a certain series of organs, but the part of this very disturbance of function, and a most important part, a part which exerts the greatest influence over the progress of the disease and the life or death of the patient, consists not in the weakened, but in the augmented strength and the increased activity of the vascular system. To designate the ultimate result upon the system by a term which gives an entirely false view of the individual processes in the economy, by which that ultimate result is produced, must, we repeat, arise either from an ignorance of the true nature of those processes, or from not reflecting on the influence which words exert over the manner in which the human mind conceives of things. For the sake of the progress of the science of medicine, for the sake of rendering the language of medicine the correct expression of the knowledge which the science has actually attained, and, above all, for the sake of accomplishing the great object of medicine, the preservation of human life, it is high time that these terms with which physicians have so long allowed their minds to be abused, should be banished from medical nomenclature, or, at any rate, from that part of its nomenclature which appertains to fever.'—pp. 323—328.

The seat of fever appears to be in the nervous system, in place of in the blood, the cause of fever seems to be a specific poison, and the effect is a modified inflammation. It is the peculiarity of the poison, operating upon the peculiar structure which it first invades, that gives a peculiar tinge and type to all the succeeding symptoms, and that renders the morbid action something else than pure inflammation. The cause is peculiar, the structure it attacks is peculiar, and the inflammation which it produces is peculiar. But the cause is an exciting cause, the structure it invades is excited, and the morbid product is a product of excitement. This excitement may be more, or it may be less, just as the cause is more or less intense, or as the structure on which it operates is more or less susceptible of excitement. The structure may be weak and the poison may be strong, and then the effect will be sudden and severe; or the poison may be weak and the structure may be strong, and then the effect will be gradual and moderate. The effect may thus be produced in a thousand different degrees, and the action of the heart and arteries may thus be called forth in endless varieties of power. But this effect is always inflammatory, and this action is always irregular. The poison may kill in a few hours, or require a few weeks; the heart may be instantaneously disabled, or excited into the most unmanageable force; nervous symptoms may preponderate at one period, inflammatory symptoms at another. It is this confusing intermixture of nervous symptoms, arising from the nature of the organ attacked, and of pseudo-inflammatory symptoms, depending on the nature of the action modified by the cause, which makes fever appear to many so perplexing and contradictory. All these points have been ably handled by Dr. Smith; and for simplicity of arrangement, perspicuity of view, power of argument, and practical deduction, his *Treatise on Fever* stands, we believe, without competition at the head of all that has been written upon this abstruse disease. The relation between cause and effect, between symptoms and the states they indicate, was never before so clearly pointed out; the theory of fever is laid down with unprecedented plausibility; and the variety of cases and dissections which are given may furnish him, who questions the conclusions which are drawn, with ample materials to construct inferences of his own. But the treatment proposed by Dr. Smith, and the important question of contagion, must be discussed on another occasion.

ART. XVI.—1. *A Treatise on Fever* By Southwood Smith, M.D. Longman and Co. London. 1830. pp. 436.

2. *Pathological Observations on Continued Fever.* By W. Stoker, M. D. Hodges and Co. Dublin. 1829. pp. 267.

IN pursuing the Review of the Works of Drs. Smith and Stoker, we address ourselves as directly to the public in general as to the medical profession. The controversy which now agitates this country upon the subject of Fever, is of equal importance to every class of society, and its issue must be looked for with anxiety by all who value the health and happiness of the community. The property of the country is of some importance, and, by revealing the dangers to which it is exposed, we have, in more instances than one, endeavoured to protect it; but the lives of the public are of still greater consequence, and we are now solicitous to prove our concern for their safety and preservation. Fever is a pestilence, as deadly in its action as it is migratory in its habits; neither rank nor fortune, neither youth nor vigour, can shield from its influence; but the healthy and the young, the helpless and the old, the rich and the poor may be alike its victims; and we can derive no consolation from the belief that this terrible malady is either generally understood or scientifically treated. The arguments about to be urged in the hope of elucidating its real nature can be understood by any person of sense, and, if they are sound, it deeply concerns every one to be acquainted with them. In too many instances the medical practitioner is called upon to perform a mental operation for which his habit and education have but ill prepared him. He has to deduce an inference on the state of diseased organs which are concealed from his observation, by signs which are appreciable by his senses, and there passes not a day in which hundreds of lives do not depend upon the skill with which this mental operation is performed. Now, the important object is to show how these signs can be successfully interpreted in fever, what dreadful consequences follow their misconception, and how easy it is to trace to this single source the rise of almost every controversy upon this subject, whether it refer to the nature or to the treatment of the disease.

In our last number many of these errors were examined with some minuteness, in the present instance it is our purpose to review a few others; and, as the points about to occupy attention are more immediately concerned in the treatment of fever, we are anxious that the public should look with their own eyes into the consequences of the errors we shall endeavour to expose, that they may see the exceeding hazard which their continuance must occasion. Were the extent of disputed territory limited to a few inches or a few feet, the value of conquest might be of little importance; but it is a wide and spacious interval which is the subject of contention. The grand point at issue is not a verbal difference, or a conventional technicality, it is an important practical doctrine. It is whether a disease, which is never absent from our cities and our villages—which

2 к 2

spares no age, nor sex, nor constitution—which comes into our families unseen and unprovided for—which creeps from house to house with noiseless progress, and covers entire countries with death and desolation—it is whether such a monster can be more effectually killed by being starved or fed.   Surely this is a wide difference, and merits some consideration.   It may be put to the good sense of the public if it can be a matter of no moment whether, in the selfsame disease we bleed and leech and purge ; or support and strengthen and excite.   These modes of treatment sadly differ, and neither of them is inert.   Each must either effect good or harm—and in many, very many, instances must save or destroy life.   If fever be an inflammatory disease, or a disease so akin to inflammation that the difference resolves itself into a mere matter of degree, it is a serious affair to nurse and fondle it with wine and cordials ; and, on the other hand, if it be really a disease of weakness, every one must allow that bleeding, purging and starvation are no children's toys.   ' To bleed or not to bleed' is a question which, in this instance, can find its counterpart only in the soliloquy of Cato ; and if the great national distress, under which we are now labouring, have not induced the public to regard life as less estimable than formerly, ' to be or not to be' ought to be their inquiry when fever enters their dwellings, and calls for the interference of the faculty.

In studying this disease the safest ground for the erection of medical doctrine is Pathology. The character of exciting causes may deceive, the nature of existing symptoms may deceive, the peculiarities of the affected constitution may deceive, but it is utterly impossible for the results of disease after death to prove deceptive ; they do not change, they cannot be equivocal.   During life there may be pain ; acute and stinging pain, and this pain may be as far from the seat of action, as it often is from being an honest representative of the nature of this action ; but, after death, both the seat and nature of this action inspection will generally disclose.   This pain may be moderate or severe, constant or intermittent, alleviated by one remedy, and aggravated by another ; yet the same action, and even the same amount of action may be present in all these instances. We may have pain without inflammation, and inflammation without pain ; acute inflammation while the pain is trifling, and trifling inflammation while the pain is acute.   Symptoms may be present indicating one stage of action, while the disease, which they indicate, exists in another, and there may be destructive, deadly disease without a symptom or a sign.

If a knowledge of external symptom were sufficient to impart a knowledge of internal action—if like parallel lines the

symptom and the action ran, *pari passu,* in company, so that the
extent of the one were the measure of the other, then it would
be as easy to pronounce upon the presence and progress of the
most insidious malady as to point out the north pole by
examining the needle, or to ascertain the direction of the wind
by looking at the weather-cock. But it must be admitted that
any such comparison is loose, if not inapplicable to every form
of disease, and that, as regards fever, it is perfectly fallacious.
If the bowels may be inflamed and ulcerated, yet pressure
over the affected organs, occasion neither pain nor uneasiness—if
the touch of a finger, or the weight of the bed clothes can
scarcely be endured over the region of the stomach, in which
nothwithstanding there is neither ulcer nor inflammation—if
the brain may be floating in water, without any corresponding
warrant of disease—if deep and spreading abscess may be
lurking within the very organ of sensation, without a warning
voice, or yet a whisper, to discover its retreat, who can say that
fever may be taught and treated through its symptoms, or that
the language of fever is unequivocal, or even articulately
pronounced. If the symptoms which do appear cannot be
entirely depended on, and if important and leading symptoms
ought to appear, which are wholly absent, then where is
the far-famed light of symptomatologists, the infallible guide to
certain treatment? If fever may be dealing destruction on the
organs it assails, if it may be preying upon life, and yet if the
path of its progress over the constitution can only be traced by the
relics it leaves behind, is it not foolish and fruitless to take
mere symptoms for our guide? The experiment has been
made, and upon a scale of fearful magnitude; its progress has
been patiently observed for many years, it has been variously
modified according to the taste of the experimenter, and it
has been brought to work upon every form of case, and every
type of constitution; yet discomfiture has been the general
result, and it is certain that nothing will, and that nothing
can, ever be the result but discomfiture. Amid a sea of such
doubts and difficulties the only ground for anchorage is
pathology. Practical doctrine can take hold in no other
bottom. If rested elsewhere it will yield—it will neither
give support nor direction; but if grounded upon this foundation a clue will be found to rescue us out of every labyrinth,
and a guide which, by conducting us to the source of evil, will
lead us to a plan of cure. When we can have an honest guide,
in the name of prudence, why should we choose a faithless one.
When we can see into the very arcana of the real and inward
action, why should we still regard only what is a mere

consequence of this inward action. A heated skin, an excited thirst, a general malaise restlessness during the day, and sleeplessness during the night, are not the constitutional elements of fever. These are not what we have to physic, and what we have to fear, any more than the vane at the mast-head is what the sailor dreads when the wind and the thunder-clouds foretell the storm. No man ever yet died of symptoms, no man ever can die of symptoms, and if fever be only a congregation of symptoms, then no man has ever yet died of fever.

If it be found upon inspection after death that vessels are gorged with blood, tissues are altered in structure, organs are inflamed, that pus and lymph, ulceration and effusion, and in a word, all the ordinary results of a disease which must during life have possessed some activity, and been characterised by some excitement, can there remain ground for doubt as to what fever is, or as to the general principles by which its treatment should be conducted ? These fruits of action are accents of disease which it is neither difficult to hear, nor, when heard, to understand. Many external signs may not, but these internal monitors must, exist; not all in every case, nor always to the same extent; but some of them do invariably exist in the present fever of this country, and each of them is decisive of the same truth which all, if present, could do nothing more than confirm. Feeling earnestly, because knowing that fever has not been generally studied under this view, and that the neglect, if not contempt of pathology has been the chief cause of the errors with which its history is observed, we are anxious to obtain from those who support opposite opinions, the results of their pathological information. If it be, that fever is weakness, that weakness stands in need of wine, and that wine cures by infusing strength; then let them adduce the proof in the fruits of fever as they are exhibited after death. Let us see the operations of this monster debility upon the organs he invades. Let us see fluids dissolved and watery, solids relaxed and putrid, a vascular system paralyzed and powerless, and that general atomy which indicates privation of strength. Let it be shown that no product of activity is met with; that we never find gorged veins, nor loaded arteries, coagulated lymph, nor extravasated serum, structures thickened by new deposits, membranes freshly formed, nor ulcers in all stages of progress. Let all this be shown, and then these symptoms, which may be adduced in favour of debility, will prove something. No indications of weakness, which symptoms alone may exhibit, entitle us to characterise fever as a disease

of weakness. Nothing can be more fallacious than such symptoms, whether they regard the duration or degree of the
disease. It is in the first instance but a weak debility which
they indicate: towards the close of the fever, indeed, this
spurious weakness becomes real, but the present argument
interferes not with the sequelæ of fever. The object is to
establish a general principle, to ascertain the primitive essence
of the disease. In the last stage, nothing can be less equivocal
than the prostration of every mental and bodily power, nothing
more awfully indicative of a wasted and worn-out fabric. But
it will shortly be demonstrated that this is not a primitive state,
but a subsequent consequence, often induced by mismanagement or neglect.

While thus contending for the necessity of teaching and
treating fever pathologically we wish not to reject the light of
symptoms during life; both sources of knowledge may and ought
reciprocally to illustrate each other. The veracity of the inward consequence may rectify the deceptiveness of the outward
sign, and the character of the outward sign may indicate
the inward state. When we are convinced that the inward consequence generally indicates excitement, to know that the outward symptom so often indicates debility cannot authorize the
inference that the cause of both is weakness. The existence
of an inflammatory product after death is incompatible with
the existence of continued debility during life, and it matters
not how far the living symptoms savoured of weakness, the
dead result is a sufficient proof that the symptoms were fallacious and that the weakness was imaginary. It is true that
patients labouring under fever do not die at every stage of the
disease, and that the same opportunities are not given to trace
the workings of internal action, with that precision with which
every change of symptom can be noted. We cannot positively
pronounce upon the moment when moderate vascularity becomes excessive, when excessive vascularity passes into inflammation, when inflammation terminates in ulceration or effusion.
But it is nevertheless true that a thorough knowledge of diseased appearances after death, in every variety of case and
constitution, of type and temperament, will form a key to
the proper understanding of symptoms during life, without
which their indications must have a greater tendency to mislead
than to guide; and he who has watched with cautious observation the various symptoms which various forms of fever have
assumed during various stages of their course; he who has
journalled these symptoms with sufficient accuracy to render
them available for future reference, and who at last has inspected

the bodies of his dead, comparing and elucidating what he discovers upon inspection with the daily history of his symptoms, will in a short time be sufficiently qualified to pronounce upon what is going on within, by watching what is going on without, and to contend with internal disease as scientifically and as successfully as though his patient were translucent, and he could witness with his own eyes the covert operations of the malady.

' Out of the hundred cases which have now been recorded, and the history of which has been made known from its commencement to its termination, take any one, or fix upon any number, in which the symptoms from being slight became moderate, and from moderate severe, or, in which the symptoms were severe from the beginning, what is found after death? Inflammation, in general, rising in degree, and increasing in extent, or both, in proportion to the intensity of the febrile affection. If this, which may be justly considered as the law of the disease, be not absolutely constant and uniform, it may be safely affirmed, at least, that there are as few apparent exceptions to it, as to any general law that can be named.—Smith, p. 397.

Since, therefore, the internal consequences of fever are inflammatory, since the external signs of fever often indicate weakness more than inflammation, since the inward consequences of fever never can deceive, and since its outward effects often do, symptoms must be esteemed as no more than the expressions of an interior agent, and safe only as far as they faithfully communicate to the spectator the operations which this agent internally carries on.

As the first question of importance in the investigation of this disease is ' in what does it consist?' the second question is 'how should it be treated'—what remedies are best adapted for its cure? The first question is preparative to the second, and when a proper solution has been furnished to the one the other can neither be difficult to comprehend, nor answer. He, who fears debility as the foe of life, will not be violently inclined to pursue such measures as are calculated to weaken the constitution, while he, who has the fear of inflammation rather than of debility constantly before his eyes, must look upon all kinds and degrees of excitement as doubtful, if not dangerous.

The treatment proposed by each will depend upon the views of each as to the character of the existing evil, and as to the nature of its future consequences. If fever be debility, and if the danger which attends it depend upon the degree of this debility, it is obvious that, as a general principle, such treatment as might tend to increase this debility would be highly injudicious; whereas, if fever be essentially a disease of excitement, and if the danger it occasions depend upon the extent of this excitement, it must be admitted that, as a general principle, such remedies as are opposed to excitement must hold out the surest prospects of relief. The following extracts will accordingly show that we are no better agreed upon the treatment than upon the nature of this affection.—

'The first principles of my practice thus appearing to be as generally received as they had before been rejected, it only remains for me to detail the remedies which I have employed ; and with respect to these, too, I might be even more brief, from having little to add to the list of remedies in typhoid Fevers, which may be found at the 18th page of my "Treatise on Fever," published in London, A. D. 1814, as well as in my " Medical Reports from the Cork-street Hospital ;" but, that as these publications may not be in the hands of the reader, some recapitulation of those remedies themselves ; and my reasons for recommending them, supported as I have been by all my subsequent experience, may be permitted. They may be arranged according to their relative importance in the treatment of fever, in the following order, viz.

IN MIXED FEVER.	IN TYPHOID FEVER.
Cleanliness.	Yeast or Barm.
Ventilation.	Wine.
Cool Regimen.	Aperients.
Plentiful Dilution.	Emetics.
Purgatives.	Blisters.
Topical Bleeding.	Tepid, or Cold Affusion.
Antimonial, or	Peruvian Bark.
James's Powder.	

Many other remedies may, no doubt, be occasionally employed with advantage for the relief of the symptoms which accompany peculiar forms of epidemics, or such as are produced by extraordinary idiosyncrasies. But these, according to my experience are more frequently applicable than any others, in the treatment of our common indigenous fever.

The beneficial effects of the four first articles of this list of remedies in the treatment of fever, it is no longer necessary to insist on, for they are no longer denied. For the same reasons, too, I need not, as on former occasions, enter more fully into explanation, why blood-letting has not a place in this list. When, however, I come to speak of topical bleeding, I shall have to state, that under the pestilential form which our epidemic fevers have assumed since the year 1823, I have found it advisable to employ even this partial evacuation more sparingly and cautiously than in my first publications on fever I felt justified in recommending.

With respect to Peruvian bark too, which I have here added to the list of remedies for typhoid fevers ; although, on former occasions, I stated, that " I had not found it necessary for the cure of the continued

fevers in Dublin," I have now to observe, that, under the growing
malignity of these distempers, I have employed some preparations, especially the sulphate of quina, with obvious advantage, even in cases
which did not partake of tendencies to remittent or intermittent forms ;
in such tendencies, however, the usefulness of that remedy was most
manifest.'—Stoker, p. 111—113.

The general reception of his practical principles, which Dr.
Stoker alludes to in the preceding extract, is thus described—

' The views taken both of the nature and treatment of fever,
by Dr. Burne, entirely accord with those which may be found
stated in my medical reports from the Fever Hospital, as well as in
my separate essays on that subject. And as (when speaking of his
denomination of Fever) I have already remarked, this leaves, I think,
no reasonable doubt of the epidemic Fevers of London having lately
become more typhoid or adynamic, than they had formerly been. It
is further satisfactory to me to find, that the treatment which I had
long since adopted and recommended in our typhoid Fevers, has been
found suitable to the prevention and cure of those in London ; and
that, too, in proportion as they have acquired more of that form, with
which I was best acquainted.'—p. 110—111.

Now, to put the reader in possession of Dr. Burne's plan of
treatment we shall quote the following passage—" Although the
judgment here wants the assistance of experience, the very
great and unaccountable debility and listlessness, with the other
signs, indicate very evidently the threatening of an attack of
fever. It is of much importance for the physician to see his
way clearly ; for if he should attribute this obstinate attack to
any other than its just cause, and be induced to abstract blood
he will inflict an injury it is not always easy to repair. The
abstraction of blood does no good, and it will now and then be
succeeded by a gradual alarming sinking of the powers of life,
from which the patient may never recover. Should the pain in
the head be so severe (it rarely is) as to tempt the practitioner to
draw blood, let the quantity be small and its effects be observed
some hours after it has been abstracted ; because patients will
appear to bear bleeding at the moment, while in a few hours its
injurious effects will be manifest." See a practical Treatise on
the Typhus or Adynamic Fever, by John Burne M. D. London.
1828. p. 200—1.

If, then, the sentiments of Doctors Stoker and Burne so
entirely correspond, and if Doctor Stoker considers these sentiments generally adopted throughout London, merely because
Doctor Burne has re-echoed them, we beg to disabuse Dr. Stoker's
fancy with the few passages from the work of Doctor Smith,
physician to the only exclusive hospital for Fever within London ;

and although we feel it a harsh and invidious undertaking to lower an author in his own esteem, by narrowing the limits of his influence, we do feel it, at the same time, to be a duty to the public and to the profession, to the advancement of truth and the promotion of sound medical knowledge, to place landmarks around the Doctor's territory that he may hereafter know it to be forbidden ground, should the boundary again be ever over-stepped.

One would think that the following paragraph was penned as an antidote to the very passage above given :—

' Bleeding in fever cannot be performed too early. The very first moment of excitement, could that be discovered, is precisely the moment when the employment of this powerful remedy would produce the greatest effect. The earlier the bleeding, the greater will be the impression made upon the disease, and the less upon the patient; or, the more effectually will the inflammatory action be stopped by the loss of the smallest quantity of blood.'—p. 382.

Both authors are describing what ought to be done at the very opening of the disease, yet the one talks of bleeding as at the very best a most precarious resource, while the other labours for utterance to express its importance !—

' The object to be aimed at in practice, then, is clear : it is to prevent, or to remove inflammation. Accomplish this, the fever will not be cured at once ; it will still go on for some time ; but it will come sooner to a close, and it will proceed mildly and safely to its termination. Fail to accomplish this, and the fever, however mild at first, will increase more and more in severity until it become truly formidable, and death take place at last, in consequence of the destruction of the organs by the process of inflammation.

' If excitement be set up in an organ which has as invariable a ten-dency to terminate in inflammation, as a stone to fall to the ground, what is the proper remedy to prevent the transition of excitement into inflammation ? Bleeding. Before we can say that inflammation is established we may foresee that it will come : if the preceding excite-ment be not stopped, we know that it will as surely come as that blood will flow from a wounded blood-vessel. Because we cannot tell the precise moment when increased vascular action passes into actual inflammation, are we quietly to look on and do nothing until we have made that discovery ? We know that inflammation is at hand ; we know what will prevent it, or, at any rate, what has a powerful ten-dency to prevent it : shall we not bring into immediate and vigorous use our means of prevention, or shall we wait until the inflammatory action shall have given unequivocal and alarming indications of its presence and operation before we interfere ? To trifle in such a manner, to lose these precious moments when we have such a fearful, such an active, and, if once it be allowed to become active, such a masterless enemy to contend with as fever, is as great a folly as it would be when a building is on fire to stand idle by as long as the fire is smouldering, and to take no measure to extinguish it until it has burst into flame, nay, not until the flame has spread from the floor to the ceiling, and from the ceiling to the roof. We may not be able to see a single spark, but if we see the smoke and feel the heat, we know that there is fire somewhere, and that however concealed at present it will soon make itself visible enough, and that it will consume not only the structure in which it originates, but others with which it may come in contact if it be not put out. With equal certainty we know that fever, though apparently mild in the commencement, will excite inflammation in vital organs, and that that inflammation, if it be allowed to establish itself, will place the fabric of the body in the most imminent danger. The physician, in the first stage of fever, armed with his lancet, is to his patient what the fireman with his engine, before the flames have had time to kindle, is to a building that has taken fire. At this early stage, the former can check inflammation with almost as much ease and certainty as the latter can prevent the flames from bursting out. On the contrary, the physician who is called to treat inflammation in the later stage of fever is in the position of the man who arrives with the apparatus for saving the house when its stories have been already consumed and its roof has fallen in.'—pp. 379—382.

This must sound somewhat like thunder in the ears of Doctors Stoker and Burne, and the gentle reader will be strongly tempted to refer to our table of errata for some solution of such discrepancies. But, verily, no solution will be met with there —the statement now given is in the *ipsissima verba* of the three originals we quote, without addition or subtraction; and did space permit, or argument require it, it would be easy, with the assistance of two parallel columns, to favor the reader with one of the most extraordinary comparisons that ever three works presented to the public. The assurance alone must, however, be sufficient with the specimens now given, and, without stopping to congratulate Doctor Stoker on the general adoption of his practical principles, we shall proceed with our train of observation, and, while it shall be our aim to expose the fallacy of these principles, it shall also be our endeavour to trace their origin.

In no one instance of fever that we recollect, have stimulants appeared necessary or useful at its commencement. When the severity of the first attack has been subdued by other measures, and when the energy of the constitution has been impaired, stimulants have often accelerated recovery ; or when the period for active treatment had escaped unimproved, and the patient had arrived at that state of atomy which ever follows unmitigated excitement, cordials have seemed somewhat to lengthen out a hopeless existence. But in the former of these cases they were merely employed to expedite a recovery, which had been previously secured, and, in the latter, their only use was, to protract a life which they were unable to preserve. In both instances, the debility against which they were directed was a mere consequence of previous excitement, a sequela of fever. It was not a primitive debility, a part and parcel of the first attack, and, therefore, they were not administered at the commencement. At the commencement of nine cases out of ten, in the present fever of this metropolis, it is not debility that we have to fear, it is inflammation. It is not want of strength that we have to provide against, it is excess of action. This bugbear-debility, is the *ignis fatuus* which has been so implicitly followed, to the neglect of every warning voice that has issued out of the groans of those who have fallen victims to its delusion. Cordials are given, because the pulse feels weak, because the strength seems depressed, because the patient complains of languor. And if the pulse were raised, or the strength improved, or the languor permanently diminished, then the effects would justify the treatment, and the treatment would verify the symptoms. But if, in despite of our stimulants, life goes on evaporating, and if, in place of alleviated symptoms, the pulse continue to sink, the strength to decrease, and the languor to be unrelieved, or if, as is frequently the case, the pulse is raised, and the strength is increased, and the languor is diminished, but all this only for a time, and if, after the subsidence of this transient excitement, the patient lapse into a state of collapse ten times more alarming than the first, out of which no amount of stimulation will resuscitate him, then, if there be not a *locus*, there should probably be a *tempus pœnitentiæ*, and it might with some shew of reason be inquired whether are we doing good or harm? The sad and invincible error of this sect, is, that they will look no deeper than symptoms, that they will see nothing in these symptoms but debility, that they will let the wind blow on and cable their bark to the weathercock. Of all plans of cure which the most profound ignorance could suggest, none could be invented so diametrically opposed to what a perfect knowledge of pathology would recommend, as that which these physicians have adopted. Wine and bark, or bark and wine, are the last remedies which any one would think of trying in a disease of excitement. To stimulate in the first stage of fever is destruction. The debility, which is looked upon with so much horror, has no existence in nine cases out of ten at the outset of fever. It may come on, and it often does come on, as the disease proceeds ; and when it does come on, we have ample need both for wine and bark. But it will not come on, it cannot come on, in nine cases out of

ten, if we discharge our duty in the first instance, and crush
that action which precedes it. When first called in to a case
of fever, we have only to remain idle for a few hours, or days to
ensure the appearance of abundance of debility. We wish to
be doing something, we have only to lay down our lancet, and
uncork our bottle, and administer our cordial, to be speedily
greeted with abundance of debility. But it may here be worth
a question to inquire, is there any advantage gained by waiting
till this far-famed debility appear? Is the disease more manageable at that period; is there a better prospect of recovery; can
our remedies be applied with more effect? If we can gain power
by losing time, then there is a *quid pro quo* to sanctify the loss,
and we may practise just as many dalliances with the
disease as we find convenient. If the enemy can be decoyed
out of his vantage ground by manœuvering, then most certainly
let us have manœuvering. Prudence calls for it, the strictest
principles of tactics sanction it, and we see no reason why Es-
culapius may not be favoured with the privilege of a *ruse de
guerre* as well as Mars or any other God, more especially when
the motive of having recourse to it is to save blood which would
otherwise be shed. When the only remedies which physicians
of this school will use are excitants, it indicates a prudent feeling of consistency to wait until the period of excitement shall
have passed away. To exhibit wine and bark before this period
is certainly hazardous, and the rationale of any useful action they can be supposed to have, it might be rather perplexing
to explain. But there can neither be hazard nor obscurity in
the plan which waits with resignation till debility appear, and
then pours in its bark and wine. The only suggestion calculated to improve a system distinguished for two such virtues as
prudence and patience, is, that there is no necessity for, no
advantage gained by, such delay, inasmuch as there are remedies as applicable to the first stage of fever, as wine and bark
are to the last. In the first stage there is excitement; in the
last stage there is collapse. Wine and bark may come safely in
at the last stage, but they cannot at the first; and as substitutes
for wine and bark it seems sufficiently reasonable to employ
leeches and the lancet. The lancet and leeches are as well
adapted to the stage of excitement, as wine and bark are for
that of depression. The lancet and leeches diminish excitement by lowering the strength; the wine and bark diminish
depression by increasing it. The dangers to be feared during the
first stage of fever are the consequences of excitement, but
bleeding and starvation are the surest preservatives against such
consequences; and the dangers to be feared during the last stage

of fever are the effects of exhaustion; but stimulants are the most certain means of obviating such effects. The *médicine expectante* cannot therefore be advised in any stage of treatment. Furnished with remedies for every period of the evil, idleness is objectionable in any. As long as the inflammation may be dreaded, starve and purge, bleed and blister, and whenever debility is the foe, stimulate, strengthen, and support. Wait for nothing but a cure. Amid many advantages by which this plan stands recommended two more especially deserve attention. The first is that the stage of excitement is much more manageable than that of depression, and the second is, that, if the treatment which is recommended during the first stage be judiciously prosecuted, in nine cases out of ten the stage of depression will never have to be encountered. The opposite plan can only remove debility, it can never relieve excitement; while this by removing excitement, prevents debility. That is favourable to excitement, which when left unsubdued, passes into such debility as it cannot cure; this obviates debility, by attacking the cause of which debility is the effect. In combating with fever it is a much more hopeful task to assail it at its commencement than at the middle or towards the close of its career. The chances of recovery are at this period numerous; but they decrease in an inverse ratio to the progress of the malady. When the excitement of the first stage has passed into the collapse of the last, when the inflammatory action has exhausted the resources of the constitution, when muscular tremor and mental confusion, functions nerveless and inefficient, organs insensible to stimuli and disobedient to control, are to be contended with, all human aid although employing in the wisest manner the most approved remedies is commonly powerless. Wine may be exhibited by the dozen, bark may be swallowed by the pound, stimulants the most concentrated may be administered, and cordials the most agreeable may be poured in; but it is of no avail. The contest is over, the constitution has ceased to struggle, and nature, worried and worn out, at length yields to the foe. In nine cases out of ten the only formidable debility which appears in this disease proceeds from excitement, which ought in nine cases out of ten to be overcome by depletion. If the debility of fever were pure debility, were mere deficiency of strength, a mere negative quality, tonics and cordials would be judicious remedies; but it is not the absence of strength so much as the presence of disease which composes it. It is deranged function, complicated with disorganized structure, which enters into its very essence, and this deranged function and structure must be repaired before that debility, which results from them, can possibly be removed.

Turgid vessels must be emptied, adhesions must be dissolved, depositions must be abstracted, ulcerations must be healed, effusions must be absorbed, and all the sequelæ of excited action must be got quit of, before such strength and tone and vigour can be communicated to the patient as shall secure his safety. Now we ask can wine and bark do this? If wine and bark can, then the advocates of the stimulating system are right. Can wine and bark cool the skin, lower the pulse, and remove head-ache? Can they arrest inflammation of the bowels, can they prevent inflammation of the lungs, can they deplete the turgid arteries of the brain? If they can, then wine and bark are superior to bleeding and starvation, and it were bad taste as well as bad practice which preferred them. But, if they cannot do any of all these things; if, on the contrary, they can do every thing else; if they can increase heat, quicken the circulation and aggravate pain; if they can excite and fasten inflammation; if they can promote and propagate ulceration; if they can encourage and increase every form of effusion from red blood to limpid serum, it is plain that bark and wine are neither suitable nor safe in the treatment of this disease. It were just as hopeful an undertaking to remove the lameness of a broken leg by pouring in wine and bark, and neglecting, as useless, splints and tapes, rollers and compresses. The fracture of the bone is the cause of the lameness, when the fracture heals the lameness will gradually disappear, but as long as the leg continues broken it must likewise continue lame. The grand secret in treating fever is to know how to prevent this debility, not to cure it. To prevent the activity of the first stage from going into the debility of the last, to subdue that excitement which, if unsubdued, will terminate, must terminate in torpor, to preserve structure and function from that state of disease which can only end in weakness—these are, or ought to be, our indications for treatment.

But, continues Dr. Smith,

'Suppose, however, the proper treatment not to have been applied; suppose the case to have been neglected or mismanaged; either not to have been seen at all, or to have been too much contemned; suppose the pain in the head to have been not severe; that no complaint was made of it; or that giddiness only was felt; that the skin was not burning hot, but moderately warm; that the pulse was neither strong, nor bounding, nor hard; but of moderate strength and soft; that the mind was tolerably distinct, and the restlessness not great: why should blood be drawn? what indication is there for the employment of so violent a remedy in so mild a case? No symptom is prominent; no symptom is urgent; the case will do well.

' Such is the view that would be taken by the great majority of practitioners of this kind of case, and their treatment, without doubt, would
be correspondingly inert.   And this is the true origin, in many cases,
of typhus symptoms; of adynamic fever.   The disease is allowed to
take its own course ; and the product of every fever, at a certain stage
of its process, is adynamia : the physician does not perform his office ;
the disease advances; the restlessness increases ; there is no sleep ;
delirium comes on ; muscular tremor begins to be perceptible; the
pulse rises; the sensibility diminishes; and stupor, if it be not already
present, is close at hand.   And now the disease, it is sufficiently
obvious, is severe ; now, it is admitted, it calls for a powerful remedy ;
and, now for the first time, the lancet is thought of.   But the bleeding
relieves no symptom; it increases some ; the progress of the inflammation is not checked ; the adynamic symptoms are more fully developed ; the patient is more prostrate, and the fever, in all respects, of a
worse character : the inference is, that bleeding is a most inefficient
and dangerous remedy in fever ; and this inference is deduced from
experience ; those who draw the conclusion, judge from what they see ;
they disclaim reason; they pretend only to understand and to respect
the lessons of experience.

' I appeal to the attentive observer, whether this be not a faithful history of the progress and termination of hundreds of fever cases; whether
such a history may not be recorded as of daily occurrence; whether
what has been stated be not commonly the view, the practice, the
result, and the lesson.

' I will not appeal to the different history that belongs to cases that
are differently treated.   But I do earnestly appeal to the pathology
that has been stated ; that, at least, is experience, and it teaches a lesson, which it is worse than foolish to despise or to forget.   Every symptom just enumerated, has been detailed over and over again in the
cases that have been laid before the reader : inspection after death
must have made the conditions of the organs, as indicated by those
symptoms, familiar to his mind.   Of what avail can bleeding be, when
the patient is brought into the condition which first excites alarm, in
the case here supposed ?   The blood is no longer in its vessels ; it is
beneath the membranes, or in the ventricles, or at the base of the
brain ; the inflamed capillaries have done their work upon the cerebral
substance and upon its membranes ; and have left proof enough of their
activity, in the thickening of the one, and the softening or the indu-
ration of the other.   What can blood-letting do in this state of the
organs?   What can shaving the head, and applying cold do ?   What
can blisters do ?   What can purgatives do ?   And above all, what can
wine do ?   Nothing can be done ; at least, nothing effectually or certainly.'—pp. 388, 390.

And, surely, it is a sad and unenviable spectacle which the
physician, who has trifled away the period for activity, is
doomed to witness when his patient arrives at the last stage of
fever, with danger undiminished, and symptoms unrelieved.

Prostrate and powerless, with every nerve unstrung, with every member paralyzed, with every function woefully deranged ; without strength to resist death, and too weak to encourage treatment, the unfortunate sufferer lies insensible to his fate, and the practitioner, infatuated by the plausibilities of a system which he can neither defend nor understand, ascribes all to inveterate debility, and heaps upon this scapegoat the consequences of his own doctrines.

If, then, in nine cases of out ten, in the present fever of this country, the first stage is unmarked by any such debility as should sanction the use of stimulants, if the debility, which is dreaded in the last stages, may in nine cases out of ten be prevented by early and proper treatment, and if the debility, which will infallibly occur in the last stages, if such early and proper treatment be not adapted, is in nine cases out of ten beyond the efficacy of stimulants, does it not follow that little can, little ought to be expected from a system of treatment, which has stimulation for its favourite if not exclusive objects from first to last ?   But further still ; if in nine cases out of ten the present fever of this country betray such symptoms of excitation at the commencement as denote activity, if this activity be what we have to fear in nine cases out of ten, and if the debility, the only formidable debility, which exists in nine cases out of ten, be a relic or result of this activity when neglected or unsubdued, does it not follow that stimulants must be greatly and generally injurious, if employed at the commencement, and that they must naturally promote that state of apathy and nervelessness which it is so desirable to prevent, because so difficult to remove ?

In thus speaking of unmixed stimulation Dr. Stoker's custom of applying a few leeches to the temples " when the head is particularly engaged" is not forgotten ; nor that of the application of leeches to the arms with the same view he " reports most favourably." If this can mitigate the offence of stimulation it were cruel to deprive him of the use of it.   But, when we find these directions shielded within the following *cavete*, that, " although topical bleeding is a remedy of paramount importance in those tendencies to unequal distribution of blood in the system, which sometimes occur when typhoid and inflammatory fevers are combined, as well as indeed also for those local inflammations which so frequently succeed the partial turgidity of blood-vessels which then takes place ; yet I feel it my duty on an occasion like the present, to state, that for several years past, but particularly since our epidemics have assumed so pestilential a character, local abstraction of blood has not appeared to me so frequently applicable for the relief of the symptoms as it had previously been," and when we find the doctor forcing upon us his views and treatment as suitable to London, it cannot be thought strange should we entertain a very indifferent notion of this leeching plan. In many instances topical depletion is very highly beneficial and ought not to be dispensed with ; but in many more instances its employment will only interfere with the adoption of an equally safe and far more effectual remedy.

But, while endeavouring to expose the practice of stimulation in fever, it must not be concluded that stimuli are never necessary, and that depletion is always useful. To each of these views we are equally opposed. Cases will occasionally occur in which bleeding to any amount or by any mode, would be certainly destructive; and cases do frequently occur, the mildness of which renders it unnecessary. Where the symptoms are moderate, the excitement trifling, and no pain is particularly complained of—where spare diet, gentle aperients and cooling diluents are all the remedies which are necessary—where, in short, to do nothing is the best treatment—then it were only to make a wanton waste of vital fluid either to leech, or bleed. The duration of the attack can be seldom shortened by it, and the convalescence of the patient it will merely protract. Again, where the constitution has been worn down by age, or wasted by disease—where the mind has been unnerved by sorrow, or exhausted by fatigue—where the exciting cause has been peculiarly active, and the powers of life have been suddenly overwhelmed, depression and debility may reign from the first moment of complaint to the last hour of existence ; and, in all such cases, even active purging, not to mention bleeding, would be ruinous. Indefinite and indiscriminate depletion is most destructive treatment. Stimulants and tonics must occasionally be tried, and the quantity employed must be measured by no other criterion than their effects.

' But instead of bleeding, the proper remedy may possibly be the very reverse : it may be requisite to afford a stimulus. The change of structure produced by the inflammatory process may not have proceeded to such an extent as to be absolutely incompatible with life : but the powers of life may be so exhausted by the inflammatory excitement that, unless aid be brought to them, they will be overpowered, and sink : afford them appropriate aid, and they will rally, and, although slowly, ultimately repair the lesion which the organs have sustained.

This is precisely the condition, and perhaps it is the only condition, under which stimuli are really beneficial in Fever. Whenever such remedies are indicated, the vascular action is weak, and there appears to be a want of due supply of arterial blood to the brain.

Of all stimuli, wine or brandy is the best. If it be doubtful whether a stimulus can be borne, or will prove beneficial, a few ounces of wine may be administered. It will soon be manifest whether it be the appropriate remedy. If the restlessness, the heat, the delirium increase under its use, it will be obvious that it cannot be borne; if, after some hours, no perceptible impression be made upon any symptom, it is seldom of the least service, given to any extent, or persevered in for any length of time. If it be capable of doing any good, some improvement in the symptoms is commonly perceptible in a few hours after it is first administered. Sometimes that improvement is sudden and most striking; more commonly it is slight, slow, but still easy to be seen. If the pulse become firmer, and especially slower, the tremor slighter, the delirium milder, the sleep sounder, the skin cooler, and, above all, if the sensibility increase, and the strength improve, it is then the anchor of hope. It will save the patient if it be not pushed too far, and if it be withdrawn as soon as excitement is reproduced, should that happen, which it often does.

No certain indication for the administration of wine can be drawn from one or two symptoms alone : neither from the state of the pulse, nor of the skin, nor of the tongue; neither from the tremor, nor from the delirium. There is an aspect about the patient, an expression not in his countenance only, but in his attitude, in the manner in which he lies and moves, being, in fact, the general result, as well as the outward expression of the collective internal diseased states, that tell to the experienced eye when it is probable that a stimulus will be useful. Depression, loss of energy in the vascular system, as well as in the nervous and the sensorial, indicated by a feeble, quick, and easily compressed pulse, no less than by general prostration, afford the most certain indications that the exhibition of wine will be advantageous: and if the skin be at the same time cool and perspiring, the tongue tremulous, moist, or not very dry, and the delirium consist of low muttering incoherence, these symptoms will afford so many additional reasons to hope that it will prove useful. On the contrary, if the skin be hot, the eye fierce or wild, the delirium loud, noisy, requiring restraint, and the general motions violent, it is as absurd to give wine, as to pour oil upon a half-extinguished fire, with the view of putting out the yet burning embers.

When wine is indicated, but does not produce a decided effect, brandy may be substituted. I have seen no benefit arise from giving either in large quantity. When the condition is really present in which alone it can be useful, a moderate quantity will accomplish the only purpose it can serve. In every other condition, wine may be administered to any extent, (and I have given half a pint every hour) until the stomach return it, by vomiting, without the slightest impression being made upon the disease, or any, or scarcely any, upon the system. The malady is in possession of the seat of sensibility; it has destroyed the organ; it has abolished the function : what advantage can result from the application of stimuli?—The spirit that could feel their impression, and answer to it, is gone : organs destroyed by over-stimulation, cannot be regenerated by the application of additional stimuli : the apparatus is broken ; the wheels are clogged : the obstruction lies in that part of the mechanism in which the main power that works the machinery is generated ; that obstruction cannot be removed ; the movements of the machine must cease. Even when the case is not thus utterly hopeless, wretched is the physician whose only dependence for the safety of his patient is in wine.'—pp. 389, 391.

All this is intelligible, all this is rational. But when we are told by one that bark can cure continued Fever, the continued Fever of London, nearly, if not quite, as certainly as it can cure ague, and by another that venesection is not called for in nine cases out of ten of Typhus Fever, and by a third that transfusion of blood into the systems of those labouring under Fever is a promising resource, what are we to think or say when we look at Doctor Smith's 100 dissections, and see nothing strewed over the bodies of the dead but vestiges of inflammation and proofs of activity !

' I may state from my experience, that small quantities of wine, diluted with water, according to circumstances may be often given advantageously, even at the commencement of malignant Fevers of a decidedly typhoid character. In most cases, therefore, of that kind, especially such as I can ascertain to have been produced by contagion, I have prescribed from the commencement, from two to four ounces of wine, diluted with water ; this to be given in divided portions, in the course of twenty-four hours; commencing from the time the patient was placed under my care ; but the quantity and the time to be regulated by its effects; *e. g.* if found to excite distress, the interval between each dose to be increased, and the succeeding dose to be diminished; and *mutatis mutandis,* to administer it more frequently, and in larger doses, according to the urgency of circumstances. Wine thus administered, need not interfere with such evacuations, as are deemed necessary in typhoid Fevers. The due evacuation of the bowels should be attended to at the same time ; and in mixed cases of Fever, where the urgency of symptoms of inflammation, local or general, demands local or general blood-letting, I often find the cordial support of wine to promote the beneficial effects of such evacuation, and to counteract the consequences that would otherwise succeed. It is of the first importance, however, in determining on the early employment of wine in Fevers, to ascertain whether they are or not decidedly of a typhoid character ; and this is so difficult, during the first three or four days from the attack, that I have rarely ventured even on the small quantity just mentioned, excepting in cases attended with positive signs of debility, or such as I know to be the consequence of exposure to contagion. In such cases, indeed, I have found it highly beneficial, in relieving headache, tendency to delirium , restlessness, and even other symptoms, which, under other circumstances, I would have deemed counter-indications of wine.'—pp. 128-9.

What it has been our anxious effort to prove is, that all such cases constitute the exceptions and not the rule, and that while the exceptions should be studied with as much attention as the rule, such importance only as exceptions ought to have, should be ascribed to them. The rule is, that the general and abstract character of the Fever of this metropolis is excitement, that such measures are necessary for its treatment as are opposed to excitement, and it matters not in what climate or constitution, in what stage or under what circumstances, this excitement appears, when it does appear it should be assailed with an energy proportioned in its degree, that those doleful consequences —helpless debility and hopeless disorder—which ever follow it when unsubdued may be effectually avoided. The various remedies which may be employed for this purpose, it is not our intention to detail. To state how often the lancet must be unsheathed, how many leeches must be applied, or how many purgatives must be administered would be entering into minutiæ of no interest here. Our business throughout has been with prominent principles. If they can be settled it will not be difficult to adjust the detail, and those who wish to extend their knowledge into minute statements, will find in the work of Doctor Smith every necessary particular, and to its careful perusal would we earnestly recommend them. Again, let the disciples of Brown produce their facts, their arguments, their cases. General statements, vehement assertions, abstract deductions will not do: individual descriptions, minute particulars: symptoms of every case from first to last; the daily results of daily treatment in different constitutions at different stages of disease, the circumstances which show the marked evil of early and judicious depletion, contrasted with those which establish the marked good of early and general stimulation, and, finally, a description of the relative appearances of those who die after such modes of treatment, this is what we ask. Such information has been given on the other side, and it is now again given in the fullest manner in the works of Doctor Smith. Again, those who say to the disciples of the school of Brown, explain it to us, why our bleedings are almost invariably followed by relief, when we are intrusted with the management of the first symptoms ? inform us why the pulse does not sink, why the functions are not weakened, why the powers are not impaired ? Tell us why the blood which we draw, is in nine cases out of ten, inflamed, why the pain which we draw it to relieve is in nine cases out of ten relieved, and why, in very

many instances, the symptoms are so moderated after depletion, performed at the proper time and prosecuted to the
necessary extent, that little is afterwards left for the physician
to do, beyond preserving by prudence the vantage ground
which his activity has procured ? Explain to us all this, and
when your commentary is complete then take it to our dissections, and make it harmonize with all that is there revealed.
Make it account for our coagulated lymph, our recent
adhesions, our new membranes, our spreading ulcers, and our
loaded vessels. And after you have satisfied yourselves that
your harmony is made out, then require of us why we bleed;
and if we cannot show cause, we leave you at full liberty to tax
our practice as unscientific, and our language as intemperate.

If we are to follow the directions of Doctor Stoker, and never
employ our lancet in any case, in any constitution, in any climate, under any circumstance, and by any chance—if we are to
look upon leeches as upon lions, with fear and trembling—if we
are to regard " disappointment generally, and irreparable injury
sometimes, as the result" of free purgation, it is only fair to give
us something in the form of argument, with the weight of truth.
We maintain that this something of proof and argument has not
yet been given. If in the treatment of the Dublin-fever we are
to be hedged in by such precautionary death-warnings, be it so ;
but we would recommend it to the doctor to watch over the
firstlings of his own flock, for in the persons of Mills and Cheyne
and a few other unbelieving bleeders, we verily believe him to
have wolves in the centre of his own fold. Let his admonitions
be directed towards them, and, in as far as in him lies, let him protect the lives of his devoted countrymen from the consequences
of their frightful sytem of depletion. As for this metropolis it
must needs, we believe, select its creed from another liturgy,
and until the evidence of sense shall cease to outweigh that of
testimony, we must not only persevere in heterodoxy, but be perverse enough to enhance our guilt by endeavouring to convince
others we are right. We must believe that the London-fever
requires both leeches and the lancet—that moderate purgation
is always necessary and free purging often beneficial—that a
total removal of all stimuli from all cases is incomparably safer,
as a general rule, than that the lancet is inadmissible in any—
that every mean, which Doctor Stoker would employ against an
ordinary attack of inflammation, may be employed to a certain
extent in the present fever of this metropolis—and the only reason
we can advance for the faith that is in us is, that a very similar
action is going on in both, and very similar consequences are to
be feared from both. The action and consequences of both differ

we believe, principally in degree, and the means necessary to cure both must differ nearly in the same respect. All this we believe in nine cases out of ten, and he, who requires more argument than the limits have suffered us to advance in support of this opinion, has only to consult Doctor Smith's work to procure it. We solicit the attention of the public as well as of the profession to this work. If it advocate error, the error is of such magnitude that it ought to be exposed, and the earnestness and plausibility with which it is advocated arms its intrinsic evil with tenfold mischief. But, if the doctrines it contends for be founded in nature, and be derived from the study of nature, the author merits the reward of a double service—by arriving at important truth amid much popular error, and by laying this truth before the world in a diction, and with a demonstration which most powerfully recommend it to the judgment. It brings forward the opinions of conflicting sects with equal candour and perspicuity—it subjects to the ordeal of reason what experience cannot reach, and it tests with experience what reason has approved—it neither devotes itself to empty speculation on the one hand, nor to abstract dogmatism on the other. Its business is with practical truth. Where novel opinions are hazarded, the arguments which convinced the writer are laid before his reader—where old opinions are impugned, the reasons for objection are fully stated, and whether its theme be the exposure of error or the support of truth, no doctrine, however roughly handled, is condemned by merely brandishing the wand of magisterial authority, and no assertion, however feasible, is suffered to go forth unsustained by evidence. And when the mass of information which the work contains, is considered with relation to the source from which it has been obtained, it can scarcely be said that the inferences to which it arrives are rashly drawn or feebly advocated. The London Fever Hospital has been the principal field of observation. Into this valuable establishment no disease is admissible but fever, and no other hospital exists in the metropolis, which gives indiscriminate admission to this disease. It is obvious, therefore, that if the amplest opportunities for observation can give weight to the results of experience, it is from such an institution that the most authentic knowledge should be looked for. If anything can be certainly known of this pestilence—if seeing it in every form of constitution, in every stage of progress, in every change of atmosphere, and under every variety of cure—if watching it daily and carefully from its commencement to its close, where every medicine can be seasonably prescribed, and every prescription judiciously administered—if attending the sick under the salutary discipline of a rigid police, where every injurious influence can be effectually removed, every promising remedy advantageously applied, and every direction implicitly obeyed—a well-conducted hospital for the cure of fever, like the Fever Hospital of London, is the fountain from which the purest information should be found to emanate. Upon such neutral ground nothing may be omitted which it is desirable to do, nor any thing done which it were better to omit. There every symptom can be carefully traced, every change of symptom instantly noticed, medicines can be exhibited with a precision and surveillance which the ignorance of attendants cannot frustrate, nor the prejudices of the patient counteract. The diseased are thus rescued out of the baneful influences of vulgar prejudices, the disease is rooted up out of its disadvantageous localities, and the constitution is placed upon a vantage ground, which infinitely multiplies the chances of recovery by adding to the efficacy of the remedies employed. Such establishments, when ably conducted and amply endowed, are productive of advantages which can be adequately appreciated only by the poor; but were their usefulness even limited to the important benefit which we have already specified, their value, as schools for the initiation of the profession into the mysteries of fever, were more than a sufficient recompence to the public for the expenses they incur. It appears strange that London, so overgrown, so overpeopled and so obnoxious to fever, should consider a hospital, containing no more than between sixty and seventy beds, sufficiently spacious to answer all the purposes of such a charity; and it must appear stranger still, that this little solitary hospital, which admits upwards of six hundred patients annually, and annually expends a sum no greater than two thousand pounds, should be annually obliged to appear as a petitioner before the public, for the means of support. It is a duty which the affluent owe to themselves as well as to the destitute, to place this benevolent institution above the influence of poverty, that the sphere of its usefulness may not be unnecessarily contracted by any pecuniary disabilities; for let them be assured that the most effectual mode of preserving their own families from the scourge of fever is to facilitate, by every means in their power, the speedy removal of the destitute poor from their crowded and filthy habitations into the wards of a comfortable and well-conducted hospital.

There still remains one other point connected with the works of Doctor Smith, which it was our intention to have included within the present paper—namely, the subject of contagion as connected with fever;—but the very great importance of the points in which we have been engaged has tempted us into a minuteness, which was not originally contemplated. We hope, however, at no distant period to take up this question, when we shall attempt to establish two positions—the first of which is, that it is as much unsettled as it ever was ; and, in the second place, that it may be for ever set at rest by some such plan as shall be then detailed.

ART. XI.—1. *Die Asiatische Cholera in Russland in den Jahren* 1829, 1830, *und* 1831. Von Dr. J. R. Lichtenstädt, &c. Berlin. 1831.

2.—*Die Cholera Morbus ; ihre Verbreitung, ihre Zuffälle, &c.* Von Dr. Schnurrer, &c. 1831.

3.—*Rapport au Conseil Superieur de Santé sur le Choléra Morbus Pestilentiel.* Par Alex. Moreau de Jonnès, &c. Paris. 1831.

4.—*Mémoire sur un Nouveau Traitement du Choléra Morbus, et des Affections Typhoides, &c.* Par H. F. Ranque, &c. Paris. 1831.

5.—*History of the Epidemic Spasmodic Cholera of Russia ; &c.* By Bisset Hawkins, M. D. &c. London. 1831.

6.—*Cholera ; its Nature, Causes, and Treatment, &c.* By C. Searle. London. 1831.

7.—*Papers relative to the Disease called Cholera Spasmodica in India, now prevailing in the North of Europe.* Printed by authority of the Lords of his Majesty's Most Honourable Privy Council. London. 1831.

8.—*Trattato delle varie specie di Cholera Morbus.* Di Michele Buniva, M. D. Turin. 1831.

In this detail of the evidence brought forward by the advocates of terraqueous miasmata and of contagious influence, we have studiously abstained from expressing any opinion upon a subject that every one, who reflects upon the facts and statements which have been here collated, may be equally competent with ourselves to decide upon. The profession, as well as the public at large, are sadly divided upon the contagiousness of Cholera. Even those who have witnessed it in different countries, and at all periods, who have traced its progress upon the field of its operations, have studied its character in different stages and constitutions, and have had the very amplest opportunities of drawing truth from the fountain, are opposed in sentiment; and, therefore, to whatever side our private opinion may be disposed to lean, both the settlement of this controversy and the cause of science may be more judiciously consulted, by leaving the question, for the present, to the unbiassed discretion of the reader's judgment, Should this malignant pestilence ever land upon our shores, and give us a personal opportunity of confirming, or of modifying the views which we entertain, it will then be our duty to lay the result before the public; but if the evidence now before them cannot lead to some conclusion, in virtue of its own merits, no deduction drawn by us could in any measure fill up the deficiency.

Having thus endeavoured to sketch the history—causes—and character—of Spasmodic Cholera, it only remains for us to make a few observations upon the means found best calculated to prevent its approach, and the treatment found most effectual in accomplishing its cure. We have seen facts sufficient to convince us, that however rapid and extended the progress of this epidemic has hitherto been, it is by no means beyond the control of judicious and active interference. While it swept the Mauritius from one shore to the other, it was incarcerated within St. Denis, in the isle of Bourbon. These two islands are placed in all respects under the same physical and moral circumstances, and no reason can be assigned why the disease did not spread to the same extent in both, but that in the Mauritius a blind adherence, in the first instance, to the doctrine of non-interference permitted it to follow unchecked the laws of its own nature, while in the neighbouring island the governor was taught wisdom by the sad result of this experiment, and used the necessary means for limiting it to the spot where it first appeared. The towns of Sarepta and Tripoli are equally striking illustrations of the effects of a well-conducted quarantine; and it is a fact which well merits the notice of our government, that in every country, city, and town, which Cholera has as yet visited, the extent of its ravages has been uniformly in an inverse ratio to the general health of the inhabitants, and to the perfection of the means employed for its prevention. Those classes of society, whose habits, occupations, and rank in life render them most obnoxious to pestilential agents, have been beyond all proportion its most frequent, its earliest, and its easiest victims. In India it preyed with peculiar violence upon the natives, who are restricted by their religion to a vegetable food, are generally employed in all menial offices, and are necessarily exposed to more privations than the European population. In Arabia, Persia, and Syria, the poor, aged, and debilitated, were always the first cut off; and in Russia and Poland but few of the upper orders of society have become its victims.

Little reliance, it would appear, is to be placed in any of the disinfectants which have as yet been tried. A chemist at Moscow, M. de Kartzoff, is said to have preserved a family of thirty individuals, even while in close intercourse with their neighbours, by employing the chlorides of soda and lime; and a vessel from Bordeaux is reported to have remained uninfected at Calcutta, in the centre of vessels which had been decimated by the disease, by keeping her decks sprinkled with a solution of these salts. Dr. Albers, the head of the Prussian commission, however, speaks in very moderate terms of these chlorides; and sir W. Crichton asserts that fumigation with chlorine had been abundantly tried, but without any favourable result. These salts can be procured from any of the chemists; and if fumigation with chlorine be preferred, it is easily performed, by pouring six drachms of oil of vitriol on a mixture of four drachms of powdered manganese, and eight drachms of common salt. These articles should be placed in a china cup, and the doors of the apartment to be fumigated should be kept shut for two hours; after which the fresh air should be freely admitted. In Moscow fumigation is generally performed with spirit of juniper and burnt litter; but free and frequent ventilation is certainly more to be depended on than any or all of these modes of purification.

The stomach and bowels should be preserved in a natural state; extreme or sudden vicissitudes of temperature should be religiously shunned; raw fruits, adulterated beer, sour wines, and all kinds of indigestible food should be strictly prohibited. Regular hours are indispensable; the mind should

not be suffered to despond; unwholesome localities, such as
the neighbourhood of low and marshy grounds, close and ill-
ventilated habitations, condensed and over-crowded districts
should be as much as possible avoided; and all degrees of
intemperance, whether in food or drink, are especially destructive. In short, every thing which can add tone to the general
health should be pursued, while whatever tends to weaken the
powers of life should be counteracted. In many respects no
town which Cholera has yet visited, can furnish an easier conquest than our own metropolis. The hundreds of starving paupers
who come to London for relief, and are compelled from want to
herd together in much less cleanliness and comfort than the
lowest orders of the native Indians, are ever predisposed to the
invasion of such an epidemic; and the over-peopled condition of
many of our streets, courts, and alleys, will strongly co-operate
with the intemperate and filthy habits of many of their inhabitants, in giving a facility to its propagation, which the wisest
and most rigid quarantine may be unable to neutralize. A
medical commission should be appointed to investigate the
health of the metropolis, and every thing, which in their opinion
would tend to encourage either the entrance or progress of this
pestilence, should be reported on. This precautionary measure
should be adopted now, and in the event of the dreaded arrival
of Cholera upon our shores, the town should be divided into districts, each district should be placed under the surveillance of
a medical sub-commission, which should have erected for their
use a temporary hospital centrally situated, and severe penalties
should be inflicted upon all who did not inform the members
of this commission the moment symptoms of the disease were
detected. It was some such preventive plan as this which
was adopted at Moscow; and when Cholera was ravaging
Madras, two men were stationed in every street to carry the
sick to the hospitals as soon as they took ill, and to each street
was appropriated a lazaretto, sufficient to accommodate as
many as required its assistance. Experience, however, has
demonstrated the difficulty of so effectually isolating the diseased, as to place the healthy beyond the reach of attack; and
in such a country as England, where the means of communication are so numerous, and the expense of travelling so
moderate, unless our quarantine arrangements entirely prevent
its introduction, we strongly fear that no prophylactic measures
which can be afterwards adopted, will be found sufficient to
circumscribe it within any given space. This was evidently
the fatal error which the Russian government at first committed. Finding that their exertions had arrested it on its

first appearance in Astracan, they permitted it on its re-appearance, in 1830, to pierce into the very heart of the empire, before the active measures which were afterwards employed, were carried into operation. So universal, consequently, has the disease spread through Russia, that no place being now left which it has not visited, the government have no longer continued the system of quarantine. But should it unfortunately visit our shores, we have good reason to anticipate that it will make much less havoc among our population, than it has done either in India, Russia, or Poland. Our people are better clothed and better fed; our habitations are more spacious and better aired; our charities are more numerous, and conducted on a more generous scale; and our long connexion with the east has made the faculty generally well acquainted with the nature of the disease, and with the various remedies which have exerted the greatest influence upon its progress and mortality.

Like every other malady of a very fatal character, the variety of medicines which have been recommended for the cure of Spasmodic Cholera, is only equalled by their conflicting properties. Dr. Joechnichen and Moreau de Jonnés entertain a very moderate estimate of the powers of the healing art in the present instance; but by comparing the mortality of those who have received no treatment with that of those who have, there seems to be no ground to despond. "In one district," says Mr. Kennedy, the "population of which is about 200,000, 15,945 were attacked with Cholera. Of these 1294 had no medical assistance, and there is reason to believe, that of that number every individual perished; whereas 166 were attacked on the estate of Count Guriev, in Saratov, and out of 147, who were attended to from the first, twenty-six only died, or one-sixth of the whole, while the remaining nineteen, who received no treatment, perished without one exception." As a general statement we have reason to say, that when the disease has been abandoned to itself, it has usually destroyed one-half, and not unfrequently two-thirds of those whom it has attacked; whereas, when it has been early combatted by proper remedies, its mortality has been rarely one-third, and sometimes not more than one-fifth of the diseased. Cholera is principally a disease of function, and not of structure. Beyond slight inflammation of the stomach and small intestines, and considerable vascularity of the brain, no marked appearances of any consequence are discoverable after death; consequently, if these deranged functions can be restored to their natural state, there exists no organic lesion to obviate or retard the cure. Hence is it, that

when the Cholera-patient recovers, his symptoms are as rapidly
banished as they at first appeared; and the constitution, which
was apparently on the eve of breaking down beneath an accumulating mass of wretchedness, regains in a few hours its
wonted elasticity and vigour. The medical world are, however,
most unfortunately unsettled in their arrangement of the
means best adapted for the treatment of this disease. One
physician says, that nothing can be done without the lancet,
and another contends that bleeding is little better than to kill.
Opium is given in enormous quantities by one practitioner,
while it is denounced by another as decidedly injurious; and
whether we speak of oxyde of bismuth, calomel, magnesia,
glauber salts, castor oil, cajeput oil, oil of turpentine, olive oil,
nux vomica, ether, ammonia, brandy, or wine, we find almost
the same distracted state of medical opinion. "But," as
Dr. Kennedy observes, " it is now high time for the profession to come to some decision, if possible; for there need
be no hesitation in supposing that, of two opposite systems,
both cannot be harmless; and some difference of result must
be expected, when one bleeds to relieve oppression of the brain,
and another to relieve congestion of the liver; when one gives
the most acrid stimulants as excitements, and another simple
doses of calomel and laudanum by tea-spoonfuls as sedatives;
and finally, when one declares that opium alone is to be
depended on, and another that it is the worst medicine which
can be exhibited." Where, therefore, unanimity is not to be
found, we must be guided by the judgment of the greatest
number; and in following the majority of the best informed
upon this disease, it would appear that the following is a summary of the treatment which has been found most successful
both in India and upon the Continent.

   If the patient be seen as soon as he is attacked, a vein should
be opened in the arm, and blood should be abstracted in proportion to the violence of the symptoms, and the powers of the
patient. At the same time a pill, composed of twenty grains of
calomel and two grains of solid opium, should be taken, and
instantly followed by a draught, composed of one ounce of
camphor mixture, one drachm of laudanum, and one drachm of
œther. The entire body, but more especially the extremities,
should be rubbed with warm flannel, or flannel steeped in spirits
of turpentine; and bottles, containing hot water, are to be applied to the feet. If these measures succeed in affording relief,
the pill and draught may be repeated in the evening, and half
an ounce of castor oil should be given on the following morning; after which no further danger need be apprehended. But

if the symptoms remain unabated, and, as often happens, no blood can be obtained by the lancet, from twenty to thirty leeches should be applied to the pit of the stomach ; the pill and draught should be repeated every two hours, until the spasms relax, and after the leeches have done bleeding, the bowels should be covered with a mustard poultice or a blister. As soon as bile appears in the evacuations, strong hopes of recovery may be entertained, and half a drachm of compound jalap powder, mixed up with two ounces of peppermint water, may then be given to solicit this secretion, and be repeated if necessary. The attack, if violent, seldom continues longer than from twelve to twenty hours ; but inflammatory action is not unfrequently set up afterwards in the brain, stomach, or other important organs, which requires both skill and watchfulness. As medical assistance, however, can always be procured before the case has progressed so far, these accidental consequences may in general be avoided.

Mr. Corbyn gave his calomel in powder, and washed it down with one dram of laudanum, twenty drops of oil of peppermint, and two ounces of water. He bled freely in the early stage, and supported the heat by friction, warm-baths, and cordials. Mr. Scott advises laudanum and ether, of each one drachm, joined to half an ounce of brandy and one ounce of water. This he gives, after every attack of vomiting, and afterwards, in the same way, twelve grains of calomel, three of camphor, and one of opium, joined together with three drops of oil of peppermint. Dr. Burrell, of Calcutta, asserts, that opium is indispensable ; and cases are recorded, in which immense quantities of this drug were administered with almost uniform success. When blood can be obtained, the lancet is also admitted to be invaluable. Dr. Kennedy says, " I always feel it a subject of regret when I cannot bleed ; it is, in my mind, next to signing the patient's deathwarrant, when I decide that the critical moment is passed, and he no longer capable of undergoing it." Dr. Burrell states, that out of 100 patients, eighty-eight were bled, and twelve not bled. Of the eighty-eight, two only died, while of the twelve, eight perished. In many instances, however, more especially when they have been long neglected, the circulation upon the surface of the body is so languid, that no pulse can be felt at the wrist, and when a vein is opened, no blood flows. In such cases, an ounce or two of brandy, or some cordial stimulant, may excite the circulation ; and as soon as a few ounces of blood have been obtained, the symptoms gradually moderate. All forms of drink were once prohibited, but this precaution is found no longer necessary, and water, either cold or warm, acidulated with some vegetable acid, is given freely.

This is the Indian mode of treatment ; but, as the Russian practice has been modelled on the experience of the East, it is not essentially different. The Russian physicians, however, seem to depend most upon the application of heat ; and some of them, as sir W. Crichton, go so far as to assert, that calomel and opium are not so beneficial as medicines which elevate the temperature, and excite perspiration. " The exciting of copious diaphoresis," says Dr. Hermann," " is the only efficacious remedy against Cholera, and no patient recovered in Moscow, without this critical secretion." At Warsaw, poultices of hempseed, rung out of warm water, are wrapt over the entire body as warm as they can be borne, and renewed as they cool, until a profuse perspiration is produced. M. Ranque, of Paris, eulogizes, in no very measured terms, the employment of epithems, the principal ingredients of which are hemlock, camphor, sulphur, and tartar emetic. Plaisters, composed of these substances, are laid over the stomach and bowels, and the extremities are well rubbed with a liniment, composed of sulphur, ether, Belladonna, and laurel-water. In Batavia, according to M. Reveille Parise, a kind of family specific, which the natives call " cholera water," is kept ready made in the shops, to which immediate recourse is had on the first manifestation of the disease. This medicine is composed of one part of laudanum and two parts of spirits of mint, taken in doses of one table-spoonful frequently, until the spasms are overcome. It is said to prove very efficacious.

In the absence of more official information on the treatment of this formidable pestilence, we have considered it our duty to close this article with a brief abstract of that remedial plan which experience has most approved. But it were highly desirable that the Board of Health should lay before the public, in a plain and unprofessional style, the substance of the information which has reached them upon this interesting point. In such a disease as Spasmodic Cholera, where minutes are as valuable as hours, and where the loss of an hour may be the loss of life, the public at large cannot be made too well acquainted with the symptoms which characterize, the measures which may prevent, and the remedies which may cure it. Should the present pages in the least contribute to this important end, the object for which they were written will be obtained.

Art. X.—*Gatherings from Grave-yards, particularly those of London, &c.* By G. A. Walker, Surgeon. Longman. 1839. pp. 258.

WHAT a mass of unimaginative, unthinking beings, forms the genus man. Fill the mouths of thieves and paupers with wheaten bread, the whiteness of which does not quite rival that on the Queen's table, but which is exceedingly wholesome and nutritious, and very much better than that which is eaten by the greater part of the self-sustaining labourers of all Europe, and both Houses of Parliament are in throes of humane agony at the wrongs of the poor. The difference of colour can be seen with mortal eyes; it is a subject of most obvious comparison. Fill, however, the lungs of thieves and paupers—fill their prisons and poor-houses—fill the Sunday-schools of the young, and the churches and chapels of the virtuous, and the workshops and pent-up dwellings of the industrious—fill the lordly mansions of the rich, and the very palace of royalty itself, with the deadly poisonous emanations of burial-grounds and charnel-houses; let these pestiferous gases saturate the air where crowds of coroneted worshippers are assembled in our churches, or where multitudes of little children get their Sabbath-day's brief dole of learning; let half a city be corrupted with human putrescence, and so long as these matters do not seize violently and continuously by the nose the people of quality, no public commotion is raised, no Parliament is petitioned, no sound is heard about the neglected health of the community. The chief reason of this is, that to convince the judgment, thought and consideration are needful—to prove that such evils exist, and that they are unwholesome, facts must be collected, experiments performed, and conclusions carefully deduced; all which are matters of some trouble and difficulty. The simplest biped that walks, will not, with his eyes open, jump into a break-neck hole, or run straight upon pointed spikes; and yet men, the great and the learned even, are so blind, that they surround themselves, by day and by night, with equally certain although more slow instruments of death. It is only educated men,—it is only a highly-instructed class, who take rational care of their health. When ill, people in general take physic to be sure, and they get well or die; but they do not know nor consider that the preservation of their health, and the defence against disease, are very much in their own power, and that when tolerably put together by nature, it is in general only by a violation of some of her laws that they become diseased. Had it not been for the neglect of this most useful knowledge, the cities of England, and particularly the metropolis, would not have remained up to the present time without sanatory regulations, especially respecting the burial of the dead, the neglect of which are among the most certain causes of unwholesomeness. In this country, the Government rarely takes the initiative; improvements are effected only when the people clamour for them, but it is a tedious and difficult thing to educate a people up to the appreciation of new and wholesome regulations. In other countries, as in France, the Government *moves:* here it is moved; there it is sufficient for a few instructed men to show the need and usefulness of a law, and it is likely to be introduced.

The unwholesomeness of inhumation in cities, especially when densely peopled, caused governments in ancient times to prohibit its practice. " Plato, in his republic, did not even permit inhumation in fields fit for tillage; he reserved for that purpose dry and sandy ground, which could be employed for no other use." Indeed, the practice was little known or scarcely allowed in Europe until after the Christian era. Wealthy and pious persons sometimes, as an especial favour granted by the ecclesiastical authorities, were buried within churches, or in chapels contiguous to them; by degrees the exception became the general rule: " the prerogative, originally reserved for emperors, became the portion of the lowest class of citizens, and that which at first was a distinction, became at last a right common to every one."

Much curious matter has been collected by Mr Walker respecting the funeral rites of people in different ages, and in different parts of the world. He cites the practice of the Jews, the laws of the ancient Greeks, Romans, and Carthaginians, all of whom strictly prohibited interment within their cities. Many extracts are given in Mr Walker's book from Orders in Council, and letters of bishops and others, against the renewal of this pernicious practice in later times, which practice had gradually increased, " until the churches had become almost cemeteries." The French have nearly abolished the practice, not without difficulty in some of the provincial towns, where superstition and private interest have arrayed themselves against measures of the most obvious utility.

" The Parliament of Paris, in 1765, required the cemeteries in that capital to be closed against future burials, and their present contents to be removed (with great labour and cost) to the well-known catacombs, excavations which extend under a great portion of the southern faubourgs. These immense caverns (deserted stone quarries) were consecrated in 1786, and the removal of the bodies commenced ; the bones were conveyed by torchlight in funeral cars, followed by priests chanting the service of the dead.   It is certain that the remains of more than three millions of human beings are entombed here—some writers have estimated them at six millions! In 1790, the National Assembly passed a law, commanding all towns and villages to discontinue the use of the old burial-places, and to form others at a distance from their habitations.   This has been completely carried into effect in Paris by the formation of four large cemeteries without the barrières, including Père-la-chaise."

All that belongs, however, to the history of the subject, either ancient or modern, is rather curious than useful, except in as far as too many persons are influenced, rather by authority than evidence, and they prefer to know that the institution they are urged to adopt formerly existed, and has only fallen into abeyance, rather than to take up with something quite new, or with an innovation, which, however useful, is supported merely on the ground of recent experiments and demonstration.   People are inclined to do that which others do, or which others have done, rather than to do that which is strictly but merely useful.

It is one of the conditions of health, that atmospheric air should be in a certain degree of purity ; its component parts of oxygen, nitrogen, with a little carbonaceous and aqueous matter, must be in definite ratios, and without further commixtures, to be salubrious.   Air in motion is more salubrious than air at rest ; human lungs deteriorate the air, which is more readily relieved of its corruptions by being moved about, for it then mingles with the purer masses which are in the upper and surrounding atmosphere, and becomes infinitely diluted.   Low and moist places, by sending forth their peculiar gaseous products, injure the air for the purposes of animal life.   Even the process of tillage, with the manure that is used, and the vital and chemical influences of vegetable growth, as well as vegetable and animal decomposition, injure the air ; certain soils even, by their chemical and physical properties, alter the salubrity of the air.   Some localities are eminently healthy, where there is the exact adaptation of soil, heat, wind, and dryness, and freedom from excessive cultivation.   An examination was made some time since, respecting the comparative salubrity of certain districts, and the most healthy were found to be those where there is little tillage ; upland tilled lands were found more healthy than low verdant flats; but of all places, densely-peopled towns were found to be the most unhealthy. The mere aggregation of multitudes of people, causes a rapid deterioration of the air. Although London is but a small speck in the vast aerial ocean above and around it, and although it occupies but a few feet of vertical elevation in an atmosphere which is said to rise many miles, yet it is found practically that flowing through its sinuous streets, and pent up in the countless little cells where its myriads toil like clusters of coral-insects at the bottom of the sea, the air, by constant inspiration, as well as other causes, is polluted and deteriorated faster than it can be purified, by commixture with the circumambient mass. It is found that some parts of London are less healthy than others, and that those kinds of fever which are produced by corrupt air, abound more in those parts where there is the greatest aggregation of human beings, in narrow streets, and in blind courts and alleys. It is not possible, chemically, to measure the relative insalubrity of the air; though it will vary from being the means of certain and speedy death, as in the instance of the black hole at Calcutta, up to a scarcely appreciable tenuity of degradation, as in the metropolitan parks, where the air is *comparatively* good, but not nearly as salubrious as that which wafts to our noses the delicious perfume of the wild flowers on Hayes-Common or Chislehurst. The very presence of the living crowds of the metropolis is cause enough of corruption of the air, even although all the inhabitants should be the best ordered and the most cleanly. It is, therefore, the supreme duty of a municipality to be strenuously vigilant that there be no other agents to taint the air but those which are inseparable from the circumstance of crowds of living beings constantly using it. The most trifling addition to the causes of such deterioration is worthy of attention. The mere straightness and the direction of streets have much to do with the purity of the air. Streets should be continuous, and not terminated at short distances by other streets blocking up the ends by passing at right angles. Compare the New road with York street, which runs parallel to it at the distance of a few yards. The former is continuous, and open at either extremity, while the latter is crossed by houses at both ends. The air in the one will be clear, and the sun bright, at the same moment the other is filled with smoke and fog. No buildings should on any account be constructed without efficient sewers, and closed places for the reception of offal; no exposed surface of decomposing matter should be suffered to eliminate its gases into the air, which the next moment will be imbibed by human lungs; no houses should be built to which there is not a constant supply of good water; nor should dwellings (not even workhouses or prisons) be placed, under any circumstances, in a locality of known and unquestionable unwholesomeness. We remember walking with a surgeon in a country town, for its size one of the most unhealthy in England, when, pointing to a row of houses then in the course of erection, he said, " Those houses are being built without hollow foundations, or any kind of drainage, on the clay land near to the river—plump upon the wet earth ; and I shall have plenty to do when they are occupied, for the inhabitants will have fever in abundance." People are not now allowed by law to abide in out-houses and shambles, nor should they be permitted to reside in dwellings unwholesome to themselves, and prejudicial to the public health; or rather, the law should not allow builders to erect any but such dwellings as are wholesome, as far as present knowledge and art will admit. There would then be fewer houses in the metropolis, and fewer families, but they would be much more healthy, and consequently more happy. The salubrity of London, in addition to those agents which have been mentioned, is impaired by its being built on a clay sub-soil, occupying a portion of the broad and moist valley of the Thames. Its coal-fires too, emitting a mass of smoke, which, sustained by the heat of the city below, and condensed by cold at a variable elevation above, stretched and hovering over its whole extent (from Greenwich even beyond Hammersmith), lies like a huge pall, which confines and represses the unhealthy emanations from beneath, and keeps the air well nigh saturated with them. The burial-ground is the most decided place of maleficent influence. To the necessary degradation of the air by the living, is wantonly and unnecessarily added, the decomposition of the dead, whose gaseous products in the open country would be directly neutralized by mixing immediately with the surrounding atmosphere, or they would be seized and fixed in the processes of vegetable action, and become less unhealthy and much more agreeable, which in a city lie accumulating and lurking at the base of the walls which confine them, rise slowly into the upper air, or rather disperse themselves horizontally into the streets, alleys, houses, and finally into the lungs of the people. In the city there is no living laboratory of vegetable organism to convert the poison of the dead into the healthy tissues of life, but it floats about freely, and becomes to animal life, when combined with it, the cause of disease, decrepitude, and death.

The process of decomposition is so minute, and is carried on so secretly, in the molecules of the body, that its rationale is not very well understood. " On peut assurer que leur histoire est encore à faire malgré les travaux isolés dont ils ont été l'objet," says a French chemist. Its ultimate results are, however, obvious enough.

" The chemical constitution of the soil seems to have little influence in retarding or accelerating decomposition, the two most active agents in hastening this process are air and moisture. Accordingly we find that the greater the depth from the surface at which a body is interred, the longer it resists putrefaction, and it will remain unchanged for a considerable period if enclosed in a leaden coffin, so as altogether to exclude the air. The action of the earth depends in a great measure on its power of absorbing and retaining moisture : thus, in sandy soils, through which the water drains quickly, decomposition goes on slowly, and is sometimes altogether prevented, as in cases where people have perished in deserts, and have been overwhelmed by the drifting sands, in which their bodies have been found long after, dry and shrivelled, but without any sign of having undergone putrefaction. In clayey soils, which retain water, putrefaction readily takes place, and quickly proceeds, to the destruction of all the soft parts, unless transformation into *adipocire* takes place, which stops decomposition. Bodies may change in three ways, as the result of decomposition; first, the putrefactive process may go on uninterruptedly till the soft parts are destroyed, and only the skeleton remains; secondly, the flesh may be converted into adipocire; thirdly, the body may become dried, and preserve its form, and be converted into a sort of natural mummy. This last change sometimes takes place in very dry and elevated situations, but more frequently in dry vaults and caves."—('Penny Cyclopædia,' Art. 'Interment.')

The gaseous products of decomposition diffused through the atmosphere are not, it is true, appreciable by chemical tests, for even air collected on the tops of mountains, and in the foulest corners of a town, shows the same proportion of oxygen and nitrogen, yet this only proves that our tests are not sufficiently delicate. The living human heart and lungs are a much more delicate test than any inanimate matter, and when these are rendered abnormally susceptible by disease or other causes, the very slightest change of air is detected by them. That remarkable being, Caspar Hauser, whose organization was very much more susceptible than that of other persons, and who afforded a test much more delicate than an air thermometer or a torsion balance, affords a striking exposition of the effects of corrupted air. It is related in his life, that when he passed on one occasion, in the autumn of 1828, near St. John's Churchyard, in the vicinity of Nuremberg, the smell of the dead bodies, of which his companions had no perception, affected him so powerfully that he was seized with an ague, and began to shudder. The ague was soon succeeded by a feverish heat, which at length caused a violent perspiration, by which his linen was thoroughly wetted. When he returned towards the city gate, he said he felt better, yet he complained that his sight was obscured. What would have been the effect produced upon this being, of so delicate a nervous susceptibility, had he passed by the crowded burial-places in the most densely-peopled districts of London ? Although these violent effects are not produced upon people in general, yet the same gases are eliminated in greater abundance from the thousands of dead bodies in London, which become mixed with the air, and are breathed by the people, incorporated with their blood, and thus the very putrefactions of the dead become parts of the living. In the case of Caspar Hauser, a living chemical test was applied, of such exquisite sensibility, that the presence and noxious qualities of these agents were manifested. The difference between the effects produced upon him and upon other human beings, is one rather of degree than of kind; the emanations are equally poisonous and destructive to health, but most persons are better able, being less sensitive, to withstand them.

The pestiferous effects of decomposition have been demonstrated by " Dr Majendie, who has shown, by experiment, that this decomposition produces a poison which, when concentrated, produces instant death by a single exhalation ; and that even when diluted by the atmosphere, and spread over a large extent of country, it is the fruitful source of disease and death. By cold and other agents he condensed some of this poison, and found that by applying it to an animal previously in good health, he destroyed life, with the most intense symptoms of malignant fever. Ten or twelve drops of water containing this matter, were injected into the jugular vein of a dog ; in a short time it was seized with acute fever, the action of the heart was inordinately excited, the respiration accelerated, the heat of the surface increased, the prostration of strength extreme, the muscular power so exhausted that the animal lay on the ground unable to make the slightest movement ; after a period it was seized with the black vomit, so characteristic of yellow fever; and what is still more remarkable is the fact, that by varying the dose of the poison, he could produce fever of almost any type. When diffused in the atmosphere, this poison taken into the lungs, or absorbed by the larger surface of the skin, enters the blood, and produces diseases of varying malignity, modified by the producing causes, as they are of animal or vegetable origin. Thus, when the poison from marshes, or decayed vegetable matters, is employed, intermittent fevers, as ague, and remittent fevers, are produced ; but when the poison from decomposing animal matter is employed, typhus, and the class of fevers which are marked by a diminution of power in all the functions of the body, and a general disposition to putrescency, both in the solids and fluids, invariably follow."

Dr Armstrong observes, "I believe that putrid matter, introduced into the blood, produces an affection so exactly resembling typhus fever, that I should think no individual could confidently pronounce that it differed from typhus fever."

Dr Mead, speaking of Grand Cairo, says, " This city is crowded with vast numbers of inhabitants, who live not only poorly, but nastily; the streets are narrow and close; the city is situated in a sandy plain at the foot of a mountain, which keeps off the winds that might refresh the air; a great canal passes through the city, which, at the overflowing of the Nile, is full of water; on the decrease of the river, this canal is gradually dried up, and the people throw into it all manner of filth, offal, &c. &c. The stench which arises from this and the mud together is intolerable, and from this source the plague every year preys upon the inhabitants, and is stopped only by the return of the Nile, the overflowing of which washes away this load of filth. In Ethiopia the swarms of locusts breed a famine by devouring the fruits of the earth, and when they die, create a pestilence by the stench of their putrefying bodies. The Egyptians of old were so sensible how much the putrefaction of dead bodies contributed towards breeding the plague, that they worshipped the bird Ibis for the services it did in devouring great numbers of serpents, which, they had observed, injured by their stench when dead as much as by their bite when alive."

Mr Walker adduces the following cases in illustration of the effects produced by the gases generated during the *first periods* of decomposition:—

"In the month of June, 1825, a woman died of typhus fever in the upper part of a house in Drury lane. The body, which was buried on the fourth day, was brought down a narrow staircase. In order that the coffin might pass the more easily into the street, it was placed for a few minutes in the doorway of a room on the second floor, inhabited by Lewis Swalthey, a shoe-maker, who was sensible of a most disgusting odour, which proceeded from the coffin. He complained almost immediately of a peculiar coppery taste, which he described as being seated at the root of the tongue and the back of the throat: in a few hours afterwards he had, at irregular intervals, slight sensations of chilliness, which before the next sunset had merged into repeated shiverings of considerable intensity; that evening he was confined to his bed; he passed through a most severe form of typhus fever; at the expiration of the third week, he was removed to the fever hospital, and recovered. This man had been in excellent health up to the time he was exposed to this malaria.

"A patient of mine was exposed some years since to a similar influence. A stout muscular man died in his house in the month of June, after a short illness. On bringing the body down stairs, a disgustingly fetid sanies escaped from the coffin; Mr M. was immediately affected with giddiness, prostration of strength, and extreme lassitude; he had a peculiar metallic taste in his mouth, which continued some days; he believes that his health has been deranged from this cause.

"I offer the following proofs of the effects of the gases produced by the extreme degree of putrefaction :—My pupil, Mr J. H. Sutton, accompanied by an individual for many years occasionally employed in the office of burying the dead, entered the vaults of St —— Church ; a coffin ' cruelly bloated,' as one of the grave-diggers expressed it, was chosen for the purpose of obtaining a portion of its gaseous contents. The body had, by an inscription on the plate, been buried upwards of eight years; the instant the small instrument employed had entered the coffin, a most horribly offensive gas issued forth in large quantities. Mr Sutton, who respired a portion of this vapour, would have fallen, but for the support afforded by a pillar in the vault. He was instantly seized with a suffocating difficulty of breathing, giddiness, trembling, and extreme prostration of strength; in attempting to leave the vault he fell, from debility ; on reaching the external air, he had nausea, vomiting, accompanied with frequent flatulent eructations highly fetid, and having the same character as the gas inspired. He reached home with difficulty, and was confined to his bed during seven days, and for many days his gait was very vacillating. The man who accompanied him was affected in a precisely similar way, and was incapacitated for work for some days; his symptoms were, prostration of strength, pains in the head, giddiness, and general involuntary action of the muscles, particularly of the upper limbs : these symptoms had been experienced by this person on many previous occasions. I myself have suffered from the same cause, and have been compelled to keep my room upwards of a week."

" New Bunhill fields, in the New Kent road, is a private speculation, and belongs to a Mr Martin, an undertaker. At its entrance is a chapel, arched with strong brick-work, containing one thousand eight hundred coffins, and not more than twelve, I believe, are of lead. Iron gratings are placed on each side of the vault. A strong ammoniacal odour pervades it, not so offensive as in most other depositories of this description, which I attribute to the constant transmission of the noxious vapours through the open gratings to the circumambient atmosphere," that atmosphere which is the food as it were of the passengers, and inhabitants of the many houses that surround it.

In what state of neglect are the municipal regulations of London, when burial-places are under no official control, and when any private speculator may prepare a cellar for the packing away of dead bodies (the burial-place just described is only a cellar), and let off the gaseous decomposition into the streets? If a dye-house, chemical or gas works, were to let off matters into the streets much less prejudicial, but visible, the law would soon stop the nuisance.

It seems that even the lordly and royal inhabitants of Westminster are not less infested with ill-conditioned burial-grounds than their poorer subjects, for *close upon Buckingham Palace* is a chapel, the vaults and grounds of which send forth in abundance pestiferous exhalations to mix with the air, and lurk over the dainty viands of the rich and luxurious, the royal and the noble. A poor shepherd on Salisbury Plain, sitting beside a hill, eats a morsel of bread permeated by no such offensive particles as those which penetrate the food of the royal palace.

One of the most striking examples is afforded by the death of two men (one a grave-digger) in the church-yard of St Botolph's, Aldgate, September, 1838, who were seized with instant death in a grave about twenty feet deep. It was a pauper's grave,—commonly kept open until there are seventeen or eighteen bodies interred. " It was not the custom," said one of the witnesses, " to put any earth between the coffins in such graves, except in cases where persons die of contagious diseases: grave-diggers could not sometimes go down, owing to the foulness of the air; they are then in the habit of burning straw, and using other means to dispel the impure air." Such is the stench arising from this burial-ground, that in hot weather the inhabitants are obliged to keep their windows closed, thus *shutting in, and again and again breathing air, poisoned by their own lungs, that they may escape a stronger and more malignant poison lurking outside their windows, emitted from the rottenness of a crammed-full ground in the very heart of the city,* and within the jurisdiction of the Corporation of London.

The condition of Enon Chapel is hardly fit for publication; yet how else can sufficient disgust be excited in the mind of the public, so indifferent as yet about its best interests? " This burial-place is surrounded on all sides by houses, crowded principally by poor inhabitants. The upper part of the building is used as a chapel,—the lower part as a burying-place, separated from the upper by a boarded floor, and is crowded at one end even to the ceiling with dead. The rafters supporting the floor are not even covered with the usual defence of lath and plaster. Vast numbers of bodies have been placed here in pits dug for the purpose, the uppermost of which were covered only by a few inches of earth; a sewer runs angularly across this burying place. Soon after interments, a long, narrow, black fly is observed to crawl out of many of the coffins; this insect, a product of the putrefaction of the bodies, is observed on the following season to be succeeded by another, which has the appearance of a common bug with wings. The children attending the Sunday-school held in this chapel, in which these insects were to be seen crawling and flying in vast numbers during the summer months, called them ' body-bugs.' The stench was frequently intolerable: one of my informants states, that he had a peculiar taste in his mouth during the time of worship, and that his handkerchief was so offensive that immediately on his return home, it used to be placed in water. Some months since, handbills were circulated, ' requesting parents and others to send the children of the district to the Sunday-school,' *held immediately over the masses of putre-faction in the vaults beneath.* Residents about this spot in warm and damp weather have been much annoyed with a peculiarly disgusting smell; and occasionally, when the fire was lighted in a house abutting upon this building, an intolerable stench arose, which it was believed did not arise from a drain. Vast numbers of rats infest the houses! and meat exposed to the atmosphere after a few hours becomes putrid!"

Affectionate relatives consign their dead to burial-places (to be devoured, in all probability, by rats), who would be excited to riots and violence by interested men, were it proposed by government to remove the dead from this shameful place—known among undertakers as the "dust-hole"—to a place of decent security.

" The effluvia proceeding from the burial-ground in Portugal street, known as the Green-ground, is so offensive, that persons living at the back of Clement's lane are compelled to keep their windows closed; the walls even of the ground which adjoins the yards of those houses, are frequently seen reeking with fluid, which diffuses a most offensive smell. Who can wonder that fever is here so prevalent and triumphant?"

It is really extraordinary, if no other persons had been disposed to take up the matter, that the clergy of the metropolis, and especially that vigorous prelate, the Bishop of London, should have allowed these appalling practices to exist; it is to be feared that they will not interfere till they are constrained to remove the evil from another cause, for their churches and chapels are likely to be deserted as places of worship by timid people who take much care of their health, when it is fully known that the most deadly agents are there present in all their virulence.

In as far as Mr Walker has executed a nauseous task for the public good, he deserves the highest honour ; nor would it have been just, either to him or to the public, to have suppressed his evidence because it might appal the sensitive ; but it must be reiterated, and added to, until public clamour calls for the extirpation of the evil, and until the sluggish legislature shall stir itself to action, and the clergy—too exclusively occupied with the spiritual health of the people—shall cease to offer opposition.

The remarks of Mr Walker on the " management," as it is called, of burial-grounds, show that decent regard to the remains of the dead,—respect for the coffins, with their emblematic garniture,—all those outward and tangible signs of respect which have been bestowed at so much cost (oftentimes ill afforded), are violated and set at nought equally with the public health itself. The claims of the public health, with respect to sepulture, are hardly less strong than are the claims of surviving friends and relations to decent regard for the remains of the deceased. " Men pay funeral dues, under an implied assurance that the dead shall be respected. The grave is still insecure; grounds accustomed to be held sacred are unceremoniously cleared under official superintendence, and that, too, with such ruthless indifference and wanton publicity, that even passers-by complain of the indecent profanation." Mr Walker quotes several communications to newspapers from persons who have witnessed the conduct and practices of the managers and their agents.

" In this ' management,' former occupancy is disregarded, coffins are remorselessly broken through, and their contents heaped together. On one occasion two men and a boy were observed exhuming the bodies in one part of the burial-ground of Globe-fields Chapel, and hurling them in a most indecent manner and indiscriminately into a deep hole which they had previously made. The police interfered, and as they were about to enter the ground they met a lad with a bag of bones and a quantity of nails: proceeding to an obscure corner, they found a great number of bodies packed one upon another in a very deep grave; the uppermost coffin was not more than seven or eight inches at the utmost from the surface; the breastplate and nails were removed from the lid, so that they could at once remove the latter; and from the appearance of the body as well as of the coffin, it appeared to be the remains of a person above the middle rank of life, and to have been interred about a month or six weeks. The ground was the property of an undertaker, and owing to the low rate of fees, and protection afforded against resurrectionmen (being surrounded by high walls), a great number of burials took place; but as few would select the remote corner as a place of rest for their friends or relations, it was used for the purpose of receiving the disinterred bodies of those buried in the better and more crowded part of the ground, to make room for others. The officers said, that the dreadful stench emitted from the half-decomposed bodies placed in the hole before mentioned, was sufficient to engender disease in the neighbourhood ; upon which, the men immediately set about covering them.

" In making a grave in a burying-ground in Southwark, a body partly decomposed was dug up and placed on the surface, at the side slightly covered with earth; a mourner stepped upon it, the loosened skin peeled off, he slipped forward, and had nearly fallen into the grave. At another place, amongst a heap of rubbish, a young woman recognised the finger of her mother, who had been buried there a short time previously. On another occasion the workmen, digging a grave, broke in upon a common sewer, and deposited the coffin there. The more endurable parts of the human fabric are 'managed' away by sending them on shipboard to the north, where many tons of bones are crushed in mills constructed for the purpose, and used as manure."

A superficial observer might suppose that so soon as such a public nuisance had been exposed, the Government would have taken immediate steps for its abolition. The British Government, however, has other fish to fry, and so it has had for many a long year past; its members are, and have ever been, men of aristocratic habits, who have large salaries to spend in the purchase of various pleasures, and who spend their energies, which ought to be devoted to the public service, in sustaining themselves against their political enemies. The British people have constantly the shameful spectacle before them of public men, who ought to be counselling together for their good, exhausting themselves in a scandalous war for the places of power, and for the profits of place. The evil expounded by Mr Walker, like a multitude of others, will therefore continue, unless some active men shall be urged by a sense of public duty to neglect their own private business, and, by a great expenditure of time and money, stir up the public clamour, and thus enforce a sluggish administration to do that which ought to be undertaken by its own promptings. Were not the profession and the practice of the Corporation of London known now to be widely different, it might be a matter of surprise that a body so immensely rich (expending altogether, for ostensibly local purposes, 540,000l. per annum) should have allowed the catastrophe in Aldgate church-yard to have passed without making some attempt to stop the burial of the dead within their city.   Mr Deputy Tyars and Sir John Cowan, however, in the true spirit of corporators, merely started a joint-stock cemetery for the north-eastern end of London, by which no doubt some pecuniary advantage was expected.

Any proposed improvement, without some caution, will receive much opposition from the metropolitan clergy. Let, however, the value of their fees* be secured, and there is little

* The following article appeared in the 'Examiner' a few months ago, and indicates the preliminary measures that must be taken to stop powerful opposition:—

"INFLUENCE OF CLERICAL FEES ON HEALTH.—At a late meeting of the Geographical Society it was stated, that 'among the diseases of the Indians in South America, the small pox was the most prevalent and destructive, and out of a population of 240,000 souls no less than 30,000 fell victims in four months. This prevalence is attributed to the circumstance that the clergy will not encourage vaccination, because great part of their revenue is derivable from burial fees.' The influence of clerical fees is also very per-

doubt that the support may be obtained of that astute and vigorous prelate, the Bishop of London, who does not gratuitously resist the improvement of society, although he resolutely supports the interests of the clergy under all circumstances.

The metropolis is of so vast and progressively increasing an extent, that suburban cemeteries, such as those at Paris, will not comport with complete salubrity. We do not quite agree in the unqualified praises bestowed by Mr Walker on the projectors of joint-stock cemeteries; several of those already formed are too near the homes of the living, and they will soon be enfolded within the extending rows of dwellings. They are objectionable also because they occupy some of the most high and beautiful localities, which, where there is so scant an allowance of room, should be appropriated to the habitations of men, or rather set apart for the relaxation of the living, and not walled in as places of sepulture. Had the health and comfort of the dense population of London and its environs been protected by intelligent and honourable municipal bodies, such beautiful spots as Norwood, Highgate, and Kensal green would never have been seized by projectors, and for their profit have been devoted to the worm of corruption;—private cupidity has misappropriated for the dead places which should have been sacredly preserved for the living.

There are now four or five railways diverging from various parts of London : some of them pass through, or are contiguous to, districts admirably adapted for burial-grounds. The Government should take advantage of this fact, and construct at least four cemeteries on a magnificent scale, some eight or ten miles from the centre of the metropolis. The Southampton railway passes through a great extent of almost worthless land, some of which at Wimbledon, or even beyond Kingston, is admirably suited for the proposed purpose. Funeral carriages duly prepared, should start at fixed hours and days, by slow trains. The cost of transit and of inhumation should be fixed, and at a very low price; indeed, so important is it that the actual cost of the burial of the dead should be of small amount, and that all excuse should be removed for persisting in the use of any, even suburban cemeteries, that we think it desirable that it should be paid for by the state, allowing families to expend any sum they please additionally, for the purposes of taste or splen-

nicious on the public health in London, where the horrid and pestiferous practice of burying the dead in the most crowded districts is persevered in, to perpetuate their burial fees. Future ages will discover some singular examples of the civilization of the nineteenth century in several parts of the world.

dour; but the removal of the dead body itself should be a matter of police or of state regulation. All the burial-grounds in and about the metropolis should be cleared of their contents in a decent manner, and the present horrid nuisance of sepulture be abolished for ever. Let reasonable compensation be given to all parties,—shareholders, grave-diggers, clergymen; but the *salus populi* demands, *at any cost*, the *immediate* adoption of some such plan as is proposed.

Interested and misguided persons may raise a cry about the sacredness of sepulture which the proposed plan would outrage. That sacredness is already violated, and in the most disgusting manner,—which violation it is proposed to abolish, and instead of the indecencies committed under "management," to make the needful removal once and for ever, and that in a solemn manner, under the control of clergymen and proper officers. Surely, all the emotions of piety and affection, all the steady, lingering remembrances with which we regard the grave—the last home of our mother, our wife, our child—are now sadly offended, when the place to which we have consigned the remains of those who in recollection still continue part of our own being, is in a back yard of some miserable street, or among workshops, smithies, laundries, brewhouses, bakehouses, butchers' shambles (see p. 149), close upon taverns, down in some cellar, abutting upon our stores of various merchandize, or in the midst of the clatter of omnibuses, carts, and drays, and in the very densest throng of thousands of pedestrians.* A metropolitan burial-ground is as offensive to our most delicate sentiments as it is to our bodily health. Martin Van Butchel exhibited a poetic refinement when he embalmed his wife, dressed her neatly, placed her in a smart coffin with a glass plate in front, and kept her in quietness in an attic of his house,—compared with the citizen who deposits his spouse in such a back yard as has been described, whence she is likely to be ejected after a few weeks or months of tenancy, cast about the ground to be mutilated or trodden upon, or pitched into a corner, or carted away as rubbish; her coffin chopped up for fire-wood, its cloth and garniture sold for the profit of grave-diggers. It is proposed to stop this horrid desecration of the dead, and to serve at the same time some of the highest objects of

---

* An advertisement appeared some time since in the 'Morning Chronicle,' stating that the church of St Bartholomew will be taken down, and that the governor and company of the Bank have proposed to erect a mausoleum on a part of the consecrated ground. How poetic must be the imagination of the Bank directors! Erect a mausoleum at the corner of Threadneedle street!

public utility; and yet against all this, no doubt, loud clamour will be raised.

Mr Walker is one of the few useful men who have performed an investigation where little or no glory can be obtained, and where the rewards are few, other than those derived from the consciousness of doing good. Speculative reformers, the bold and abstract schemers for new-modelling society, may display a grandiloquence that will fill the public ear, and bring much glory to themselves. Those who, like our author, would destroy a tangible evil or remove a local nuisance, will get little or no public approbation, but will raise up a host of determined and unflinching enemies, whose interests are assailed, and who will be much more resolute to defend and sustain the wrong done to the public, than the public is resolute to rid itself of the wrong. Every man takes care of himself, no matter at what price to the public. The public has neither time nor inclination to look after matters which are, however, really and truly its own business, as, for example, the protection of the public health and comfort.

The subject has been well opened, and it ought not now to be dropped. Some member of Parliament (who more fitting than Mr C. Buller or Mr Hawes?) should move the appointment of a committee or commission of inquiry, and bring forth an additional body of evidence that should shame into silence the superstitious and the mercenary. If the Government forget its duty, the intelligent and honest members of Parliament should do theirs, and show to the world where the neglect lies, and for what small services the public money is expended in princely salaries.

J. H. E.

Art. IX.—*Report from the Select ommittee on Improvement of the Health of Towns, together with the Minutes of Evidence, Appendix, and Index.*

(*Ordered by the House of Commons to be printed, June* 14, 1842.)

THE tyrants of antiquity were accustomed to despatch a criminal by binding the doomed wretch to a corpse : leaving the exhalations from the dead man to kill the living. While we shudder in contemplating this refinement in the philosophy of cruelty, we perhaps congratulate ourselves that in these days such things cannot be; but a little observation will convince us that the same ancient mode of extermination still flourishes, and to an infinitely greater extent than in former times, though in a modified form. Our modern law, associated with religion, permits the continuous application, to thousands and hundreds of thousands of our population, of the same revolting principle of death which formerly was concentrated upon a few miserable individuals; and this, with the concurrence of parliament and the clergy, throughout all the towns and cities of the United Kingdom. Cathedrals, parish churches, church yards, burial yards, and all kinds of grounds, consecrated and unconsecrated, have been for centuries permitted to be used as receptacles of the dead, in the midst of our places of habitation, until at length earth and walls have become so saturated with putrefaction, that, turn where we may, the air we breathe is cadaverous, and a man often *feels* that sublimated particles, perhaps of his next door neighbour or nearest relative, enter his lungs at every respiration. Thus, in truth (though in a different sense from that of the Apostle), in the midst of life we are in death.

Setting aside the question of what must be the influence on the mind from a consideration of such sickening facts, the effect of this general state of atmospheric infection upon the public health must be evident. It is physically indubitable, and those upon whose senses the truth has not yet forced itself, may soon trace its course by physical demonstration. Many of our most popular diseases are referable to this source. Medical and scientific men have often denounced it, and given warning ; but the impression upon society has been of a vague startling character, here and there giving rise to the formation of a suburban cemetery, which was, not unnaturally, recognised as a speculation, undertaken with the motives common to all joint-stock projects, rather than as an attempt to diminish or counteract an evil of which the shareholders had any serious alarms, notwithstanding all that their prospectuses might affirm on that head. While those who could comprehend the dreadful extent, and the actual and impending consequences of the system, have stated their view, local individuals who could understand, but would not act, have shaken their heads, and then dying, have been buried respectably, *more majorum*, perhaps under their own drawing-room windows.

It is strange that the practical people of Great Britain should be amongst the last to retain this disgraceful and dangerous relic of Christian barbarism. Burial in towns has been long forbidden in France. It is upwards of twenty years since the clergy of Spain concurred with the Cortes in abolishing the practice. In many parts of Italy, in Switzerland, Denmark,

Germany, and other nations of Europe, which we are apt to look upon as vastly behind ourselves in the march of intellect, burial in towns has been abolished by law. Why, then, does the system continue to prevail amongst us? Because, no doubt, the public mind has not been sufficiently aroused to a contemplation of its indecencies, horrors, and dangers ; and there is no hope of suppressing this consecrated nuisance until a feeling of disgust, indignation, and resolution takes possession of all classes of society. This can only be produced by setting before their minds a picture, local and general, of their present dreadful position.

A few scientific men having impressed Parliament with the necessity of inquiring into the causes affecting the health of towns, a Committee was appointed, which commenced the investigation by taking evidence upon our burial system as a predominating evil. Their Report has since been presented to the House of Commons. The facts which have persuaded the Committee will doubtless influence the public. We esteem it, therefore, a duty, though not certainly a pleasing task, to submit a digest of the evidence, and so assist in hastening the general legislative movement that shall do away with one of the most disgraceful and perilous conditions of English society.

Since the Report was presented, we learn, from a conversation in the House, arising out of a question put to Sir James Graham by Lord Robert Grosvenor, that further evidence has been collected by Government on the subject, and that an additional report, embodying more carefully-considered suggestions than the former, is now lying in the office of the Home Secretary. If this be the fact, we would ask why the publication of the additional report is delayed? Sir James has declined supporting Mr Mackinnon's bill, founded upon the recommendations of the Committee: why should the public not be made acquainted with the recommendations which have influenced his judgment? It may be true that his mind is not yet wholly made up—that he cannot at present clearly see his way to a sound practical measure; but the greater, therefore, is the reason for making the new evidence and accompanying suggestions public, that the country at large might assist in the discussion. Waiting these (and it would seem, from the result of the present session, that on all questions of practical improvement we must be content to wait, possessing our souls in patience), we confine ourselves to an analysis of the report of Mr Mackinnon's Committee, the statements of which, as will be seen, are sufficiently startling to demand the most serious attention of every class in the community.

The first witness examined was Mr Henry Heldson, a collecting clerk to Mr James Bingon Cooper, ironfounder, Drury lane. Mr Heldson has acted as assistant-minister of the Baptist persuasion at the City-road ground, called Bunhill fields, but chiefly at the New Bunhill fields, in the same district, the space being almost exhausted, in the former, by two hundred years' sepulture, and also rendered unpopular by increased fees.

" How were the graves generally made?—The plan on which the grave was opened was quite in accordance with that generally observed or adopted throughout London; that is, the opening, what is called a public grave, thirty feet deep, perhaps; the first corpse interred was succeeded by another, and up to sixteen or eighteen, and all the openings between the coffin boards were filled up with smaller coffins of children. When this grave was crammed as full as it could be, so that the topmost coffin was within two feet of the surface, that was banked up, and that piece of ground was considered as occupied.

" The largest number of burials I have ever attended on one day was during the raging epidemic called the influenza, I think, in 1837. On one Sunday afternoon I buried twenty-one persons myself; that was in Holywell Mount ground, situated about a quarter of a mile distant, in the Curtain road."

Sometimes this dead hole is left open a fortnight, or covered only with planks, before it is full ;* it is then covered over with earth, to be opened again in rotation at the end of a year. Speaking of the 'sequel' in New Bunhill fields, Mr Heldson observes :—

" After the first year had passed away, for I officiated in that ground about four years during the heat of the summer, when those graves were re-opened on the Sunday afternoon, when most of the funerals take place, in consequence of their being chiefly among the Irish and the lower classes of society, by reason of their burying rather cheaper than at other grounds, they were exceedingly offensive ; the swarms of some kind of black fly, which I am not able to explain the nature of, but I suppose generated in this house of corruption, were certainly so offensive, and the noisome stench arising from those deep graves was very unpleasant, so that it was difficult in the heat of the summer for any man of sensibility to discharge the duties necessarily devolving upon him.

" I have known a grave-digger obliged to be drawn out of those very deep graves after being in half an hour or three quarters of an hour, in consequence of his being overpowered with the heat and the stench accumulated there, and more particularly in opening those graves where ten or twelve corpses had already been interred ; and where they began to run, the stench was dreadful. Every subsequent summer this offensive effluvia increased, and even the sight of the coffins ; for the fact is, that as the coffins lie one on another in succession from the bottom to the top, the next grave that is opened alongside of that, to make the very most of every inch of the

* As far as the writer's observation goes, this is the official mode of burying paupers. Mr Wakley lately complained in the House of Commons, that having occasion to hold an inquest on the body of a pauper buried at Hanwell, on proceeding to exhumate, the deceased was the fifteenth in downward succession. The effluvium arising from the removal of the overlying coffins was dreadful.

speculation of any proprietor of such ground ; nay, I have been witness, from Sunday to Sunday, of my certain knowledge, of from sixteen to eighteen coffins being placed all in succession, rising one above another, and the horrible stench arising from those, and the swarms of flies and insects accumulated, it is horrible to conceive, and I have gone away sometimes so loathed and disgusted, as scarcely to be able to endure myself."

We are now in the very worst part of London. Mr John Irwin, house painter, says,—

" I live in Clement's lane, Clare market, overlooking Portugal-street burying-ground, belonging to the parish of Saint Clement Danes. Neither I nor any one of my family have been in good health since we came there, now three years since. The mortality of the neighbourhood has been very great; all the symptoms are generally those of typhus fever. I had a lodger of the name of Britt, a ruddy-complexioned man, who chose my house because it was a quiet place, but he became ill of fever almost immediately. His wife also caught it, as did Mr and Mrs Rosamond, who also lodged with me. Three out of the four went to the hospital; they all died. Rosamond died in the hospital, Britt in my house. Britt was buried within *ten feet of my wall.* The grave was opened, and a fortnight after there was another put atop of him ; but previous to that the smell was so nauseous I could hardly contain myself; I was obliged to keep my window down. ' If this be the case,' said I to the grave digger, ' well may typhus fever rage in this neighbourhood. There is *a workhouse* on the right hand.' "

We now come to the worst. Mr Samuel Pitts, cabinet maker, residing at 14 Catherine street, Strand, says,—

" I used to attend as one of the Baptist congregation at Enon chapel, Clement's lane. The surface of the floor was fifty or sixty feet by forty. The cellar below was used as a burying place, the corpses having no covering but the coffins, and nothing separating the living congregation from the dead ' *but the thin boards between the depositary and the chapel,* and there were openings between, owing to the shrinking of the boards.' The chapel and vault were owned by the late Rev. Mr Howse, who preached there. I attended from about 1828 for six or seven years. There have been on the whole about twelve thousand persons buried here ; the depth is about six feet. I have heard, when it got too full, a great many have been removed to make way for others. I did hear, and it came through a woman who used to wash for Mrs Howse, living close by, *that they used to burn the coffins under the copper, and frequently in their own fireplace.* I do not know what became of the remains unless they were *shovelled all together,* which I believe to be the case. The fees were small, and were part of Mr Howse's emoluments. As many as nine or ten have been buried there one Sunday afternoon."—" While I attended the chapel," proceeds Mr Irwin, " the place was in a very filthy state; the smell was *abominable,* and very injurious ; also there were some insects, something similar to a bug in shape and appearance, only with wings. I have seen in the summer hundreds of them flying about the chapel ; I have taken them home in my hat, and my wife has taken them home in her clothes. We always considered that they proceeded from the dead bodies underneath."

Mr Howse must have been rather a powerful preacher to draw a congregation in such circumstances. He has now followed the majority of his congregation. There is no more preaching there, and we believe the abomination of the burials below is given up through the interference of Sir James Graham. In the beginning of this year the chapel was converted into a Catholic school; but the facts were exposed in a petition to the House of Commons, and we believe the poor children are shown the way to the other world elsewhere.

" I believe," continues Mr Irwin, " the minister would not have had room for the twelve thousand bodies if he had not burned the coffins. The fee varied from 8s. to 15s., as the deceased was a child or an adult. I have frequently gone home from the chapel with a severe headache. It was a common thing to see some of the congregation removed in a fainting state. There was a sewer also running through the vault. I believe, when the wood of the coffins was taken away, the remains would in many cases fall into the sewer; but the commissioners compelled Mr Howse to build an arch over it."

Mr Moses Solomons, of Vinegar yard, Drury lane, gives us a clue to the plan which the proprietors adopted to keep room in that venerable, quiet-looking churchyard above-named. He says,—

" I have seen a grave digger take a coffin out, that coffin not being quite decayed, and take the body out; and he has taken the spade and *chopped the head from the body, so that he could take it out of the grave.* I have seen a great many coffins broken up; I suppose he puts them in the bonehouse, and the bones too. My impression is, that the coffins were taken away to be burnt."

Mr Burn had also been employed to remove rubbish from St Mary's in the Strand, and St Clement's. " They are more careful of the bones, but there is the same smell." There is another Baptist burying chapel near Lincoln's inn fields, behind Little Wild street, where the interments are more decent, but the smell is so bad that the people cannot bear it in the summer time.

The grave-diggers of London are a wonderful though little-known class of men ; and see things dreadful and strange. To form a correct idea of them they must be allowed to describe themselves. John Eyles, a grave-digger in " that spot in Portugal street," is examined as follows :—

" What is the shallowest depth at which you have known a coffin placed ?—Since I have been there they have had a tremendous deal of ground brought in when the college was being built, and they took it from one part of the ground and put it on another. There was a pauper buried out of the house which I remember quite well; nobody followed it ; it was buried out of the bone house, what they call the dead house, and it was put down where the carpet ground was, and I believe, if the earth was at the same height then that it is now, it would be under a foot, but I will say a foot ; I would rather say more than less.

" Have you ever, in passing over there, smelt any offensive smell ?— I cannot say that I have ever noticed it particularly, but there must be a smell, because neither lead nor wood will keep the stench of the body in ;

it will fly out of lead as well as out of wood; a great many coffins are now made of mill lead.

" Has it affected you in health?—It has a great deal; I nearly at one time lost my life through it.

" How did it affect you?—When I went down the grave I went down a little way, and it smelt as if it was brimstone or some sulphury stuff, and when I reached the bottom my sensation was taken away altogether, and I could hardly make my way up to the top; and when I got to the top I dropped on the boards, and then I went home and got some shavings and an old bed tick, and burnt it down the grave to get the foul air out.

" How were you affected; did it make you vomit?—It did a great deal; it was a trembling sensation over me, and a nasty coppery taste in my mouth.

" Did you lose your appetite?—I did not lose my appetite, but in the afternoon I was again taken at the same grave; I went down in the afternoon; a child was buried, and the webbing that checked the coffin had turned the coffin over, and it was my duty to unfasten the webbing. When I reached the bottom I could not make anybody hear, and I grasped hold of the webbing, and they pulled me up; and when I got out of the grave I walked to the side of the church, and there I lay for half an hour.

" What church was it?—St Clement Danes, in the Strand.

" Have you seen coffins cut through?—If you have orders for it you are compelled to do it; if you are to dig a grave in a certain place, it is your duty to do it, and if not you are told directly, ' I will get somebody else to do it.'

" Then you have cut through coffins?—I have.

" Have you ever cut up the lead of a coffin?—Yes, I have once.

" By orders?—By orders.

" What became of the lead?—I do not know; it was not in my time; I went away soon after I cut it up.

" What did you do with the lead when it was cut?—I left it there.

" What burial ground was that?—In St Clement's church.

" Is it a matter of common occurrence to do so?—I do not know; but if I must speak my mind, I think there is a tremendous deal of lead taken away, both in the churchyard and in the vaults; but I think it is a common thing for the old original coffins to be taken and chopped up; and I think it to be nothing else but the duty of any gentleman that has got any authority, to go into every church vault, and to have the books brought forward to prove how many coffins there ought to be, and to make them account for how many coffins are missing. The lead I believe is a hundred and a half or two hundred in each coffin; I should say there were about two hundred and a half, and it would fetch 1½d. a pound.

" What quantity of wood have you seen taken away, or do you know has been taken away from this churchyard? How many wheelbarrows full in a week?—I could not say, sometimes more, sometimes less, sometimes none; it all depends upon the work; sometimes we get as much out of one grave as you may out of six or seven others; sometimes you may have a bag full in a week.

" What do you mean by a ' grave,' what depth do you mean?—Five feet is the common depth for a grown person, and three feet for a child, when it is five feet that leaves four feet from the surface of the earth, but I do not think four feet is enough to keep the effluvia out.

" You think the gas gets out of the ground at that distance?—I am sure it does, because the gas will penetrate through anything; it will penetrate through the strongest man; if he happen to hold his head over the place where the gas is flying it will make him ill; and I think that people going by at the time when a grave is open must breathe some of the gas, as well as persons working in the grave, for when the gas is out you can smell it quite strong up above.

" How far from the grave will the smell of the gas extend?—It depends upon the wind.

" Supposing the wind is blowing towards you, how far will it take it? —If the corpse is about five or six feet below the ground you may smell it six or seven yards from you, but you do not smell it if you are standing by the side and continually in it.

" The vaults in St Clement Danes are close to the street?—Yes, the gas escapes from the vaults into the church through a grating cullett, and many persons who go to the church on Sunday, when they come home are taken ill and are dead soon afterwards, through the gas in the church; I do not think the lead is of any use to keep the gas in.

" You would not like to go to a leaden coffin and tap it?—Yes, I should not object to it; if you keep underneath the coffin, you would not have so much of the gas then; if you keep underneath, the gas flies up; if you tap it underneath, if there is any dead water, or any 'soup,' as it is called, it runs into a pail, and then it is taken and thrown into some place or another, perhaps down a gulleyhole. I have been, before now, compelled to put my clothes out of the window, because the stench has been so great that they could not bear the place.

" Has it ever occurred to you to go into a public house, and to find the smell of your clothes offensive to people there?—Yes, many a time; when I have been doing rather dirty work, when I have come in, I have noticed the people smell and get away on the other side of the place; there is sure to be plenty of room when we come in; they are sure to say, ' These chaps have been emptying some cesspool.'

" Is the smell of these graves more offensive than that of a common cesspool?—I emptied a cesspool, and the smell of it was rose water compared with the smell of these graves.

" Has it ever happened, to your knowledge, that the men have declined digging through the coffins, and that they have been induced to do so by the sexton?—Yes; that is the word: ' If you do not like to do it, I will get somebody else.'

" You, or some of the men, have felt a repugnance to cutting through coffins?—It is not a pleasant thing to chop away when it is not fit to chop away; when the body is decayed it does not matter taking that away.

" And you have found yourself, and other workmen with you, obliged to cut through, whether you liked it or not?—If you are paid for doing it you must do it, whether you like it or no; if you do not like it you must go.

" Is your father interred there?—Yes, he is: I did not want him to be buried there.

" Did anything occur to his remains?—I saw them chopping the head of his coffin away; I should not have known it if I had not seen the head with the teeth; I knew him by his teeth; one tooth was knocked out and the other was splintered; I knew it was my father's head, and I told them to stop, and they laughed; and I would not let them go any further, and they had to cover it over. It is time that something was done to stop it; and there is a slaughter-house close by, in St Clement's lane, which is enough to breed any fever."

" Have you ever hesitated, when ordered to dig a grave, in cutting down through coffins?—Yes; I have said, ' There is not room to put down;' but it is said, ' You must make room:' but the sexton will not stop over the grave while that is being done; our sexton I know is fonder of pastry than standing over the top of a grave; he goes and has a shilling's worth of pastry while it is being done.

" Then, when the sexton orders you to dig a grave, he goes away himself?—Yes, and leaves you to do the rest.

" Do you know anything of the burial-ground under the windows of the almshouse in St Clement Danes?—I know that the bodies ought to be removed from there; it is not fit for anybody to live in the adjoining houses; I could go there and take a carving knife, and almost take some of the lids off. They are in a deal box half-an-inch thick; there is a great heap, and if that heap was taken away within nine inches from the top of the earth, you would have to take half of the sides of some of the coffins away.

" Do you know anything about the health of the people in the neighbourhood?—Some are ill; some are better than others. I do not know how the people in the almshouses feel. If it was a hot summer you would see the ground smoke, the same as if there was boiling water put over it.

" Have you seen that yourself?—I have not noticed it particularly myself, but I know those that have, and if you take the ground up in your hands it is the same as taking ink into your hands.

" The ground is so saturated with the remains of dead bodies?—Yes, it is.

" Is this in Portugal street?—No, it is in St Clement Danes: it is what they call the pauper ground, where the people that are buried by the workhouse are put.

" Have you ever observed anything of the same kind in the burial-ground in Portugal street?—Yes, I have seen the ground smoke and reek on a summer's morning; about five o'clock you will see it smoke the same as if there had been hot water poured down.

" Is a grave ever left open at night?—If you are going to dig a deep grave, you cannot do it all in one day; perhaps you may be four or five days over it, and then it is left open: sometimes we put a tarpauling over it.

" Then the smell must come up?—It does."

Michael Pye, a brother-practitioner, being asked whether his health was ever affected by his trade, answers—

" I have. I have been taken with sickness and spitting, and with a nasty taste in my mouth. In one grave in particular I struck a coffin accidentally with a pickaxe. As soon as I struck it it came out the same as a froth from a barrel of beer and threw me backwards, and I was obliged to stand some minutes before I could recover."

Speaking of the doings at St Clement Danes' church, he says—

" To my knowledge the coffins are cut up in the vaults and removed. In one case that I can speak to, the sexton, Mr Fitch, told me to select two coffins out, which I brought him out into the middle of the vault; and after they were brought out there another man was sent for and I was sent out of the way. I suppose that I was not trusted to perform this duty; another man cut them up. But I thought it a curious thing that I should be sent away, being the regular man there at the time, and I crossed over to the Fore-gate, that is, the pillars opposite the church, and I stood there some considerable time, and about five o'clock in the afternoon I saw a stonemason's truck come down Clement's lane and go inside the church, and the lead was loaded on the truck, and two men drew the lead away of those two coffins that I had selected out, and some lots of lead and copper remaining in a large chest at the bottom of the vault went away at the same time on the truck. They went down Fleet street, through Temple bar.

" *Mr Vernon.* When the lead was taken away, do you know what became of the wooden coffins and the bodies?—The remains were put into a basket, and next morning there was a hole dug on the south side of the churchyard, and the body was put down there without anything on it.

" *Chairman.* Is it the common practice to break up the wooden coffins? —Yes, it is the common practice of late; because the ground has been so full, that in fact you cannot get a grave without doing it.

" If you come to a coffin lately put in, how do you cut through it? —If we come to one that is very fresh we can tell by a searcher; but frequently we come to one that feels very soft with the searcher, but when we get on it the coffin is full, and then we are compelled to cut through it to make way for the coffin that is coming.

" What do you do with the remains?—The remains are put down at the bottom of the grave, and the coffin that is coming is put on it.

" The remains are put at the bottom without any coffin?—Yes; there is just a small piece of ground put over it to hide it.

Bartholomew Lyons, grave-digger of St Anne's, Soho.

" How do you manage, when you descend one of these deep graves, to avoid what you have stated affects you so much?—First we put down a long ladder, twenty feet six inches long, and I go down first myself; I go down as far as I can to see if I feel anything of the effect of the foul air; and if I go down and feel it coming, and I have got a funeral to bury, I burn it out, so that I can go down.

" What do you mean by burning it out?—We have got something similar to a plumber's stove, what the plumbers have in the street, and I make that full of shavings and wood, and make a strong fire, and gradually lower it down into the grave by degrees till the foul air catches hold. The foul air, when it is strong, will put it out, and I pull it up again till I get it a-light again, and so I go on till I get it under, and when I get it under, I chuck a lot of shavings in and set fire to it, and there let it burn till it burns out, and then I go down myself and get the earth out as quick as possible.

" Do you usually find this gas and foul air coming to you from other coffins on each side of you?—At times, very soon after I have burnt it out, I shall have to burn it out again.

" And if you were to stay there, what would be the effect?—It would kill me, or any one else."

Here is an incident that equals anything in Euripides.

" In digging this depth and taking away the wood of these coffins, has it ever occurred to you that any bodies have fallen upon you?—I never had one in a deep grave, but I had one once; before I was there a man of the name of Fox had the ground; I succeeded him; he is now dead; he was a bad character; he is dead about three weeks. I dug a grave on a Sunday evening on purpose to get ready for the Monday; that Sunday evening, and it rained, I was strange in the ground at that time; and when I went to work on Monday morning I finished my work, and I was trying the length of the grave to see if it was long enough and wide enough, so that I should not have to go down again, and while I was in there the ground gave way and a body turned right over, and the two arms came and clasped me round the neck; she had gloves on and stockings and white flannel inside, and what we call a shift, but no head.

" The body came tumbling upon you?—Yes, just as I was kneeling down; it was a very stout body, and the force that she came with knocked my head against a body underneath, and I was very much frightened at the time.

" You were at the bottom of the grave, and as you were digging at the bottom, the body of this woman without a head fell upon you?—Yes.

" From the side?—Yes, from the side.

" Out of the coffin?—It had never been in a coffin; it is supposed that they took the head off for the purpose of sale.

"How long had this body been interred?—Not long; because the clothes upon her appeared to be quite fresh.

"Do you believe that the lead of the coffins has been taken away?—I cannot say anything as to myself, as I never did anything of the sort myself; but the man that is dead has done most wonderful things in the vaults; he stripped the lead off the coffins in the vaults; he has been the biggest brute of any grave-digger in this earth, and he suffered for it at last; he died in the Strand Union Workhouse at last ; he died actually rotten.

"What salary do you get?—Eighteen shillings a-week, and then of course there is a little what we call pickings-up, perquisites; may be 10s. a-week.

"Still you would give up the situation if you could get anything else?— If I could get anything with half the money ; my wife has been making home-baked bread, and we now find that we have got enough, so that by persevering a little we shall be able to get our living, so that I am about to leave in a fortnight or so."

Mr George Whittaker, an intelligent undertaker, confirms much of the foregoing evidence generally. He says all the churchyards in the metropolis are in a very dreadful state, and that the gas which issues from a coffin is of the most deadly quality, while it is so powerful that it will raise all the lids of a treble coffin and burst them.

" I once," says he, " after many attempts, got some gas from a coffin in the vaults of St Clement Danes. I bored a hole through the lid of a coffin; I then held an India rubber bottle to the hole until it was quite full. This was from a coffin buried eight years. I tried some time after again, and I was nearly killed."

The gas that Whittaker obtained he took to Mr Walker, a neighbouring surgeon, who had requested him to procure it; but Mr Walker states that he was obliged, in consequence of the intolerable stench, to pass it through water, instead of through mercury, not having his process ready ; he therefore lost a great deal of it, but it made its way through the house in two minutes, and actually forced some relatives who were in one of the highest floors to run out of doors. This gas differs from ordinary gases, there being animal matter suspended in it. The first bubble that passed through the water left a greasy pellicle on the surface ; Mr Walker was very glad to get rid of it, but it made him so ill that he kept his bed for a week afterwards. The gas generates as soon as decomposition takes place, and it will retain its virulence for a thousand years if confined; but no covering of earth, wood, iron, stone, or lead is a security against it.

So much for the details of churchyards and grave-digging in London. It is not too much to infer from this, that the practice of all resemble those which we have already described. Mr Walker, a medical practitioner in Drury lane, affirms that the emanations are poisonous to those living in the neighbourhood of the metropolitan churchyards.

" Most of those I am about to name I have personally examined; they are, the burying-ground in Portugal street; Enon chapel, Clement's lane; St Clement's church, Strand; and the vaults of *St Martin's in the fields;* Drury lane; Russell court, Drury lane; St Paul's, Covent garden; St Giles's burying-ground; Aldgate churchyard; Whitechapel church and vaults; St Mary's Catholic chapel, Moorfields; Spitalfields ground; Bethnal-green old ground; Stepney burial-ground; Mulberry chapel, St George's in the East, Ellinore Swedish Protestant church; St George's church, Cannon street East; Ebenezer chapel, Ratcliff highway; Sheen's ground; Shadwell churchyard and vaults; Trinity Episcopal chapel, Cannon-street road; the Mariners' church, Wellclose square; Bunhill fields, City road; St Luke's, Old street; Clerkenwell church, four burial-grounds and vaults; Spa fields; St James's burying-ground, Clerkenwell; St Ann's, Soho; Elim chapel, Fetter lane; St Saviour's church, Southwark; the Cross Bones, belonging to the same parish; All Saints, Poplar; St Andrew's, Holborn; St Anne's, Limehouse; Bermondsey; Christchurch, Surrey; *St George's, Hanover square; St George's, Middlesex;* St George's, Southwark; *St James's, Westminster;* St John's, Hackney; *St John's, Westminster;* St Leonard, Shoreditch; *St Luke's, Chelsea; St Margaret's, Westminster; Kensington;* Islington; Lambeth; Newington; Rotherhithe; Paddington; *Pancras;* and many others."

"*Mr Denison.* Will you state whether you have seen disease arising from that cause?—I have; but it is sufficient to state that the neighbourhood to which my attention has been especially directed is surrounded with graveyards; and that there are hundreds of tons weight of human bodies resting temporarily in the earth until displaced to make room for a succeeding tenant. Bodies, in many situations, are placed within six inches of the surface. Martin's ground, in the Borough, measures two hundred and ninety-five feet in width and three hundred and seventy-nine in length. If we multiply these together, we shall make 111,805 superficial feet. If we allow twenty-seven feet for the burial of an adult body, and divide this (the product) by that number, we shall obtain a quotient of 4,140 and a fraction. The vault is one hundred-and-eighteen feet long and forty-one feet wide. If we take the main width of a coffin, or the space it will occupy, I think, speaking of adults, we shall be able to place on the surface four hundred-and-three bodies. According to the best information I can obtain from a man that has worked there ten years, it appears that 14,000 dead bodies have been deposited in this ground and vaults during the time he has been there.

"Can you say whether, in your immediate neighbourhood, there is any disease traceable to this cause?—Yes; and I shall prove, by a very intelligent witness, that he has known persons affected by this cause. They prepare graves in many graveyards in London for ten or twelve funerals on a Sunday, the day on which funerals mostly take place; there is the most unseemly haste during the time of the burying; I have seen a clergyman go hastily from one to another, reading the service at each; a number of mourners come depressed with grief; their power of resistance is weakened; they may not have eaten for some time previously; they breathe the gases given off, and have been seen to stagger both in the vaults and on the edge of the grave, and in many instances have, within a week, been deposited in the grave themselves.

"You have mentioned the circumstance of burials taking place only six inches from the surface; from what cause is that; is it to save trouble?— It is frequently done to save trouble; but in many instances they cannot go lower. There is an utter disregard of consequences; and I know the working clergy are so careful not to breathe this air, that a direction has been given to the sexton to place the box at a considerable distance from the grave, so as to avoid it.

"*Chairman.* You have mentioned two sorts of gases, one sinking to the bottom, and the other rising up, and you stated that you considered that there was some animal matter floating in the gas?—In the compound mixture I have no doubt there is.

"How do you distinguish the two gases?—There are several gases intermixed with an oleaginous compound; and I am quite certain there is an animal matter floating in that mixture; having passed a quantity of this through water, on one occasion, a pellicle arose; there is no doubt a very large portion of animal matter is present in a suspended form.

"You form your conclusion from the greasy sort of matter found in the water?—Yes; the gas will be absorbed, to a certain degree, by the water, and this fatty matter will be found on the surface.

"What is it that sinks to the bottom?—The carbonic acid and other gas; these are the gases which destroyed the men in Aldgate churchyard in 1838. If the man had been on his guard, and held his breath during the time he endeavoured to render assistance, I do not think he would have died; but he unfortunately leant over the body of the dead man, inspired the gas, and fell down lifeless."

Mr Walker, who has devoted a meritorious attention to this subject, repeats, in a variety of forms, his conviction that the burial of the dead in every one of these places is injurious to the living. We have underlined some passages for the purpose of impressing on the aristocracy, who in the parts referred to have their own world, that they are just as much in danger as the poor man in Limehouse; the vaults and yards in all the fashionable churches, whether for marriage or prayer, being crowded often to within six inches of the surface.

It is as bad as anywhere else next door to the Queen, Lords, and Commons in Parliament assembled, as appears from the following extract from the 'Lancet' for June 13th, 1840 :—

"William Green, a grave digger, while employed in his vocation in the churchyard of St Margaret, Westminster, was suddenly seized with faintness, excessive chilliness, giddiness, and inability to move his limbs. He was seen to fall, removed home, and his usual medical attendant was sent for. The poor fellow's impression was that 'he should never leave his bed alive; he was struck with death.' He was subsequently removed to the hospital, where he died in a few days. No hope was entertained, from the first, of his recovery. Mr B., the medical attendant, was seized with

162 *London Churchyards.*

precisely the same symptoms. He was attended by me. I apprehended, from the first, a fatal result; he died four days after the decease of the grave digger. The fatal effects of this miasm did not end here; the *servant was seized* on the day after the death of her master, and she sank in a few days. There can be no doubt *that the effluvium from the grave* was the cause of the death of these three individuals. The total inefficiency, in the three cases, of all remedial means showed the great power of the virus, or miasm, over the animal economy from the commencement of the attack. —(Signed) J. C. ATKINSON, surgeon, Romney terrace, Westminster."

Let it be remembered that if this cadaverous gas comes into undiluted contact with the lungs of a man for an instant, his life is in the most imminent danger, and his health may be destroyed for ever. No length of time can be a warrant that a coffin does not contain this gas. Mr Walker states that a short time ago a portion of the old graveyard of St Clement's in the Strand, was dug up to make a sewer, which was much needed in that neighbourhood. One of the men employed struck his pickaxe into a coffin; the body it contained had been buried in the year 1789; the gas was clearly perceptible— it issued from the coffin like the steam from a teapot spout, and the stench was insufferable.

When the republicans of Paris were plundering and devastating the vaults of the Kings of France, in the church of Saint Deny, a gas issued from the coffin of Francis I, the contemporary of our Henry VIII, of so dreadful a nature that it nearly killed the depredators; nor would they venture near the Royal corpse again for some days.

"It has been vainly thought," says Dr Farran, of Dublin, in a letter to the Chairman, "that when the body has been committed to the tomb all disease will moulder with it. We have many instances to prove the contrary to be the case: even when it has lain for years, and returned to its kindred dust, on being disturbed and exposed to the air, the disease springs up, renovated as it were by the rest it enjoyed in the grave, to recommence its havoc. We have the example which Eyam affords; in this place the plague broke out afresh from the inadvertent opening of a grave, after a repose of ninety-one years, and cut off to the extent of four-fifths of the inhabitants of a populous town."

It will be observed by some that this gas, especially carbonic acid, though undoubtedly mortal in its undiluted state, is still heavy and sluggish, and keeps about the graveyards. This certainly is its tendency; but the grave diggers will not let it alone—they force it into circulation.

The Chairman of the Committee asks—

"Is it only that gas which evaporates in air which you consider to be noxious to the population?"

Mr Walker answers—

"Undoubtedly the heavy gases also become diffused, are mixed with the atmosphere, and breathed by the dwellers in the locality, or those passing

by. In very many graveyards they are obliged, when they dig deep
graves (and in most instances they are compelled to do this), to throw
down lighted straw, or paper, or shavings, or water, to absorb the gases
before they descend. Thus these gases are rarefied, driven up, and diffused
in the atmosphere, and the next current of air may pass them into the
street or into a house. There are many places I am acquainted with in
the vicinity of a graveyard where they cannot keep their windows open
in warm weather. I consider this a source of illness in the metropolis."

We have now taken a pretty fair survey of the burial-grounds
of the metropolis. We have omitted the names of several ; but
it is enough to repeat that the condition of them all is horrible,
atrocious to the dead and dangerous to the living. Colonel
Acton, Mr Ainsworth, and Colonel Fox, members of the Committee, visited Enon chapel and some of the burial-grounds
about Lincoln's inn fields, in company with Dr Walker, after his
first testimony, and from what they saw, but still more from
what they felt was *concealed* from them, they assured their honourable colleagues that they might rely on his testimony as not
at all exaggerated. The specific amount of injury done by this
state of things to the health of the population cannot, of course,
be precisely stated ; but the general opinions of Dr Walker, who
seems to have more practically investigated this question than
any of his contemporaries, are confirmed by the testimony of
other eminent authorities.

Sir James Fellowes, who was physician to the army in the
peninsula in 1804, says, that

" Even the bigoted people of Spain were convinced, by the fever that
devastated their chief cities about that time, that the burial of the dead
amidst their towns always killed more or less of the living, and that since
1810 the practice has been suppressed by the Government."

Sir William Clay then observes—

" You are clearly of opinion that even in this climate the effluvia arising
from decomposition of dead bodies might become a generating cause of
pestilence ?"

The answer of Sir James is—

" That is my opinion, and it always has been so. When I returned
from Spain I saw some account of the fever in Andalusia, and I mentioned
my opinion of the extreme danger of burying in towns, and that it was
high time that we should give up that system in our country.

" *Chairman.* It is your conviction generally that the decomposition of
corpses is capable of generating disease in the human frame, which disease
may in its turn become an epidemic?—Sir James : Yes, it might be so,
from the extrication of gases ; that was the opinion in Spain."

It would appear, from Sir James's testimony, that his repre-
sentations in 1804 had a considerable effect in urging the
Spanish Government to the enlightened resolution it adopted ;
for, though we were at war with Spain then, he had a passport

from General Castanos to go where he pleased ; the authorities gave him all facilities ; they then adopted the determination to suppress burial in towns, and he was present in 1810 when it was confirmed by the Cortes.

Dr George Frederick Collier, of Spring gardens, says—

"My impression is that the interment of persons within large towns must be one cause, *inter alias*, of fevers. I believe that no single cause produces fever, but that the effluvium given off from the human body tends to depress, impair, and enervate the human frame ; and I look to this as one cause, *inter alias*, of fevers ; for my experience of twenty-three or twenty-four years tells me it is so."

He adds, that the greatest care will not render vaults harmless ; —that even in the case of royal funerals in this country, it seldom happens, where parties descend too curiously into the tomb, but that some person or other is affected with cold or fever ; but other causes are co-operating in addition to the effluvium of the vault.

Mr G. D. Lane, surgeon, of Wilson street, Drury lane, having given an account of a case thus caused, which he had cured with great difficulty, then relates us the following little professional incident :—

"I was at the burial of a friend about six weeks ago in St Giles's churchyard ; the corpse was not in the ground more than three feet down ; the clergyman who officiated was a sensible man ; he was as far off as that window, so that there being a little wind up you could not well hear him, and he got partly under the lee of the church ; but there was a very strong effluvia from the grave ; I tasted it ; and when I saw him keeping so far off that I could scarcely hear him, I thought he was a sensible man,* but out of respect to my friend I stood near it and bore it ; I would not leave my post out of respect to the deceased, but if I could have been alongside the clergyman I should have been glad of it."

Dr Copeland, Censor of the Royal College of Physicians, states, that

"Burying in large towns affects the health of individuals, in the first place by emanations into the atmosphere, and in the second place by poisoning the water percolating through the soil."

How many pumps are there standing right under the churchyard walls, as in the case of Aldgate pump, Shoe-lane pump, St Bride's pump, the pump in the pavement around St Martin's in the fields—not to talk of other fountains—the streams of which we may imagine rippling their dark course amongst bones and coffins, and oozing through the ribs perhaps

---

* A week before this, however, the Rev. J. E. Tyler, the rector of St Giles's-in-the-fields, assures the Committee that " we have never, in any one instance, found any effluvia from the churchyard. On the contrary, it *is a decidedly healthy spot.*"

of the late churchwardens and the highly respectable chairman of the vestry!

If you quench your thirst in the river Hoogly, into which the dead Hindoos are thrown, you may swallow a dysentery or a putrid fever.

Dr Lynch supports Dr Copeland. Sir Benjamin Brodie informs the Committee that he has always considered the crowded state of the churchyards as one cause of fever or disease.

It must be admitted that exceptions are taken to the emphasis of some of the foregoing testimony. For example, Dr R. B. Todd, of King's-college hospital, which adjoins the burial-ground in Portugal street, of which we have often spoken, declares to the Committee that " no inconvenience whatever " has been felt in the hospital from the contiguity of the graveyard. The danger is more than compensated by the ventilation afforded by the space, and the patients, officers, and pupils, have been, he adds, remarkably free from fever.

The Lord Bishop of London, while entertaining a very strong opinion of the necessity which has long existed for some change in the present system of interment in towns, especially the metropolis, observes—

"I still must think that the actual evils which have resulted from it have been considerably exaggerated."

This is not unlikely : when we cannot measure the exact amount of an evil it is as natural that we should overstate as understate it ; but a bishop can know but little personally of the horrid details which are the work of the second and third grave diggers, whenever the sexton who orders them "to make a grave" and " to cut through " turns his back upon the operation, and goes to eat pastry. However, his lordship is decidedly anxious that an end should be put to the system. Whilst the Bishop assures us that he never perceived any bad smell while residing in the churchyard of St Botolph, Bishopsgate, as rector, the Rev. Dr Knapp, vicar of Willesden, who had been twenty-seven years curate of St Andrew's Undershaft, in the city, declares that the " abominable exhalations " at length ejected him out of the rectory house, and finally from the living, which was worth 200*l.* a year, to a very inferior one.

In all the private burial-grounds something in the shape of a burial-service is read over the corpses. The proprietor is generally an undertaker, the " minister " some low tradesman who lives close by, and receives a yearly allowance from his master. When the poor see this man approach with his surplice, they never think of inquiring by whom he was ordained, and per haps, at the only time when the words of an educated pious clergyman would make a good impression, they are disgusted or hardened by the demeanour of this sham parson—perhaps even his " pernunciation " sends the mourners laughing to the public house. In a private ground in Globe fields, Mile end, belonging to a brute named Tagg, where the dead are soon dug up and crammed piecemeal into pits, the coffins being burnt in order to make room for more, we have a " chaplain " of this sort, a shoemaker of the name of Cauch. Hoole and Martin have another " clergyman " to go through the service at their horrid place in the Borough. Haycock, the grave digger, says his name is Mr Thomas Jenner. He is a dissenter and a patten-maker; he lives close by, and gets 20*l.* a year. " So it suits him very well." The fees are 11s. for a grown person, 8s. for a child. In all these places the fees are low " to suit the poor."

But we have already overloaded our pages with evidence of the condition of the metropolis, allowing every possible deduction for the influence which bad ventilation, dirty and crowded houses, lanes, streets, and alleys, obstructed sewers, uncleansed privies, bad feeding, and filthy personal habits must have upon the health of the inhabitants, if there were not a corpse buried within ten miles of London.

Let us take a glance at the "state of the country." Excepting Liverpool and Glasgow, where the evil has been mitigated to some extent by the opening of well-managed cemeteries a little way out of town, the system seems to cry aloud for a remedy as well as in the metropolis. In Liverpool they have an excellent cemetery, but every one is not buried there ; and in some of the other churchyards they persist in the evil practice of accumulating a pile of coffins in the same pit. Even in Glasgow, Dr Bowring says, " It occurred to me, some time ago, to *see corpses absolutely visible* on the surface of the churchyard ! "

CARLOW.—Dr Shewbridge Connor states, that

" The churchyard in Carlow is in the centre of the town, and so closely surrounded by tenements, that in some places the wall of the dwelling house, often loosely built, alone divides the bed of the occupant from the perhaps newly-tenanted grave."

OXFORD.—Alderman Sadler states—

" Eight out of our twelve churchyards are inconveniently filled ; and in 1837, when I was called to the office of chief magistrate, I convened several meetings of the local clergy and parish officers, to endeavour to establish a cemetery near the city ; but petty jealousies prevailed, and the subject dropped."

Dr Randall adds, that

" In some cases decency has been outraged by the revolting exposure

of the remains of the dead ere yet the grave has fully done its task, as well
as by the laying open to view the circumjacent coffins in digging fresh
receptacles for the corpses of the parishioners."

CAMBRIDGE.—Mr Fisher, the mayor, states, that in most
of the churchyards there is no unoccupied space, yet more
bodies are rammed into the ground every day. Dr Hairland
confirms this, adding—

"The state of the burying-grounds in this town is most offensive,
demoralising, and injurious to the health of the inhabitants."

DUBLIN.—Dr Fitzpatrick writes a letter to the Chairman,
too brief and interesting to be abridged :—

"Park street, Dublin, 25th April, 1842.

"Sir,—As in an investigation such as you are prosecuting every
authentic fact bears some value, I beg to bring under the notice of the
committee the following circumstances demonstrative of the abominations
consequent on the frequent re-opening of graves. In 1835 I attended the
funeral of a lady to St Bride's churchyard, in this city : on arriving there
I was surprised to see a coffin on the ground tied with ropes, and in so
shattered a condition as to permit a partial view of the body which it contained. On making inquiry, I ascertained from one of the attendants,
that owing to the crowded state of the churchyard, it was necessary to lift
up this coffin in order to make room for that of the lady, and while they
were removing it to a short distance it broke asunder, and the body, in an
advanced state of putrefaction, fell to the earth, creating so disgusting an
effluvia as obliged the grave diggers to retire to a distance. On the occasion alluded to, a gentleman and I recognised the head of a friend who
had been interred in the same grave two years previously ; the muscles
and the lower jaw were removed, but the scalp being perfect, the peculiarity
of the hair and the formation of the skull satisfied us of its identity. Thus,
sir, independent of the question as to the influence of noxious emanations
from decomposed bodies on the already loaded atmosphere of cities and
large towns, some of the best feelings of human nature are outraged by such
profanation of the grave, and by the indignities offered to the remains of
those who during life were esteemed and loved. Every man of well-regulated
mind must wish for the prevention of such abuses, and this object can only be
attained by the establishment of extensive cemeteries, thereby removing
the necessity of re-opening graves, until at least such changes were effected
as would prevent identification of the body, or the production of noxious
effluvia.   I have, &c.

                          "THOMAS FITZPATRICK, M.D.

CARLISLE.—A letter from Mr Mounsey, the mayor, contains the following paragraph :—

"In Carlisle there were, until within a very few years past, only two
burial-grounds, the crowded state of which frequently caused most revolting
exposures, and in hot weather very disagreeable effects. Two small additional burying-grounds were provided, eight or ten years since, in the
suburbs ; but they are filling very rapidly, and the town extending around
them."

SOUTHAMPTON.—Mr Dickson, the mayor, describes the
general burying-ground in St Mary's parish as in a very crowded

and disgraceful state. The Town Council has offered a gift of twenty-two acres for a cemetery, " but the Radicals in vestry assembled refused this boon." The worthy mayor gives no opinion as to these Radicals, but we have no hesitation in saying that they ought to be buried alive.

LEEDS.—This place is in a dreadful state. Mr Robert Baker, surgeon, being examined before the Committee, speaks generally of the ground as being extraordinarily full. The parochial ground, consisting of three distinct pieces, has been filled and refilled, diffusing fever around. The burial-places are surrounded by inhabitants.

"I was in the ground last Wednesday collecting information, and the sexton took me to a grave which they were then digging for the interment of a female ; two feet below the surface they took out the body of a child which was said to be an illegitimate child, and it had been buried five years ; below that, and two feet six inches from the surface, were two coffins side by side, the father and the brother of the person who was then going to have the interment ; the father was buried in 1831 ; the coffins were opened, the bones were in a state of freshness ; the matter had been putrified off the bones, but they were perfectly fresh ; they were thrown on the surface, and at that time the person came in who was going to have the interment ; he spoke to me about it, and made use of this expression, ' Look ! these are the skulls of my father and my brother, and the bones of my relations, is not this a bad business ?   It cannot, I suppose, however, be helped ; I must have a family grave.' He was very much shocked ; he stayed a short time, and then went away a little distance.

" That the parish churchyard, Sheffield, is in the centre of the town, surrounded by retail shops, offices, and respectable private dwellings ; that graves are continually opened, from which offensive smells are emitted, especially in particular parts of the burial-ground ; and at one corner resides a family who are so annoyed as to be under the necessity of keeping their windows constantly closed. I am myself often obliged to give orders for my windows to be shut when the grave digger is at work, and the wind from the south. On the south side the land is very wet, and frequently buckets of black water, of a most pernicious and unpleasant odour, are emptied at or near to the principal street of the town. It is not unusual to see old coffins, in which bodies appear to be in a state of decomposition, taken out of graves, and secreted in what is termed the bone-hole, until a funeral has taken place, in order to make room for another interment, where scarcely it is possible to deposit another body, so crowded are many and most of the graves. I frequently see human skulls and bones strewn about the graveyard in a most disgusting manner, and very often graves are opened only just deep enough to cover the coffins. I can only account for this, that either the parties were too poor to pay the full fee of interment or that the grave was full.

" That St Paul's churchyard is in a thickly-populated part of the town of Sheffield, and the land there is also very wet, and when graves are opened much annoyance is experienced by the inhabitants. In the summer, after a heavy shower of rain, the nuisance of the drains into public street channels is intolerable, so much so, that one of our most active and respectable magistrates has complained.

" That St George's churchyard is situated in one of the best parts of the town, but this graveyard is a complete nuisance to the tenants of the respectable dwellings around it ; and I have often heard one of our most respectable medical practitioners complain of having to pass this, as one of the greatest nuisances to the public health in the town of Sheffield."

But why make a circuit of general grave delivery through every town in the United Kingdom? The reader is perfectly safe in the conclusion that many other towns are in a similar condition to those to which we have adverted, and he may infer thence the sepulchral grievances of the country at large. We may, therefore, cut short our dismal tour of inspection, and proceed at once to consider the immediate and prospective *remedies* that have been discussed by the Committee.

The first class of remedies is merely mitigative and temporary, not interfering with vested rights, and so far easy, but running contrary to popular prejudice, pride, and human affections, and therefore very difficult of execution.

The first evil in the present system of treating the dead is, that the corpse is kept in the house of the family much too long. This fault extends through all classes, but to an excess amongst the poor.

Mr Robert Carr, of Duke's court, Bow street, London, an undertaker, who is 'thankful that he has lost the sense of smelling,' tells the Committee that the most deleterious odours are the consequence of this practice. "I am not sensible of what I inhale," he says; "but I have had a very bad taste in the throat." We subjoin the continuation of the dialogue :—

"*Mr Ainsworth.* After you have been at one of the interments have you had an unpleasant taste in the throat ?—Yes, if the body happened to be very bad, which is too frequently the case among poor people. If a person dies, we will say on Wednesday, the following Sunday is the convenient day. The first Sunday is too soon for them ; they keep it till the Sunday following, when you can hardly go near the body, it is so bad.

"*Chairman.* Have your children been afflicted with illness ?—My little boy was ill some time ago, in consequence of a body that I had in the house : and it made me ill also.

"Why did you have a body in your house ?—A man died at the King's-college hospital, and I removed the body to my house, the people not having convenience to take it to their own home ; then it was not convenient for them to bury it in a reasonable time, and at last it became so offensive that we could hardly bear the place. The body was placed on a bench in the shop. My little boy works a little in his way, and this body was on his bench ; it was very much in his way ; he kept puddling about at his little bench, and I really believe that his illness was occasioned by that, in consequence of being myself so ill ; he was more about the coffin than I was.

"What was his disorder ?—He was taken ill very suddenly ; he breathed very quickly, and I supposed that he would not live long. I went to Mr Walker ; he came, and he said he was very bad, and if something was not done very quickly he would have a most severe illness, but he would do what he could.

" Did he cure him ?—Yes, to my astonishment, and of every person who saw the child.

" I suppose that has been a lesson to you, never to have a dead body in your house again ?—Yes ; and if ever I should have another, if it is not buried within a reasonable time, I will go to the overseer and insist on its being done.

" *Chairman.* Now you, as an undertaker, have great opportunities of seeing the customs of the poor ; have the kindness to state to the committee your opinion as to the custom they have of keeping bodies so long before interment ?—In many instances persons say, ' We cannot bury under a week ;' that is from custom. Others have not the means of getting a black gown, and they cannot follow in a coloured one ; that is their bit of pride ; then it is put off, it may be, two or three days on that account. They will not have their relatives buried by the parish ; they would rather do anything than that, saying they wish them to be buried respectably ; and then the end of it is, that myself, and other people like me, often bury for nothing, not intending to do it. They cheat us ; and if they would do away with their little pride, and let the parish do it, the bodies would be removed in a reasonable time, and such men as myself would not be imposed on as we frequently are.

" *Mr Ainsworth.* Does any drinking go on ?—It is generally a drunken job ; it is too frequently so.

" *Chairman.* From what you have stated, as to this dead body being in your house, making you and your boy sick, your impression is that it is very injurious to the health of people keeping bodies in that way ?—I am sure of it.

" And you attribute it to the two causes you have mentioned ?—Yes, keeping bodies above ground too long ; and it would be a very good thing if it could be altered, so that a body should be compelled to be buried within six days."

The following example is taken from Mr Walker's subsequent correspondence with the Committee :—

" In the month of June, in the year 1835, a woman died of typhus fever, in the upper part of the house, No. 17 White-horse yard, Drury lane. The body, which was buried on the fourth day, was brought down a narrow staircase. Lewis Swalthey, shoemaker, then living with his family on the second floor of this house, and now residing at No. 5 Princes street, Drury lane, during the time the coffin was placed for a few minutes in a transverse position in the doorway of his room, in order that it might pass the more easily into the street, was sensible of a most disgusting odour which escaped from the coffin. He complained, almost immediately afterwards, of a peculiar coppery taste, which he described as being situated at the base of the tongue and posterior part of the throat ; in a few hours afterwards he had, at irregular intervals, slight sensations of chilliness, which, before the next sunset, had merged into repeated shiverings of considerable intensity. That evening he was confined to his bed ; he passed through a most severe form of typhus fever ; at the expiration of the third week he was removed to the fever hospital, and recovered. He had been in excellent health up to the instant when he was exposed to this malaria."

The poor operatives dressed in black, whom the undertakers employ, suffer dreadfully from this custom when they attend a " walking funeral."

The Chairman to Mr Whittaker, the undertaker :—

"What is the practice employed in walking funerals ?—There are men underneath ; the pall covers them, and they convey the body to the ground.

" Is not that likely to be unhealthy to the men who convey the bodies ?—Yes ; I have been affected very much myself by a walking funeral before now.

" Is not the gaseous matter that escapes from the coffin, being shut up under the pall, likely to affect the coffin-bearers ?—Yes, particularly the men at the shoulders ; they are closely covered by the pall, consequently they inhale more of it than the men at the feet.

" Have you found that affect their health ?—It has affected mine.

" *Colonel Fox.* In what way has your health been affected ; what have been the symptoms ?—I have lost my appetite, in the first place, with severe sickness ; I have not been able to follow my work. In some cases, where I endeavoured to get some gas at one time from one of the vaults, I was laid up then for a week, or nearly a fortnight, and was not able to follow my business.

" Did you consult any medical man on that subject ?—I consulted Mr Walker.

" Did the medical gentleman that attended you attribute your complaint to that occupation ?—Yes ; and I am certain it was that.

" *Chairman.* According to your impression, is that gas exhaling also injurious to the houses in the vicinity of the graveyard ? — I should certainly think so.

" You judge so from the effect which it has had on yourself ?—I do."

The Rev. E. James comes forward with the following dreadful testimony :—

" I was asked, on my former examination, whether I had experienced anything offensive issuing from the tombs in attending Stepney churchyard, in answer to which, I said, no. I beg to repeat that ; but though I say that, at the same time I have suffered dreadfully from effluvia issuing from bodies interred, where parties have kept their friends till they were in such a state of decomposition as literally to render it impossible for any person to approach near the coffin. I recollect on one occasion distinctly, where the corpse was brought into the church between the services on a Sunday, no language can describe the scene I witnessed ; the undertaker's men all covered over with that which ran from the coffin, and such a scene in the middle aisle of the church it was enough to poison a person, and I was obliged to send for chloride of lime to disaffect the church to enable persons to come to afternoon service, which they could not have done unless I had taken that precaution.

" *Lord Mahon.* What period of time after death had the corpse to which you allude been kept ?—That I cannot answer ; but that, I presume, depends very much upon the state of the weather.

" *Chairman.* It is your impression that it is very injurious to the living to keep bodies too long uninterred ?—Certainly.

" What time do you think they should be allowed to be kept unburied ?—I should say generally five days.

" *Lord Mahon.* In practice does it happen, except in very rare cases, that anybody is kept from burial longer than one week ?—In the summer time it very often happens."

No wonder, then, it should be an observation amongst

172 London Churchyards.

undertakers that those who attend a funeral one Sunday are often brought to the same churchyard on the following Sunday as corpses! Even the protections of embalming within three coffins are not always sufficient. Mr Bunn, one of the gentlemen-at-arms, states in the ' Stage, before and behind the Curtain,' that while doing duty around the remains of his late Majesty, he could scarcely endure the odour that evaporated from the royal corpse.

This great preliminary evil can only be effectually checked by an Act of Parliament compelling the interment of a corpse within a period of from twenty-four hours to six days, according to the nature of the disease or accident that had produced death. It is as reasonable that Parliament should interfere on this point as that it should have done so in the enactment enjoining the burial of the dead in woollen, and commanding that the depth of a grave shall not be less than five feet. The grave diggers, however, seem to treat this latter law as a " dead letter." The new restriction could be easily carried into operation in towns by the addition of a medical supervising officer to the local division of police, and of course by the attaching heavy penalties to cases of non-compliance.

The next proposed improvement is in the fabric of the coffins ; —the desideratum being not that they should be better, but that they should be *worse* than those now in use. Mr Walker says,—

"I think there is a great deal of unnecessary expense as to coffins. The French are wiser than we. They seldom pay more than five or seven francs for a coffin.* The public will perhaps think that they do a very clever thing in putting the body of their friend into a leaden coffin, but it is not the least protection. The elm is more durable when in the ground than deal ; therefore it is desirable that deal should be substituted for elm. The coffin should be as light as possible. The cheap French coffin is made of the pine. It is exceedingly similar to an orange chest, in the form of a roof to the top. The city mark is placed on it."

This intelligent witness adds, that a body placed in an ordinary coffin will be decomposed in seven years. The inference is that in the lighter proposed deal coffin decomposition would be much quicker. An elm coffin placed in moist ground will last for a great number of years. Dr Navier, a French physician, states that upon examining three bodies, one at seven, another at eleven, and another at twenty years after interment, he found them all in a state of active putrefaction. In dry, well-ventilated vaults, as in St Patrick's, Dublin, and the cathe-

* Mr Harker, undertaker, of St Stephen's, Coleman street, states the cheapest coffin, made for a grown person, to cost about 14s.; that is for elm, but a slight deal coffin could be made for 9s. or 10s.

dral at Vienna, bodies become mummies, and endure longer than any coffin.

As long as we must have burials near a dense population, and in grounds over-occupied, it is admitted that the introduction of every method that can accelerate decomposition will be a public advantage. Next to the light coffins comes the consideration of quick lime as an agent of dissolution. The committee frequently advert to the Neapolitan plan, and ask whether a modification of it would be practicable here ? The practice referred to is one of the wonders of Naples, and is carried on at the Campo Santo, which is situated outside the city, looking towards Mount Vesuvius, and is used exclusively for the burial of the poor. A low wall encloses a quadrangular area, which contains three hundred and sixty-five deep pits, one for every day in the year, each covered with a slab, to the centre of which is fastened a massive iron ring. When the anniversary of one of these holes arrives the slab is removed; in the evening come one or two carts laden with the bodies of the poor. They are brought without clothes or coffin, or distinction of sex, but thrown and pressed over each other with infinitely less care than a farmer would bestow on the carriage of half-a-dozen dead pigs to market. Two or three athletic brutes, almost naked too, are engaged in pulling the corpses out of the cart. Each assistant sets the body on his shoulder, or sometimes astride on both his shoulders, according to its weight and size, and then, trotting to the mouth of the pit, bends his neck, and allows the burthen to fall over, exactly as a porter at the wharfs dispatches a sack of grain. When the last of the dead is flung in, an immense quantity of quick lime is thrown over the bodies. The dark cavern is then closed up, and, when it is again opened that day twelvemonth, nothing is seen but a heap of bones at the bottom !

Mr Walker says, " I do not think the public would submit to that ; I think the old Roman plan of burning would be preferable." Unquestionably. But as to the practicability of a modification of the plan, there is considerable difference of opinion amongst the witnesses. Colonel Fox asks—

" Might not that objection be obviated by doing it in a more decent manner than it is done at Naples?—Mr Walker : I think it might ; the English are a very sensible people, and they might be brought to anything reasonable."

Dr Copeland thinks the opposition to the introduction of quick lime into and about coffins would not be material ; the practice would be beneficial. But Dr Bowring doubts this :—

" In Portugal, where, generally speaking, quick lime is used for the purpose of destroying the corpses of the dead, I recollect some of the churchyards in the city were exceedingly offensive."

If lime be laid on the exterior of the coffin the effect on the corpse will be little or nothing ; but quick lime neutralizes the carbonic acid gas : for the purpose of neutralizing other gases the chloride of lime is best.   The fact is, quick lime is already used in most, if not all, of the metropolitan graveyards.   Mr Whittaker says it is merely strewed or intermixed with the ground, or the sides of the coffin are taken out and the lime is strewn over the body.   We have had repeated evidence that it has been in abundant use in Enon chapel.   Quick lime, as an accelerative, is too slow, and, as a neutralizer, a mere palliative when brought to act upon the immense amount of mortality which our grounds and vaults contain.

The next immediate partial remedy suggested is, that the bodies should be buried side by side, and not one over the other, as is the present practice.   Mr Walker observes :—

" I have examined upwards of ninety graveyards, and am decidedly of opinion that coffins should be placed side by side, even as a matter of economy, and not as they are in Barbican and other places, where they have twenty or twenty-five bodies in one grave.   We have had the old graveyard of St Clement's turned up within these few days, and given to the street ; this was necessary, for the purpose of a sewer ; the stench was abominable, though it is forty years since that was used as a graveyard ; if that place had been opened in the summer, it might have produced an epidemic.

" Suppose a case," he continues, " where it is necessary to exhume a body for judicial purposes, as happened at Chelsea in 1840.   A poor man died in a wretched hovel in Paradise row, Chelsea, and was buried in the usual way by the parish.   A judicial inquiry was instituted, and it was necessary to exhume the body.   The grave digger opened the hole, and after searching for some time, he declared his inability to find it.   The coroner (Mr Wakley) inquired of the summoning officer the precise number of bodies interred in the same pit ?   The officer replied, to the best of his recollection there were twenty-six bodies.   The coroner wished to be informed if they *rammed them in with a rammer ?*   The officer said he was not aware that they resorted to such a process, but the bodies of paupers were packed together as closely as possible, in order to make the most of the space. The coroner observed that such a system of burial was revolting to humanity, and reflected the highest disgrace on a Christian country.

" With regard to the burials of the poor, it will be difficult to say how they should be provided for ; but if we go upon the old system of putting eighteen or twenty bodies in a grave, we shall leave a source of disease which may be acting for a long period.   In Paris they have an excellent mode for the interment of the poor.   The 'fosses communes' of a cemetery was dug to a depth of four feet, the earth being thrown up on either side by the fosse for a considerable distance.   The bodies are deposited side by side, but not one upon the other.   The mortality of the day being received, the earth is thrown on the coffins thus deposited until the fosse is filled, when another place is dug and occupied in the same manner.   This ground, as required, may with safety be again employed for burial after a period of five or seven years."

But, admitting Mr Walker's theory of the economy of space

to be true, it will not be carried into practice in the metropolitan graveyards or in those of country towns. The crowded, or rather crammed state of the grounds, the urgent demands of our present mortality, and the vested rights of the grave diggers, will continue the deep pits.

It cannot be denied that the institution of suburban cemeteries has, in some slight degree, checked the practices of which we complain; but their benefit is hardly sensible—in fact, the inadequacy of what they have done, or can do, only demonstrates the enormous extent and inveteracy of the present means of burial, and the necessity of the Legislature stepping in as the only power able to afford us general relief and protection. Most of the cemeteries established out of town are joint-stock speculations, and we do not see why we should speak more harshly of this kind of scrip than of any other; we must give them credit for every advantage they offer, and then remember that the shareholders are as anxious for the public accommodation, and their own, as are the "honourable proprietors" of any railway or steam-packet company, or, in short, of any other undertaking. The Highgate cemetery is beautifully situated; but Sydney Smith says we use for our tea the water that percolates through it. Mr Walker observes, that the Kensal-green cemetery is flanked by a canal, " and here they follow the very objectionable practice of placing several bodies in one grave." The Rev. Mr Knapp fears that some of the cemeteries will soon be too near London, as they are already beginning to be built round. The situation of the Norwood cemetery seems amongst the best; but we are not sure whether it is consecrated. Mr Walker thinks cemeteries ought not to be nearer than two miles to town; Dr Knapp thinks five miles; but a preference should be given to an elevated situation, as there the gases would pass off with the currents of air.

It being admitted then, on all hands, that burials in towns should cease, that cemeteries should be established outside towns, and that Government ought to take the question into its own hands, we have now to proceed to consider how this is to be done.

The Bishop of London thus addresses himself to the difficulties of the case :—

" Feeling, in common with other persons, the necessity of applying some remedy for the evil complained of, I am at the same time interested in the subject for another reason ; looking to the interest of the parochial clergy of my own diocese and of others, but especially of my own, as being involved in the question. I am sure that the clergy, generally speaking, would be willing to make some sacrifice for the sake of effecting so great an improvement as is contemplated ; but you cannot expect men, the principal part of whose subsistence in some cases depends upon the fees arising from a practice that has hitherto not been complained of, willingly to give up the whole source of that income without some compensation. In some of the parishes, as I will shortly prove by instances, a considerable proportion of the incumbent's income arises from burial fees ; and whatever measure is adopted with a view to remove the interment of corpses from cities and crowded towns, to cemeteries placed in the neighbourhood, it will scarcely be possible to prevent considerable loss to the clergy ; because, even if you can secure to them the fees to which they are now entitled by law, for every corpse which is carried out of their parish to be buried in a cemetery, they will mostly lose the complimentary fees, and what are called 'the fittings,' that is to say, scarves and hatbands, which in some parishes amount to a very considerable sum annually ; these are only given, of course, where the clergyman attends in person, and unless he himself performs the ceremony in person he cannot expect to receive what are called the complimentary fees. All I can say with reference to that part of the subject is, that I hope that in any legislative measure, some care will be taken to diminish the loss to the clergy, as far as consistent with the public interest ; and that such a thing may be done, though I am afraid not without some difficulty. In the first cemetery established in the neighbourhood of London, that of Kensal green, when the whole question was new, and the effects of the cemetery could hardly be calculated, a fee was reserved, I forget the amount,* upon each funeral coming from certain parishes, to the incumbents of those parishes, which, however, proved to be an utterly inadequate compensation, and the incumbent of Paddington, whose income arises principally from fees and Easter offerings, informs me, that in consequence of the opening of that cemetery he considers himself to have lost at least. 200*l.* a-year ; that from one parish ; and the loss to the rector of St Marylebone, I am sure, cannot be less. The next cemetery opened was that at Highgate. That bill was passed at a time when I was prevented by severe illness from attending to public business ; and by the Act which was passed, a small fee was secured to the clergymen, and there again they are great losers. The third cemetery near London was that of the West London and Westminster Cemetery. In that case the company are obliged by law to pay a fee of 10s. for every funeral to the clergyman from whose parish it comes. That sum was considered by the clergymen, whom I consulted upon that occasion, as being a fair compensation, taking an average, for the losses they were likely to sustain. I may here remark, with respect to that mode of compensating the clergy, that it makes it necessary for them from time to time to go round to the different cemetery offices to look over the books, and to see what funerals have been brought from their respective parishes, to calculate the amount, and then to demand it of the officers of the company, which is not a very agreeable, nor, at times, a very easy task for the clergyman to perform ; and, upon the whole, I fear that it will not be possible to secure the interest of the clergy effectually, but still it may be done to a considerable extent. While I am on the subject of cemeteries, I would remark, that a provision ought to be made (and this will be one of the difficulties of the case) for the funerals of the poor ; as it is, they are much too expensive for poor people, and if they are obliged to carry the bodies of their friends to a distance in the country, in the present mode, it will become more so. There is, however, no expense so little thought of by the poor as the expense of a funeral. I have known repeated instances where they would deprive themselves of

* Dr Knapp says it is 5s. for a vault funeral, and 18d. for a common grave funeral.

the necessaries of life for the sake of paying respect to the bodies of their departed friends ; and I should be sorry that that feeling should be interfered with beyond a certain extent. I think, by means of a cheap and decent kind of conveyance, of a hearse, that the expense of a funeral may be reduced, and if the poor do not object to avail themselves of it, that it may be done as cheap as their funerals are performed at present, if they are willing to dispense with what is called 'a walking funeral.' I think that it is wholly impossible to pass any law, the provisions of which (unless there be a latitude of application provided) shall be applicable to all parts of populous towns in the kingdom ; what may be a very wise provision for the metropolis, or for any given populous town, may be found not to be applicable to another town with an amount of population nearly as great. I would take the liberty of mentioning one instance, that of my native town, Bury St Edmunds, where there is but one churchyard for the whole of the town, containing about 11,000 inhabitants ; and if you were to go merely by the rule of population, you would say that no funeral should take place in the town ; but then that churchyard is very large ; it is open on one side to the country, and will serve the purposes of the town for many years to come, without the slightest chance of detriment to the health of the inhabitants ; therefore I think it must be left to the local authorities, acting upon certain principles, and under certain regulations laid down by law, to determine in what cases funerals shall be prohibited, and what provision shall be made for the interment of the dead. I do not think anything else occurs to me at the present moment, which I think it necessary to state, unless the committee should like to hear the amount of burial fees in some of the parishes of London for the last three years."

The following list of burial fees was then handed in :—

—	1838.			1839.			1840.		
	£.	*s.*	*d.*	*£.*	*s.*	*d.*	*£.*	*s.*	*d.*
St James, Westminster - - -	329	0	0	298	0	0	246	0	0*
St Botolph, Bishopsgate - - -	36	1	2	42	7	2	23	9	10
St George the Martyr - .. -	70	12	6	59	5	10	59	0	8
St John, Westminster - - -	123	7	0	93	19	8	105	13	7
St George in the East - - -	101	15	0	101	8	6	74	8	6
St Bride - - - - -	51	6	8	51	2	0	81	2	4
St Margaret, Westminster - -	160	14	0	115	1	6	128	0	8
St Giles in the Fields - - -	764	16	6	608	19	6	635	13	0
St Dunstan, Westminster - -	39	9	2	24	0	8	35	5	10
St Clement Danes - - -	121	14	9	112	19	10	86	3	4
Bethnal Green - - - -	71	4	0	67	4	0	62	3	6
St George, Bloomsbury - - -	273	7	6	159	4	6	235	2	0
St Botolph, Aldersgate - - -	60	8	4	58	2	8	45	10	0
St George, Hanover square - -	597	17	0	423	8	2	488	11	2
St Giles, Cripplegate - - -	87	9	6	66	6	10	56	14	10
St Sepulchre - - - -	80	16	6	66	8	0	72	6	0
St Andrew, Holborn - - -	306	0	1	324	14	1	223	15	2
St Catherine Cree - - -	75	3	6	43	16	6	56	13	6
St Olave, Hart street - - -	60	8	0	37	4	0	32	2	0
Allhallows, Barking - - -	31	19	6	7	19	0	15	16	6
Paddington - - - - -	494	14	0	404	18	0	425	4	0
Kensington - .. - - -	216	13	6	154	9	4	254	13	6
St Marylebone - - - -	589	17	6	548	15	4	516	11	0

* In the six preceding years the yearly average was 405*l.*

The decrease is attributed to the establishment of the cemeteries in the suburbs. The establishment of general cemeteries in the country would deprive the clergy of all these fees, and also of fees upon monuments, grave-stones, and tablets. His lordship would have no objection to a part of a public cemetery being left unconsecrated, for the accommodation of those who do not belong to the Church of England : but the clergy should get no fees from the latter. If the act for the abolition of burials in towns were passed, he would be for preserving the rights of family vaults, within strict limitations, under the churches ; but he would not permit the opening of new vaults. He would extend the same principle to some family graves in churchyards, provided always that there should be a sufficient number of feet (four or five) over the uppermost coffin. He also hopes that the case of the parish clerks of London, a respectable body of men, will be taken into consideration, before they are deprived of their fees. The sextons and grave-diggers he would leave to shift for themselves.

Mr Knapp thinks that in large parishes a penny rate would cover all the expenses connected with the new cemeteries, including the fees to the clergy. But in every place it is assumed that the clergy would willingly accept a moderate compensation for their precarious fees. The expense of the decent burial of a pauper in town is about 2*l.* ; but if several bodies were carried to the cemetery in one hearse, as has been the case at St Giles's, though the bishop objects to it, the expense to the parish would be much less. Whether we refer to the " noisy declamations of the Radicals," as at Southampton, or to the factious opposition of certain Dissenters, as at Leeds, it will be seen that the local feelings of the dispassionate and enlightened inhabitants cannot act until they are protected by a general statute.

How discreditable to this country is the difference between the English and the Egyptian fashion of legislating on this subject! We find the following interesting narrative in the evidence of Colonel Patrick Campbell, late British consul-general at Alexandria :—

" I was resident at Alexandria at the time the different burial-places were removed out of the town. For each religion there was a separate burial-place ; a Protestant burying-place, a Roman Catholic burying-place, a Greek Church burying-place, a Jewish burying-place, a Mohammedan burying-place, and an Armenian burying-place ; in fact, every sect in the country had a burying-place within the walls of Alexandria ; and indeed the Turks had several burial-places, which were easily known by the marble tombs ; they generally put up a different kind of turban, according to the position of the person buried. And in the year 1835, after the severe plague, or towards the early part of 1836, I was talking to Mahomet Ali one day about it ; he asked, whether any means could be adopted to remove the burial-places : whether I thought it would be advantageous ? At that time the Roman Catholic burying-ground was completely burthened with dead inside the walls of the town, exceedingly offensive. I told the Pacha I thought there was plenty of space out of the town, one or two miles from the town, and that it would be easily arranged with the consent of the heads of the different religions, to remove the burying-places, or prevent further burials going on in Alexandria; and immediately he sent the chief of police to me. I was at that time president of what was called the Board of Ornament, which Mahomet Ali begged me to take charge of, for the improvement of the streets. Some of the streets were very narrow —very many buildings irregularly placed. I was perpetual resident. Mr Thurburn, who was British consul at Alexandria; Mr Harris, the principal British merchant; and the Greek consul-general, and another consul-general; the Turkish head of police; the Turkish president of the Tribunal of Commerce, and the Turkish military engineer. There was the chief civil engineer, an Italian; and we took everything of that kind into our own hands. The Pacha sent the chief of police to me; I told him to take the civil engineer, who was paid by the Pacha for attending on the board, and go to the chiefs of the different religions, and arrange with them about having their burials out of the town. The Turkish burying-ground was taken to Pompey's Pillar, and the others towards the Rosetta gate, about a mile off the road, and a mile and a half or two miles out of the town : each company fixed on their own burying-ground, and the ground was given up to them, and since that no bodies have been interred within the walls of Alexandria; and many of the numerous Turkish burying-places have been lately built on, so that the town has been very much improved."

As plans and suggestions innumerable will be brought forward respecting the kind and modification of cemetery that would best promote the object, it would not be fair here ·to pass by in silence the project of Mr Wilson in 1830. He objected altogether to the principle of burying the dead within the surface of the earth, as, upon this plan, if suitable accommodation were provided for every corpse, the result must be the usurpation of large and valuable tracts of land, which would be better occupied by tillage or the recreations of the community. This objection particularly applied to the case of London. Instead of a superficial-burying place, he therefore proposed a pyramid cemetery :—

" A metropolitan cemetery on a scale commensurate with the necessities of the largest city in the world, embracing prospectively the demands of centuries, sufficiently capacious to receive FIVE MILLIONS OF THE DEAD, where they may repose in perfect security, without interfering with the comfort, the health, the business, or the pursuits of the living."

This stupendous structure would occupy eighteen acres, but was intended to afford accommodation equal to one thousand acres of churchyard. The great pyramid of Gizah would be no longer one of the wonders of the world, as Mr Wilson's would far surpass its magnitude. The design of this Babylonian work covered a base as large as the area of Russell square, and towered twice as high as St Paul's cross ; four cyclopean flights of stairs ascending from the pavement to the pinnacle. The whole mass was to be faced with square blocks of granite, and surmounted by a plain characteristic obelisk, having a circular stone staircase, and terminating in an astronomical observatory. The inclosure surrounding the pyramid would contain several acres beyond its base, which might be tastefully laid out for the reception of cenotaphs and monuments. Next there were to be within the walls a small plain chapel and a register office ; also four neat dwellings for the keeper, the clerk, the sexton, and the superintendent. There were to be four terrace-walks along the four walls, each angle crowned with a watch-tower. The approach would be through a lofty Egyptian portal.

The estimate of the expense was *two millions and a half ;*—a startling sum in the days when the cost of the London and Birmingham railway was unknown ; but assuming the annual number of interments to be 30,000, and the accommodation for each to be 5*l.*, the income of the pyramid would be 150,000*l.*, or fifteen millions in one hundred years !—thus saving not less than 12,500,000*l.* of the public money in the short space of a century—and what signifies a century in the progress of a work designed for eternal duration, or for a period as long as the earth shall endure ! However, the pyramid cemetery, instead of rearing its gloomy mountain-side into the clouds, and casting the shadow of death over every part of London in succession in the course of the day, exists only upon paper : the dividends were too remote, and joint-stock people would not wait one hundred years for one hundred per cent ; though doubtless some of those gentlemen have since invested their money in Spanish scrip and in the stocks of the New World, to see a return of interest or principal from which they will have to live at least a thousand years.

The impression made upon the Parliamentary Committee is contained in the resolutions added to their Report. Having recognised the necessity of protecting the rights of the parochial clergy, whose chief source of income is in some cases derived from fees received from interments, the Committee inform the House that they have resolved :—

" 1. That the practice of interment within the precincts of large towns is injurious to the inhabitants thereof, and frequently offensive to public decency.

" 2. That in order to prevent or diminish the evil of this practice, it is expedient to pass an Act of Parliament.

" 3. That legislation upon the subject be, in the first instance, confined to the metropolis, and to certain other towns or places the population of which respectively at the last census exceeded 50,000.

" 4. That burials be absolutely prohibited, after a certain date, within the limits of such towns or places, except in the case of family vaults already existing, the same partaking of the nature of private property, and being of limited extent.

" 5. That certain exceptions, as applying to eminent public characters, be likewise admitted with regard to Westminster Abbey and to St Paul's.

" 6. That certain exceptions be likewise admitted with regard to some cemeteries of recent construction, according to special local circumstances, to be hereafter determined.

" 7. That within the dates which may be specified the parochial authorities in such towns or places be empowered and required to impose a rate for the purpose of forming cemeteries at a certain distance from the same.

" 8. That a power be given to the parochial authorities of two or more parishes or townships of the same town to combine, if they think proper, for the same cemetery.

" 9. That a *minimum* of distance be fixed for such cemeteries, from the motive that leads to their establishment—the public health ; and that the *maximum* of distance be likewise fixed, so as to secure the lower classes, as far as possible, from the hardship of loss of time, or weariness in proceeding to a great distance to attend the funerals of their relatives.

" 10. That the parochial authorities be responsible for the due and decent administration of each burial within the new cemeteries, in the same manner as they now are within the present churchyards; and that, on the other hand, they be entitled to the same amount of fees on each burial as they at present receive.

" 11. That due provision be made for the perpetual possession by the parishes or townships of the ground on which the cemeteries shall be made.

" 12. That due space be reserved, without consecration, and within the limits of the intended cemeteries, for the separate burials of such persons or classes of persons as may be desirous of such separation.

" 13. That no fees from any such burials in unconsecrated ground be payable to any ministers of the Church of England.

" 14. That, subject to the conditions expressed in the tenth and thirteenth resolutions, arrangements be made to equalise as far as possible the total amount of fees payable on burials within the same cemetery, whether in the consecrated or the unconsecrated ground.

" 15. That considering the difficulty of fixing the same date for the prohibition of burials within the limits of different towns, or the same distance for the construction of the new cemeteries, and the importance of having reference to various local circumstances, it does not appear desirable to observe in all cases an uniform rule in these respects, but that the time and manner of applying the principles set forth in the foregoing resolutions should be entrusted either to some department of the Government, or to a board of superintendence, to be constituted by the Act of Parliament.

" 16. That the duty of framing and introducing a bill on the principles set forth in the foregoing resolutions, would be most efficiently discharged by her Majesty's Government, and that it is earnestly recommended to them by the Committee."

Here we may appropriately conclude our paper. The facts and opinions which we have collected show the true state of our burial grounds, and demonstrate the necessity of a change for the sake of health, decency, and convenience. The members of the committee are entitled to the gratitude of society for the diligence and fortitude with which they performed their repelling task. Through their valuable labours we may trust soon to arrive at the time when the living shall be no longer scandalized, and the dead may rest in peace.   J.

[We were glad to learn that a further inquiry upon this subject had been set on foot by Government, for we do not entirely concur in the recommendations of the Committee, and think several of their resolutions require re-consideration. The proposition, for example, to allow every parish in London to form its own cemetery, would lead to many practical inconveniences, as nothing can be more defective for such an object than our existing parochial organization. We should lament to see London surrounded by a multitude of petty and ill-managed cemeteries, which would, in fact, be nothing more than the old churchyards removed to a greater distance. What every one would desire is a general cemetery, or perhaps at most three general cemeteries, conveniently situated in regard to access, where the best possible arrangements for interments might be attainable with the greatest economy of expenditure. Cemeteries have now been long established on the Continent, and it would be well if some pains were taken to profit by the experience of our neighbours, instead of hastening perhaps to commit the mistakes they now wish had been avoided. At the present moment the management of the cemeteries of Paris is about to undergo a thorough reform, and in some respects the system will be entirely changed. The report alluded to by the Home Secretary probably contains some information on this subject, and, since the above was written, Sir James Graham has announced his intention to present it to the House; probably about the close of the Session.—Ed.]

ART. III.—1. *A Bill* (as amended by the Committee, and on re-commitment) *for Regulating the Profession of Physic and Surgery.*

2. *Second Report of the Commissioners for inquiring into the Condition of Large Towns and Populous Districts.* 2 vols. 8vo ; or 2 parts, folio.

3. *A Bill for the Improvement of the Sewerage and Drainage of Towns and Populous Districts, and for making Provision for an ample Supply of Water, and for otherwise promoting the Health and Convenience of the Inhabitants.*

4. *An Act for the Regulation and Care of Lunatics.* 4th Aug., 1845.

5. *Taschenbüch der Civil-Medicinal-Politzei für Artze, &c.* Von Dr J. F. Niemann, Königl: Preussichen Regierungs und Medicinal Rath zu Merseburg. 8vo. Leipzic, 1828. Pp. 900.

(*Manual of Civil Medical Police for Physicians, Surgeons, and Public Medical Officers.* By Dr J. F. Niemann, Member of the Royal Prussian Council of Health at Merseburg, a Knight of the Iron Cross, &c.)

6. *A Discourse on the Sanatory Condition of the Labouring Population of New York, with Suggestions for its Improvement.* 8vo, pp. 58. New York, 1845.

7. *Uber die Nachtheile des Jetzigen Stellung des Artzlichen Standes für Staat, Kranke, und Artze, und die Mittel, &c.* Von Dr Carl Simeons, &c. Maintz, 1844. 8vo, pp. 172.

(*On the Disadvantages of the Present State of the Medical Profession, as regards Society, the Sick, and Medical Practitioners, and the Means of Removing them.* By Dr Simeons, Court Councillor of the Grand Duchy of Hesse, and Officer of Health at Worms.)

AT the close of the last session of Parliament, Sir James Graham, in reply to that part of Lord John Russell's speech which referred to the postponement of medical legislation to another session, observed, " I see behind the noble lord, the honourable member for Kendal (Mr Warburton), and the honourable member for Lambeth (Mr Hawes), and they will say that it is not possible to undertake a task of more desperate difficulty than to legislate on this particular subject." The newspapers report that " hear, hear," confirmed the remark of the Home Secretary. This observation, coming from an experienced statesman, and a member of the Cabinet, ought not to be lightly considered. From what do the " desperate" difficulties arise, which mar the persevering attempts of a Minister of State to legislate for the medical profession? With a large parliamentary majority, and with an intellectual, educated, and eminently practical profession, as the subject of his measures, how does it happen that the requisite legislation is so difficult? The questions are so important, not less to society than to the practitioner, that several pages may be well appropriated to their elucidation.

The active existence of the profession in the body politic is but comparatively of recent date. We doubt if history can afford an instance parallel to that which may now be seen in the United Kingdom. In ancient nations the political influence of medical science was ranged on the side of religion or superstition; the physician was merged in the priest. In more modern times the same arrangement was in operation so recently as the end of the middle ages. *Now* medical science is cultivated exclusively as an industrial pursuit by a large number of persons.

The returns of the last census (1841) afford us the following statistics of the medical profession in Great Britain; for those of Ireland we are indebted to a friend in Dublin :—

	England.	Wales.	Scotland.	Ireland.	British Isles.	United Kingdom.
Physicians	1,063	30	364	300	19	1,776
Surgeons and Apothecaries............	14,102	526	2,237	2,100	141	19,106
Medical Students	1,320	76	248	500	8	2,152
Total	16,485	632	2,849	2,900	168	23,034

As those who were students in Great Britain in 1841 (under twenty years of age) are now nearly all qualified practitioners, we may fairly estimate the profession of the United Kingdom at twenty-three thousand!—twenty-three thousand philosophers by profession, of that school whose proper study is man, and therefore knowing human nature, under all its varied aspects, as no other body of men can know it. The object of Sir James Graham's bill is the regulation of this profession of 23,000 educated men.

Concurrently with the rise of such a numerous and necessarily influential body, there has been a re-action of the medical sciences on society. Scarcely a branch of knowledge exists, if we except pure physics, to which the medical profession has not been a parent and protector. Botany; chemistry with its subdivisions, galvanism, and electricity; and natural history, in all its branches, have had physicians as their earliest and most constant cultivators. All these, without exception, have arisen directly from the profession. It is true, the steam-engine and its appliances, the electric telegraph and its marvels, modern chemistry with its triumphs, and natural philosophy in its vast development, are no longer under the paternal tutelage of the medical profession. But these sciences have only asserted their independence, as colonies that have grown into nations. Even yet the mother country of them all (to carry out the comparison) exercises no trifling influence upon their growth, and contributes to their development by a continual immigration of men educated in the profession and for the profession.

The science of public hygiène is still, however, under the protection of the medical practitioner; although it has, as yet, no recognised existence in the schools, and forms no part of the curriculum of study. Its intimate connexion with practical medicine has perhaps contributed, in some degree, to this anomaly, by limiting its applications and narrowing its sphere of research. The practitioner, confined to his daily practice, has applied it almost exclusively to the individual man, and scarcely considered those higher relations which the medical art, in all its branches, bears to society. In short, the political economy of medicine has been almost altogether overlooked; its fundamental principles have never been discussed or developed, and the physician and the legislator have been alike unacquainted with them. Like the kindred sciences, hygiène participates in the progress of the age; and thus when questions of medical police are brought forward in the legislature, all appears inextricable confusion, and a statesman, like the Home Secretary, is ready to despair of efficient measures being adopted or carried out.

The above remarks have been made, that the magnitude and importance of the subject of medico-political economy may duly impress the mind, and that the fatal mistake may be prevented of looking upon it as a trifling subject, or as a mere quarrel or dispute amongst the " doctors." It is because this narrow view has been taken of the whole question that so many difficulties have arisen. The layman can scarcely even conceive the gigantic dimensions of the relations of the profession to society, and would look upon the expounder of them with incredulous astonishment. It is neither our intention nor our wish to detail them minutely; but it is necessary that some reference should be made to the different branches of medical police, that those which the Government have adopted for legislation may come more distinctly into view.

The principal divisions of medical police are—1. Medical economy, or government; 2. Medical education; 3. Forensic medicine; 4. Eleemosynary medicine; 5. Medical (or more properly, health) police. Of these, the three last are altogether dependent upon the previous, and medical education could hardly be said to exist without some sort of medical organization. The organization, or external economy of the profession, is consequently the most important division, and merits preference; we will therefore inquire into the existing organization of the profession. Although so large, numerous, and influential a body, there is practically no form of government. The colleges have either no power to enforce their bye-laws, or, having the power, have *not* enforced them. The only authority is a public opinion of a heterogeneous mass of individuals, with a community of interests and pursuits, it is true, but with no common bond of union to give effect to the decisions of the majority. Its will, indeed, can never be expressed, for it has no organ of voice. The colleges are corporate monopolies, and represent private interests; the journals are ranged on the side of party. Under these circumstances, Sir James Graham has undertaken his " desperate difficulty" of organizing the profession. The first requisite to successful legislation is a clear perception of the end and the means,—of the objects to be attained, and of the mode by which those objects may be attained. What, then, are the objects to be attained by an organization of the medical profession, and by what method ought that organization to be accomplished, to fulfil the intent of its institution?

The objects are twofold. First, the statesman, having in view the good of society, will organize the profession so that the greatest good to society shall result. Secondly, the individual practitioner, seeking his own interests and contentment, will aim at those objects which will at once advance his interests and minister to his enjoyments. The former are political, the latter are municipal objects. A scheme of organization, to be perfect, must attain both.

A philosophical history of the profession would present many points of interest to the political economist, if drawn out with special reference to the action of the legislature, and the practice of self-organization in developing the institutions of the profession. The existing colleges were originally that which, in spirit and practice, they are now; namely, civic guilds. A community of pursuits and interests led to union. The study and practice of the medical arts developed within them a body of teachers, and they thus became educational establishments. The attention of the statesman was soon drawn to these. As the colleges lost their catholic character with the growth of the profession, medical societies were called into existence by motives identical with those from which the guilds originated, and from these in the provinces educational institutions have also arisen. We know of no readily accessible information as to the early history of these societies. Many probably existed which have never been chronicled. The ' Medical Essays and Observations,' by a Society in Edinburgh, first began to be published in 1733. The first volume of ' Medical Observations and Inquiries,' by a Society of Physicians in London, appeared in 1763. In 1774, a medical society was established at Colchester, and others were founded, from time to time, in the larger provincial towns. The latest development of the medical society system is exhibited in the Provincial Medical and Surgical Association, comprising nearly 2,000 members.

These societies were, and are, the results of attempts, on the part of the profession, to organize itself. The objects for which they were established are the objects which are sought to be attained by medical reformers, and the mode of their constitution is, without doubt, the mode that would be preferred in a legislative organization, because it is the mode adopted voluntarily by the profession itself. It will be useful, then, to institute a comparison between the principles on which these societies are established, and the objects of their establishment, on the one hand, and the principle and aims of the proposed medical legislation on the other.

The first object of the existing medical societies and associations is the oral interchange of ideas on subjects of daily interest to the profession. The society's suite of apartments is the medical man's 'Change. A new fact, or new idea, or new method of treatment, is there heard and discussed. A scarcely secondary object is the advancement of the material interests, as distinguished from the technical; disputes between members, on points of etiquette, are there arranged ; tariffs of fees are often agreed upon ; expensive instruments purchased for common use; books and journals provided; funds subscribed for the widows and orphans of medical men, or for the relief of practitioners visited by misfortune; and schools planned for the education of their children. The attacks of public bodies on the independence or honour of the profession are also discussed, and medico-political questions agitated. No single society or association professes to attain all, or even the greater part of these objects. Some are established exclusively for the relief of widows and orphans ; some for the discussion of scientific or practical questions ; some to maintain the dignity of the profession by a uniform scale of fees, or for protection against interlopers and grinding public bodies. It is sufficient for our purpose that practitioners *do* form permanent associations for these and similar objects (which we will distinguish as *municipal objects*), and that a legislative plan of organization cannot be expected to be successful if they be unconsidered.

A striking characteristic of the voluntary organization effected by the profession is this, that it is essentially local. The municipal principle of aggregation pervades the whole. The objects of the organization could not indeed be otherwise attained, because they are themselves of local origin. A medical benevolent society administers relief to its own distressed members. The benefit derived from the sale of books, the use of the library, the instruments, or the apartments, &c., are only by courtesy and under great restrictions extended to non-residents. A legislative plan of medical organization must then (to be successful) be thoroughly interpenetrated with this principle of local aggregation. It has shaped out the form of development which the profession has assumed; it has already given some consistence and force to these local institutions; and any plan which does violence to it may be reasonably expected to fail.

We will now examine the proposed plans of medical organization. We will not refer to Sir James Graham's measure, that being, we believe, abandoned; but take up those propounded by the consistent veteran of medical reform. Does Mr Wakley's plan render attainable the objects which the present voluntary organization of the profession has been instituted to obtain? The following are the heads of Mr Wakley's notice of motion:—

> The registration of every person who, at the time of the passing of the act, shall be legally practising, or entitled to practise, as a physician, a surgeon, or an apothecary, in some part of her Majesty's dominions.

An equality of rights and privileges for registered medical practitioners throughout the kingdom.

Representative systems of government in the Colleges of Physicians and Surgeons.

The election, by those colleges, of a National Medical Council, having for its president a Principal Secretary of State.

The introduction of comprehensive systems of education in the Schools of Medicine and Pharmacy.

The appointment of Courts of Examiners by the Colleges of Physicians and Surgeons of England, Ireland, and Scotland.

The admission of the examiners into the hospitals and other public institutions, for the purpose of enabling them to test the knowledge of the candidates for diplomas in medicine and surgery, at the bedsides of the sick.

The repeal of those sections of the charter that was granted to the College of Surgeons of England in 1843, which displaced the members of that College from the professional rank they had previously enjoyed.

The right of every registered practitioner in medicine and surgery to recover reasonable charges for medical and surgical advice and attendance, without other licence than the registry.

The examination and registration of chemists and druggists, in England and Scotland, by the Royal Pharmaceutical Society of Great Britain; and in Ireland, by the Society of Apothecaries of Dublin.

The more effectual protection of the public against the dangerous proceedings of unqualified medical practitioners and unlicensed chemists and druggists, by making the offences of such persons questions for the summary jurisdiction of magistrates.

The prohibition of the sale, by retail, of certain poisons, except by licensed chemists and druggists.

The separation of the practice of physic and surgery from the sale of drugs and medicines.

Let us suppose that Mr Wakley's plan of organization is adopted by Parliament to its fullest extent (we leave out of consideration the conjoined system of medical police); that the whole of the profession is united into one corporate body; that the president, council, and officers are elected by a universal suffrage, and that votes by proxy from provincial practitioners are received;—let us suppose further that the Colleges of Physicians and Surgeons coalesce with each other and with the examiners of Apothecaries' Hall, and that they and the united profession have a common hall and a common purse; the council, presidents, and vice-presidents are elected, and hold their meetings with due debate and circumstance, and everything is done with utopian perfection:—in what way will the *provincial* practitioner be benefited? Will the municipal objects we have before detailed be attained? Assuredly not. The voluntary organization will to him be just as necessary as ever. The council of the colleges would be simply a convention from which practically all but the metropolitan practitioner would be estranged; for as it would offer no municipal advantages to the provincial practitioner, and attain none of the municipal objects for which he is seeking, a tax for its support would be felt to be a practical injustice. It is manifest that the metropolitan institutions should be duplicate; the one belonging to the metropolis, as a medical borough, and analogous to similar provincial institutions; the other belonging to the united profession, and the seat of the medical parliament or convocation. There need not, it is true, be a Guildhall and a Westminster Hall; but the representative bodies meeting in the metropolis should be as distinct as the City Corporation and the Houses of Parliament. The form of crystallization which the medical profession should have is, in fact, already shadowed forth in the Provincial Medical Association; and if Mr Wakley would assist in obtaining a charter of incorporation for that body, similar to that of corporate towns, but which would provide for the government of the metropolitan societies, and the branch associations, as so many medical municipalities, or boroughs, he would then have a sound and the only true basis on which to erect a national institution like that which he contemplates. The union of these boroughs would constitute the medical commonwealth. Sir James Graham intended originally that his Council of Health and Medical Education should be a *quasi*-elective council. Further consideration has no doubt shown to him that its constitution was rather a ludicrous parody of the representative system. Scotland, with 2,427 physicians and surgeons, returned as many representatives to the council as England, with 16,485. Glasgow was thought of more importance than Bristol or Birmingham; and Oxford and Cambridge, with their little corps of a few score doctors, were considered of more pith than the 17,000 of workers. In endeavouring to evade the Scylla of "desperate difficulties" thrown in his way by the English corporations in consequence of this manifest inequality, by giving the nomination of members of the council to the Crown, Sir James fell into a Charybdis of "desperate difficulties" prepared for him by the popular party, to whom this step was obnoxious as an abandonment of even the semblance of government by representation of the profession in the governing body. Testing Sir James Graham's measures by our touchstone, we find that he has fallen into the general error, and confounded medical organization with medical education. But the two are much more distinct than the national universities and the bishops and clergy of England. This grand mistake has arisen in consequence of taking the Colleges of Physicians and Surgeons of London as a form or model by which to work. These colleges have a two-fold character. Firstly, they are medico-municipal institutions, and consequently *local* institutions, as their title declares, and as the *old* fellows of the colleges still strenuously assert. These latter, indeed, never considered them more than convenient medical clubs, and cannot sufficiently express their surprise and disgust at the late irruptions on their closeness and privacy. But secondly, these colleges are examining boards, through which every member of the profession must enter; and these boards are constituted by the proprietors of medical schools, or, in other words, by hospital physicians and medical professors. This scholastic and therefore mercantile character has made its way into all the colleges with more or less distinctness, and has given rise to the Dutch auction of diplomas which has formed one of the greatest blots on the character of the college authorities. It is manifest however as the day, that among the municipal objects sought by the popular party, is the power to *control the examining boards*, so that in supplying a cheap, they shall not supply a spurious article, and deluge the profession with uneducated half-bred men. They seek this power rather than the power to constitute themselves into examining boards. A medical school or a board of examiners is so far from being a necessary appendage to a medico-municipal institution, that both ought most strenuously to be kept distinct, responsible alike to the profession and the law.

Another defect in Sir James Graham's plan of organization is that it is directly opposed to the action of the organizing principle now in operation. While Sir James Graham endeavours to keep up the distinctions of pure physician, pure surgeon, and general practitioner in his collegiate institutions, that principle continually sets them aside in the voluntary municipal institutions. The slightest glance at those which have been constituted for general objects shows this. Let the constitution of the Royal Medico-Chirurgical Society, or any other society in the metropolis be examined, or that of the Provincial Medical Association, or any other in the provinces, and it will be seen that the *perfect equality* of the different grades is a fundamental requisite of their existence. If the law of specialization were acted upon, they all, without exception, would fall to pieces. This fault is the source of the most " desperate" of Sir James Graham's difficulties. The reason adduced for maintaining these distinctions is, that it maintains an aristocracy in the profession, necessary to it, as well as to other professions. It may be asked whether the physicians be now really the aristocracy, and whether the wants of so large a metropolis as London have not called into existence a class of physicians altogether distinct from that from which they have sprung. Formerly the physician was the consulting surgeon, the accoucheur, and not unfrequently the operating surgeon of the day. He was also the anatomist and physiologist. Now the London physician is rather a literary specialist than the erudite comprehensive philosopher of a past age. To *internal* diseases, as they are quaintly termed, the sphere of his practice is limited. If the physician have degenerated into a special practitioner, he is only fairly entitled to the honours which devolve on that class. If we are wrong, and he be a physician of the old school, let him take his position and maintain it. But, in fact, the aristocracy of the profession must be founded in talent and experience. There can be no aristocracy of *education.* The means of a gentleman's education are much more available than formerly; the results of a university training on the mind and character may now be effectually obtained without a university residence. There are, consequently, general practitioners who are fully equal in professional and literary attainments to any physician. This class, indeed, would be much more numerous, were it not that the higher fees and the *prestige* connected with the rank of physician not unfrequently induce the accomplished general practitioner to assume the doctorate. Hence it happens that so large a proportion of the now practising physicians have been general practitioners. It is worthy of notice that the Legislature and the Government have affirmed this equality of the classes in the profession. There is now no distinction of physician and surgeon in the army. In the Act for the Regulation of Lunatics the medical " Masters in Lunacy " may be either physicians or surgeons; the medical " Visitors " may be physicians, surgeons, or apothecaries; so also may be the resident medical attendants, and so also may be the medical practitioners signing the certificate required by the act. In the Act for the Regulation of the Profession of Physic and Surgery, any one of the three classes may act as the medical attendants of public institutions. These are important indications of the current of public opinion, and ought not to be overlooked.

The true aristocracy of the profession (for an aristocracy there must and will be) ought to consist of those who hold offices in the professional municipalities, or who have worked their way to wealth and eminence. Such is the aristocracy of the clergy, the bishops, deans, archdeacons, &c.; such the aristocracy of the bar, the judges, chancellors, and other law officers of the Crown. There are no distinctions of education at the bar or in the church.

THE REGISTRATION OF ALL MEDICAL PRACTITIONERS is pronounced by all parties to be a necessary measure. It is of so great importance that it is to be regretted an act was not passed for this purpose only. Although its necessity is so thoroughly appreciated, there may be some difference of opinion as to the mode of its accomplishment. This has not been stated, but practically it is of importance. Bringing it to the test of our municipal principle, the registration should be local, and conducted in *districts* in the same manner as the registration of parliamentary voters, and a circuit should be made by a revising registrar. Much inconvenience, both to the profession and the public, would thus be avoided. A registry with 200 names would be referred to by the public; a registry with 20,000 would be virtually inaccessible.

PROPOSED MEASURES OF MEDICAL POLICE.—We have observed that the object of the statesman in the organization of the medical profession should be the greatest good to society. The system hitherto adopted by which medical science may be made most useful to the public has had no reference to any plan of organization. It cannot but be desired that the profession itself should be placed under some internal control. The medical practitioner is almost an irresponsible agent. There is no discipline within the profession; "every man doeth that which is right in his own eyes." The only provisions for the necessary control are the 33rd and 34th clauses of the Physic and Surgery Bill. The latter provides that practitioners guilty of fraud or felony shall be struck off the register, and lose their right to practice : the former, that every registered practitioner who shall take or use any name or title belonging to any class to which he does not belong, shall be deemed guilty of misdemeanour, and punished on conviction by fine or imprisonment, or both, as the court shall award. We may here remark that there is no penalty if a person *practise* as one of a class to which he does not belong. We need not enter into medical deontology or ethics; our readers are sufficiently acquainted with the internal condition of the profession to know that there are offences against society which the law cannot reach, which are neither felonies nor frauds, but which ought to be restrained or punished as crimes. Is it no crime if a surgeon performs a capital operation, reckless alike of the life and suffering of his patient, that he may make a noise in the world ? It is a species of murder. Is it no crime to undertake the duties of medical charity, and wilfully neglect those duties to the detriment and destruction of the health and lives of the poor ? It is worse than robbery. Yet the law accounts neither to be a fraud or a felony, and there is no tribunal before which such a criminal can be summoned. Just as there is an inner ecclesiastical discipline among the clergy of every sect, so ought there to be an active discipline amongst practitioners of every grade.

The theory of the British constitution presumes a representative of each class in the legislative body. In the Lords we have a whole bench of bishops, a large portion of barristers as law-lords, and a number of military and naval officers. In the Commons scarcely a dissenting sect is without its representative ; barristers, naval and military officers, merchants, and manufacturers abound. Consequently, if questions are mooted in Parliament involving the interests of these classes, Parliament has competent advisers. It is by the merest political accident that there is *one* medical practitioner there to represent the knowledge and interests of so large and influential a profession. From the circumstance that once in their lives they have studied medicine, Mr Warburton and Mr Hume are constituted parliamentary oracles in medical affairs. Two seats in Parliament are now at the disposal of Ministers, in consequence of the disfranchisement of Sudbury, and we cannot but think they would do eternal honour to themselves, and essential good to the country, if the return of at least these two members was entrusted to the medical profession of the United Kingdom.

HEALTH POLICE.—We have from time to time noticed the authorized inquiries made by various parties into the sanatory condition of the people, especially of large towns. These inquiries were commenced by the late Ministry through the agency of the Poor-law Commissioners, and have been further prosecuted by the present Ministry by means of a special commission. The reports which have resulted from these inquiries constitute the largest mass of facts connected with public hygiène that has ever been accumulated under any circumstances. The report of Mr Chadwick, and the first report of the commissioners, have been long before the public. The second report (of which an octavo edition is also published) contains the recommendations of the commission, and special reports from the commissioners. Mr Slaney reports on the state of Birmingham and other large towns in the midland counties; Sir Henry de la Beche on Bristol, Bath, and other large towns; Dr Lyon Playfair on the state of large towns in Lancashire; Dr D. B. Reid on that of the northern coal-mine district; Mr J. R. Martin on Nottingham, Coventry, Leicester, Derby, Norwich, and Portsmouth; and Mr Smith, of Deanstone, on York, Hull, Leeds, and other towns of Yorkshire. There is also an elaborate and interesting report on the medical topography and sanatory statistics of Exeter, by Dr Shapter. These reports have each their characteristic merit. Mr Martin and Mr Slaney, as political economists, look mainly at the moral (or rather immoral) results of a low physical condition of the people. Sir Henry de la Beche notes specially the geological relations of the towns he visited, without, however, overlooking other portions of the inquiry. Dr Lyon Playfair's report is distinguished by its comprehensiveness and general excellence; but there is no reference to geology. Dr B. Reid is strong on ventilation, his views of which are illustrated by no fewer than twenty-one coloured plates, comprising ninety-one figures. Houses, mines, schools, churches, factories, houses of refuge, steam-baths, are all reviewed by this celebrated pneumatician, and the various means and modes of ventilation suitable to all circumstances are illustrated. Mr Smith, the drain reformer, sets forth the defects of the present, and the value of an improved system of drainage, especially with reference to the use of sewerage water as a manure.

The recommendations of the commission founded upon the vast mass of data collected by them are thirty in number, and refer principally to the legislative measures necessary for the better sewerage, drainage, cleansing, waterage, ventilation, and protection from fire of large towns.   The twenty-ninth recommendation is as follows:—

" The most eminent medical witnesses concur in declaring that it is by the careful observation of the causes of disease and mortality, operating upon large classes of the community, that the mode and extent of their operation may be ascertained, and the power of diminishing and preventing them be acquired. For this purpose the appointment of an officer, whose duty it would be to direct his undivided attention to such cases, would in our opinion be a public benefit, more especially to the poorer classes, and might be advantageously employed in making investigations into matters affecting the sanatory condition of the district under his charge.   We therefore recommend that the local administrative body have power to appoint, subject to the approval of the Crown, a medical officer properly qualified to inspect and report periodically upon the sanatory condition of the town or district, to ascertain the true causes of disease and death, more especially of epidemics, increasing the rates of mortality, and the circumstances which originate and maintain such diseases, and injuriously affect the public health of such town or populous district."

The Sewerage, Drainage, &c. of Towns Bill is founded upon these recommendations.   In this bill we find the following important clauses, the effect of which, should they be made compulsory, will be to lay the foundation of a system of health police. We quote the entire clauses :—

"And whereas the health of the population, especially of the poorer classes, is frequently injured by the prevalence of epidemical and other disorders, and the virulence and extent of such disorders are frequently due and owing to the existence of local causes which are capable of removal, but which have hitherto frequently escaped detection from the want of some experienced person to examine into and report upon them, it is expedient that power should be given to appoint a duly qualified medical practitioner for that purpose ; Be it therefore enacted, that it shall be lawful for the said commissioners to appoint, subject to the approval of one of her Majesty's Principal Secretaries of State, a legally qualified medical practitioner, of skill and experience, to inspect and report periodically on the sanatory condition of any town or district, to ascertain the existence of diseases, more especially epidemics, increasing the rates of mortality, and to point out the existence of any nuisances or other local causes which are likely to originate and maintain such diseases and injuriously affect the health of the inhabitants of such town or district, and to take cognizance of the fact of the existence of any contagious disease, and to point out the most efficacious modes for checking or preventing the spread of such diseases, and also to point out the most efficient means for the ventilation of churches, chapels, schools, registered lodging-houses, and other public edifices within the said town or district, and to perform any other duties of a like nature which may be required of him; and such person shall be called the Medical Officer of Health for the town or district for which he shall be appointed; and it shall be lawful for the said commissioners to pay to such officer such salary as shall be approved of by one of her Majesty's Principal Secretaries of State.

"And be it enacted, that whenever it shall be lawful for any coroner to summon medical witnesses and to direct the performance of a *post-mortem* examination, under the provisions of an act passed in the session of Parliament held in the sixth and seventh year of the reign of his late Majesty King William the Fourth, intituled, 'An Act to provide for the Attendance and Remuneration of Medical Witnesses at Coroner's Inquests,' it shall be lawful for such coroner to issue his order for the attendance of the medical officer of health for the town or district within which any such inquest shall be held, and to direct the performance by such medical officer of a *post-mortem* examination, with or without analysis of the contents of the stomach or intestines, without fee or reward; and any provisions contained in the said act for imposing any penalty on any medical practitioner for any disobedience of any order of such coroner shall be taken to extend and apply to such officer of health.

"And be it enacted, that it shall be lawful for the said commissioners, and they are hereby required from time to time to make bye-laws as they shall think fit, for all or any of the purposes following; (that is to say) For preventing nuisances and annoyances in any streets, or near thereto, and effecting cleanliness therein: For making regulations for registering and inspection of slaughter-houses and knackers' yards, and for keeping the same in a cleanly and proper state, and for removing filth therefrom at least once in every twenty-four hours, and for requiring that they shall be provided with a sufficient supply of water: For regulating the manner of keeping swine, and preventing the keeping thereof within any dwelling-house, and for describing the limits in such town or district within which it shall be lawful to keep the same: For the punishment of persons selling unwholesome meat, and for seizing and condemning the same: For regulating the duties of scavengers, and for regulating the management of public privies: For making regulations for the registering of lodging-houses, and for maintaining cleanliness therein, and keeping them in a wholesome condition: For laying down rules for cleansing filthy and unwholesome dwellings : And to ascertain and fix what pecuniary penalties shall be incurred by persons breaking such laws : Provided always, that no such last-mentioned penalty shall exceed, for any one offence, the sum of five pounds, and in case of a continuing nuisance the sum of ten shillings for every day during which such nuisance shall be continued unremedied."

REGULATION OF HOSPITALS FOR THE INSANE.—By Lord Ashley's act provision is made for a more strict and regular supervision of lunatic asylums. The principal points in this act bearing on medical police are,—first, the appointment by the quarter sessions of Visitors of Asylums, namely, three or more justices, and one physician, surgeon, or apothecary, to act in each borough or county. The infliction of a fine of ten pounds on any medical visitor, who shall sign a certificate for the admission of a patient into a lunatics' hospital, or shall professionally attend a patient so placed except officially. No house to be kept for the reception of two or more lunatics without licence. Medical practitioners signing a certificate of insanity to specify the facts upon which his opinion is founded. The form of the patient's disorder to be entered in a " Book of Admissions." Houses having 100 patients to have a resident medical attendant, and houses having less to be visited daily by a medical practitioner. A " Medical Case-book" and registry to be kept in every lunatic hospital according to a form prescribed by the commissioners. Powers are given to visitors to visit hospitals by night or by day ; to discharge patients, &c.; to visit gaols, prisons, and workhouses, where one or more insane persons may be, and inquire into their treatment, &c.

This act is of great importance ; not simply for the extensive powers granted (which are without precedent), but as an important precedent for the establishment of a strict supervision of all institutions for the sick. It is manifest that the same system may be applied, *mutatis mutandis,* to all medical charities, and to the system of medical relief by parochial medical officers.

THE REGISTRATION OF THE CAUSES OF DEATH.—An important advance in medical police has lately been made by the Registrar-General, in the steps he has taken to secure an entry in the public registers of the cause of death, by the medical practitioner last in attendance on the deceased. We hope the plan may be successful. It is certain, however, that there are several practical difficulties in the way of correct returns. There is no remuneration for the additional trouble entailed on the practitioner; an omission not likely to obviate any carelessness or reluctance on his part. This we think a serious defect in the plan of the Registrar-General, and one which he will do well to rectify as speedily as possible.

DR GRISCOM'S PLAN OF A HEALTH POLICE FOR NEW YORK.— At present New York is under the supervision of eighteen persons termed health-wardens. These are laymen of inferior rank and education. Being one of the poorest offices in the gift of the Common Council, the post of health-warden has rarely been sought for or filled by any other than the most ignorant and incompetent amongst the office-seekers. Frauds and collusions are practised by these officers solely to increase their paltry salaries; and when an epidemic breaks out they fear to enter a house where the disorder is said to exist; thus rather increasing than allaying any excitement. Dr Griscom laid his views through the mayor before a committee of the persons who have the appointment of these men; his paper was returned with the observation that they did not "profess to be judges of the subject." A city inspector is appointed, who stands in the relation of chief of the health-wardens; a layman also fills this office. On his appointment a memorial was presented to the council, signed by a very large number of medical practitioners, which set forth in a clear light the true nature of the office, and the necessity of a medical education in its incumbent. The especial committee appointed to consider this memorial insisted in reply on the propriety of their appointment, and maintained that not only was a medical or literary education unnecessary, but that *without it* the city inspector was "likely to prove equally, if not more capable and efficient!" A line of conduct not very dissimilar may be expected from the English town councils; political partisanship, and not fitness, will determine the appointments, unless means be taken to submit candidates to examination. Dr Griscom argues (and we cordially join with him) that it is the duty of the appointing powers to fill the offices having the control and direction of sanatory matters with men of the largest experience and most cultivated capacity in medical science; having regard to the important consideration, that a man may be a good prescribing physician without the kind of knowledge or the taste requisite for the due discharge of public duties of this character. It is very manifest that none should be permitted to practice as hygiénic physician without examination as to his fitness, unless he have already given such practical proof of his knowledge and fitness as shall be satisfactory to a government board. Dr Griscom proposes that the city be divided into twelve districts, that the twelve dispensary physicians shall be the inspectors of those districts, and that a law be passed enforcing domiciliary cleanliness and the abatement of nuisances. The medical inspectors would also be charged with the duty of reporting on the medical and sanatory topography of their districts, as well as with the ordinary duties of health officers.

THE GERMAN SYSTEM OF MEDICAL POLICE.—Before discussing further the organization of a system of medical police, it will be useful to refer to the example and experience of the German states. General hygiène has been more extensively applied to society in Germany than in any other country. It has been also applied by a method closely similar to that proposed for England; namely, through the instrumentality of government employés. In the work of Niemann, a closely printed octavo of nine hundred pages, we have a complete exposition of the whole subject, both in theory and practice; and although published eighteen years ago, we believe there is no volume to be compared with it for fulness and accuracy. The author himself is indeed a government medical officer of some rank in the Prussian civil service. In this work he first discusses the police of the profession itself; and commences with details of the organization of the profession and the medical police of Prussia. We shall shortly notice this. The whole system consists essentially in a series of subordinate bureaus in direct connexion with the Home Secretary, or Minister of the Interior, by means of a central medical section; the " director" of the latter being a sort of medical Under-Secretary of State. This section consists of three physicians (two of these must be medico-chirurgical physicians), two apothecaries, and two veterinary surgeons. A registrar and a library is attached to it; the latter containing, amongst other documents, copies of all laws relating to medical police adopted by foreign governments. Besides this, there is a scientific Council of Health (medicinal Behörde) whose duty is to advise the executive. It is composed of those practitioners who have attained to professional eminence. Subordinate to these are provincial boards and councils (Landes Collegien). The director is termed medicinal rath in North Germany (Niemann holds this rank); protomedicus in Austria. He superintends generally the medical police of his province, assisted by the kreis-physici, and visits all the more important medical institutions from time to time. The board has the general superintendence of the profession, and of all matters whatever relating to medical science. The kreis-physici, or medical superintendents of districts corresponding to our " hundreds," or counties, are subordinate to the medicinal rath of a province. It is their duty to transmit to the latter a quarterly report, containing, *a.* meteorological observations, or at least the maxima and minima of the thermometer and barometer; *b.* reports on the state and prospects of the crops, whether in field or garden; *c.* the epidemic constitution of each quarter, and the prevailing epidemics; *d.* suggestions for improvements in the ordinances relating to his duties; *e.* reports of all prosecutions for offences against medical laws, or for quackery (Pfuscherei). A quarterly report on veterinary practice is also required. A yearly return of all practitioners, of apothecaries, and of persons vaccinated, is also made to the Secretary of State. Niemann subjoins forms of registration and returns for medical officers, medical practitioners, midwives, and veterinary surgeons, vaccinations, state of apothecaries' shops, &c., all requiring minute details. It is worthy notice that the collection of agricultural statistics, a thing absolutely unknown in England, is provided for by the same agency. The kreis-physicus must be a surgical physician, and have passed an examination in state medicine (staatsarzneikunde) and veterinary state medicine. He must reside in the centre of his district, and must not be absent a night from the latter without acquainting the Landräth, or for eight days without leave from the provincial board. Amongst his other duties he is to advance the science of medicine, and establish a lese-zirkel, or medical book society in his district, either alone or conjointly with a neighbouring kreis-physicus. In Austria he is required to take a periodical, the " Medicinishen Jahrbücher der Oesterreichischen kaiserstaats."

The kreis-physicus, in addition to the duties of reporting, as stated above, to his superior officer, has to inspect the profession with reference to the practice of their art and calling. In particular, he is to see that the surgeons of the second class, and the midwives, do not overstep their proper line of practice. He must look after quacks: it is his duty also to inspect the shops of apothecaries, and superintend the medical topography of his district, the pauper medical relief, and all public hospitals, baths, schools, prisons, &c., with reference to their hygiènic condition. He must attend to sudden accidents, and assist surgically, or procure assistance; make *post-mortem* examinations, and give evidence at inquests.

The kreis-physicus, or district physician, has under him a kreis-wundartze, or district surgeon. This officer cannot be absent a night without the permission of his superior. He must supply himself with instruments for performing capital operations, as trepanning and amputation. His duties are as multifarious as those of his superior, to whom he acts as surgical assistant. They have both an official seal. A council of health is attached to each provincial executive, whose duties, like those of the central council, are to advise the latter. They are also a board of examiners for the province.

We subjoin examples of forms; the first is the form of registration for medical officers, the other forms of return of vaccinations in a district:—

FORM OF REGISTRATION.

Name and Surname of Medical person

Residence - - - -

Age - - - - -

Office - - - -

Religion - - - -

Time lived in present Residence -

Salary - - - -

Date of Graduation - - -

Place of Graduation - - -

Date of Approbation - - -

Board by which approved - -

Date of swearing in - - -

Board at which sworn in -

Moral conduct and fitness for his duties

Remarks - - - -

FORM OF VACCINATION RETURN.

NAME OF DISTRICT.

ON THE VACCINATION LIST FOR THE YEAR.

Brought forward from last year's list -

Newly born - - - -

Newly come into the district - -

    Total - - - -

FORM OF VACCINATION RETURN—*Continued.*

TO BE DEDUCTED FROM THE LIST.

The still-born   -   -   -

Deaths previous to Vaccination   -

Removals from the district   -   -

Total   -   -   -   -

Remains to be Vaccinated   -   -

Successfully Vaccinated   -   -

Vaccinated thrice unsuccessfully   -

CARRIED OVER TO NEXT YEAR'S LISTS.

Unsuccessfully or doubtfully Vaccinated

Unvaccinated for special reasons   -

Total   -   -   -   -

OF THOSE VACCINATED.

Vaccinated publicly   -   -   -

Vaccinated privately   -   -   -

The statistics of the profession are returned under the several heads of graduated physicians, not graduated physicians, surgeons of the first class, surgeons of the second class, or landwundartze, distinguishing the civil from the military; oculists, not surgeons; dentists, exclusively as such; apothecaries, midwives, veterinary surgeons. Various particulars are returned under each of these heads; for example, the return shows the number of physicians who have qualified as operators and as accoucheurs; the number of surgeons who have assistants; the number having pupils; number practising as accoucheurs; and the number graduated as *chirurgi forenses*, or forensic surgeons. The animal doctors (thierärtze) are divided into four ranks; thierärtze of the first and second classes, farriers, and licensed shoeing smiths.

Plans similar to the Prussian in their main features are adopted in the other German states, the principal difference consisting in this, that there is less of the military subordination and discipline which characterize the Prussian system. In Baden Baden, the physicus receives 40 guineas per annum, and 10*l.* forage allowance, besides special fees. In Bavaria, the kreismedicinal räth, or provincial physician, receives 66*l.* per annum; the district physician, or physicus, has from 37*l.* 10s. to 50*l.* per annum, which includes forage. The duties of the latter are to attend the sick poor, and perform *post-mortem* examinations, and practise as forensic physician. For the last-mentioned duties, from parties who are able to pay, he receives fees.

The system in Nassau differs very considerably from the preceding. There are no physicians practising privately. The whole population of 400,000 persons is distributed in 28 districts, to each of which there is attached a medicinal räth, with a salary of from 60 to 80 guineas, an assistant with a salary of one-half the above, and a junior assistant with a salary of about one-fourth. The latter must also serve two years without salary. In addition to the ordinary salary there is an allowance to each equal to 14 guineas for forage. As no private practice is permitted, young physicians are taken on as supernumerary junior assistants, and after four years' service without pay receive a small allowance. The fees that can be legally taken are miserably small,—from twopence to sixpence for a visit; and from 12 to 20 pence for an operation !

In Hesse there is a kreis-räth for each district containing 40,000 inhabitants, who has the supervision of the whole profession within his district, and of the whole system of medical police. He is a sort of medical rural dean or archdeacon. Subordinate to him are the physikatsärtze, or officers of health. Our author, Dr Simeons, is one of these. They are paid a salary and an allowance for forage, which, with fees for vaccination and forensic practice, produces an annual salary of 50 guineas, but out of this horse-hire and bureau expenses are to be paid, besides an annual contribution to the widows' fund (whether the officer be married or not) of 2*l.* 15s. Pure surgeons exist in Nassau, and they are obliged to keep themselves pure, not being permitted to treat any internal diseases, or to prescribe any remedies. They are literally chirurgeons, or hand-workers.

Although the systems of medical police adopted in Germany thus differ in points of detail, they have been constituted for the attainment of those objects which are sought after by the government and public on the one hand, and the profession on the other. The suppression of quackery is one of the objects sought by the latter; the executive adopts the desire of the profession, and attempts its suppression. In doing this, however, it acts impartially. If it forbids the apothecary or dispensing chemist to prescribe, it forbids the physician to compound. If it secures a monopoly of practice for qualified practitioners, it fixes a tariff of fees, that the public shall not suffer from such monopoly. If it limits the enterprise of the apothecary to the branch of compounding and selling drugs, it protects his interests by limiting the number of apothecaries' shops. While, however, it grants *this* monopoly, it again acts on behalf of the public by a tariff of charges, by a scrutiny of the apothecaries' drugs and laboratory, and by requiring of him a regular training and education. It is further to be observed that there are quacks *in* the profession as well as quacks *without* it, and a just government must restrain the former as well as the latter. For this reason, taking the division of the profession into classes as it exists, the German executive forbids the accoucheur to practise also as an oculist, unless he have a special licence, or the surgeon as a surgical operator, unless his fitness for the duty have been tested, or as a physician, until he has not only graduated but been licensed, or the physician as a forensic physician, until he has been examined in forensic medicine. A licentiate of Apothecaries' Hall, if under German laws, would be punished for practising as a surgeon, unless he had also a diploma as a surgeon, and a general practitioner would not be permitted to practise as a physician without the licence of a physician. Such conduct would be considered and punished as a quackery, which undoubtedly it is.

We present these facts to the contemplation of those who insist upon protection from practising druggists and quacks, and leave it to their consideration whether (on the supposition that the German system *could* be successfully introduced into England) such a system would not be a greater, a much greater evil, than that they would fly from. We will now, however, look at this system in its practical results.

The pamphlet of Dr Karl Simeons enables us to do this very concisely. Dr Simeons, although a government employé (a physikatsärtz) in the Grand Duchy of Hesse, with a salary of about 50 guineas per annum, is a medical reformer, and dedicates his book to the medical Under-Secretary of State of Hesse, as a warm friend of the practitioner. His descriptions, therefore, of the condition of the latter may be received with some confidence. They are melancholy enough.

The profession in Germany is quite overstocked. The number

has doubled in the Duchy of Hesse within the last 25 years. In the towns there is one physician to 800 of the population. The long war, and subsequently the prevalence of typhus fever (hospital fever) created a demand for medical practitioners. The profession was prosperous, and this circumstance induced parents to educate their children as medical men long after the demand had ceased. Many of those who had been brought up as barber-surgeons sought the higher dignity of the doctorate, and the title has become at last so common, that now in Worms, a city with 10,000 inhabitants, it is no rare thing to hear barbers and their apprentices addressed as "Herr Doctor."

As in England, so in Germany, youths are brought up to the profession as a means of subsistence, without any reference to their moral or intellectual fitness. The parents of the German student are generally poor, and get them through their examinations as quickly as possible, to thrust them forth into the world unpractised, inexperienced men. Some begin practice for themselves who have never seen such a thing as a sick child. These persons never call a senior into consultation. One of this class resident in Nassau observed to a brother practitioner, "How do you get on with your croup cases? I have had ten, and they have all died. I thought at first I must have mistaken the complaint, but it was not so." He had given these children a large dose of belladonna every two hours. There a young man of this class starts with ideas as to success of the most roseate hue ; he feels a love for his profession ; he has carefully studied it ; is energetic and enthusiastic. He settles down in a district pretty well filled, as he well knows, with medicos already ; but Dr Y. is lazy, Dr G. is uncourteous, Dr F. drinks, Dr. A. is not by any means clever ; *he* hopes confidently for success, because he is neither lazy, uncourteous, dissipated, nor unskilful. Shortly, however, he discovers that one physician is not always preferred to another for his talents or good qualities. A. calls in Dr A. because he is a relative, or an old acquaintance, or a convivial friend, or because he is related to an influential individual, or because he is unmarried, the patient having a marriageable daughter. He finds at last that the way is not open to industry and skill ; and irritated and annoyed by the petty insinuations and slanders of his colleagues, whenever he happens to get a patient, he takes to puffing. The German method of puffing differs, it appears, in no respect from the English. The puffer runs about here and there, as if he were excessively busy, goes to the houses of distinguished people, gets called out of crowded assemblies, shows sham lists of numerous patients, sets up a carriage before he wants it, affects a deeply thoughtful air, talks learnedly, relates his astonishing cures, always promises success in the most hopeless cases, represents simple diseases to be of the most dangerous character, takes care his fame is duly trumpeted forth, gets himself recommended to others'patients, or thrusts himself into families, &c. Of course, professional jealousies and pettinesses abound. Now all this happens in Germany, and happens, as our author thinks, because the public is not a tribunal fit for the estimate of a professional man's talents. " I have known," remarks Dr Simeons, " decided and well-known dunces get into extensive practice." It appears that one mode of making money is an understanding with an apothecary. If the physician may not compound his own medicines, there is no check on the *quantity* he may prescribe, or the *mode* in which he will administer them. A per-centage system is therefore easily established.

Physicians practise as general practitioners in the widest sense of the term. They will set broken legs, bleed, apply blisters, nay (and with great indignation Dr Simeons writes it) will condescend to hold their doctor's hat in the one hand, and with the other give the clyster they have themselves prescribed. They are accoucheurs *ex officio*, draw teeth (or rather break them in), couch, and sell groceries, playing-cards, and drapery goods.

The officer of health with his miserable salary is in a condition not much more respectable. He is dependent in a great degree on the apothecary, surgeon, barber-surgeon, and nurse, over whom he has to maintain a strict supervision, for what private practice he can pick up. " One hand washes the other," our author observes, " and the badly-paid health officer overlooks the grossest contraventions of the law that he may not lose his practice by the shrugs of the apothecary when reading his prescriptions, or by the unfavourable opinions of the petty practitioner and midwife." Besides his intra-professional duties, he has to take care that the druggist does not act as apothecary; that the grocer sells no poison ; the butcher no diseased or tainted meat; the baker only sound bread ; that the brewer is honest with his beer ; that no unripe potatoes or fruit come to market; that no manufactories dangerous to health are erected on unsuitable sites, &c., &c. As forensic physician he must decide impartially on the importance of the wound which rich Mr A. has inflicted on poor John B. ; must determine the fitness of the men in his district for military service, &c. In short, there are numerous occasions in which his duties as an officer of the government come into collision with his interests as a private practitioner, and he has to balance the duty and small pay as the former with his neglect of duty and greater gain as the latter. Dr Simeons does not deny that there are many high-minded men in the profession who do their duty at all hazards, but there are not a few infirm minds who yield to the temptation.   At all events, the system is a bad system which tempts to evil conduct and presents no encouragement to good.

On a more particular analysis of the preceding statements, we find that the objects of the ordinances made by the German executive have been both municipal and political.   The attempts made to diminish the number of medical men, as well by a direct limitation of the number, as by an increase in the length and cost of the requisite studies, were made for the municipal object of elevating the profession, or at least maintaining its respectability. The establishment of book-societies, and of tariffs of fees ; the restrictions as to the practice of the various grades, &c., are all examples of municipal objects.   It is to be noted, however, that although the German governments have almost despotic power to carry out their views, the whole system seems to have *failed as a system*.   With the exception that vaccination is universal, and small-pox scarcely ever known, we know of no one branch of state medicine in which we English are practically inferior to the Germans.   The sanatory condition of our towns is superior to that of German towns ; our sanatory reports are generally superior ; our vital statistics will bear comparison with the best on the continent; our unsystematic method of medical education, however inferior in scientific results to the German (and we freely acknowledge that it is inferior), produces a class of men equal, if not much superior, in gentlemanly bearing and practical skill, to those we find in Germany.   We have no encouragement, therefore, to adopt the German system as a model for British state medicine ; it would seem a far better and wiser plan to note the defects of our own system, compare them with those of the German, and see whether the causes thereof have not a common origin.

The defects of the German system originate partly in the defects of the individuals making up the professional body.   Enterprising and talented men force their way into it from a low station in society.   These individuals, however praiseworthy for their energy, perseverance, and practical tact, carry with them all the traits of character which arise from low breeding and defective general education.   They disgust the higher and more polite classes of society by their plebeian deportment and rudeness. Society in consequence becomes tabooed to them as a body ; and as a necessary result, members of families of the higher ranks join the church, the army, or the bar, in preference to entering the medical profession.   Dr Simeons' remedy for this state of things is the remedy applicable to our condition : he recommends a more complete education in general literature, the languages, philosophy and mathematics, natural history, chemistry, and physics.

Poverty and idleness have also an evil effect as well in Germany as in England. The medical profession is selected by the poor parents of a clever boy as a bread-winner, incited to the step by a solitary example of some individual who has risen to wealth and eminence from as low and poor a condition. Their hopes are baseless; the youth comes into the press and the throng: he must toil: more than half the time that ought to be devoted to his studies is probably occupied as an assistant in return for board and lodging; he then craves for his examination, and hurries away to struggle for the pittance of a union and five-shilling mid-wifery fees. Having no capital, he has no alternative between this humiliation and starvation.

These are the results of poverty; those of idleness and dissipation are not much dissimilar. Practically the influences on the respectability of the profession are more noxious, for the poor student tries hard to be honest and respectable: his poverty and not his will consents. The dissipated and idle student becomes an ignorant, shameless, mean practitioner. Dr Simeons' remedy for this state of things is applicable to our own. It is a more strict supervision of the studies of the medical student; more numerous examinations; suitable punishments for idleness; exclusion for incapacity; in short, scholastic discipline.

The general defects of the German system, as stated by Dr Simeons, are so like those of our own, as pointed out by Mr Chadwick in his able sanatory report, that we quote them.

" 1. That the generality of medical persons are not sufficiently supervised with reference to their official and professional duties, and the necessary means are not given to the state to maintain continuously their technical and scientific development.

" 2. That generally (with the exception of Nassau) the health officers (physikatsärtze) receive too small stipends: consequently they are in a great degree dependent on their private practice. Hence they do not give the necessary guarantees, neither as health officers, nor as supervising boards of the profession in their districts, because their impartiality is doubtful.

" 3. That the number of physicians (with the exception of Nassau) is everywhere unlimited, and every one is left at liberty to choose his own place of residence, in consequence of which, while no provision is made for the due supply of practitioners to poor districts on the one hand, the more populous places are crowded with them on the other, with the evil results previously stated.

" 4. That the examination of practitioners does not offer the necessary guarantee for their practical knowledge, and that after his examination he can practise as he likes without the least control.

" 5. That the division of the profession into physicians and surgeons leads to many inconveniences."—P. 96.

Dr Simeons' remedies are to appoint a professional man to the office of referent or medical under-secretary of state ; to establish a medical council (of which the referent shall be president), consisting of four physicians, a veterinary surgeon, and an apothecary; to institute a kreisphysicus for every 400,000 of the population ; to limit the number of practitioners to one for every 2,000 of a city population, and 5,000 of a rural population ; to have junior or unattached physicians; a medical assistant (heildiener) trained for his duties and the practice of petty surgery, for every 1,000 of the population; an apothecary for from 6,000 to 8,000 of the rural population, and for 4,000 of that of the city, and to have the necessary number of midwives. In populous governments there should be deputy referents and provincial medical councils in the proportion of one to every million of inhabitants. In addition, he would have a public operator, who being in a central part of his district, shall exclusively practise the operations of surgery.

The duties he allots to the kreisphysicus are those which we have previously described as belonging to this officer. The supervision of the profession, of professional institutions, and of the sanatory police of all public institutions, of dead-houses, of epidemics, of epizootics, vaccination, orphans, the insane, schools, factories, and localities with reference to their sanatory condition, food and drink, recruits. This officer would make returns to medical inquiries from the superior board, undertake the medical jurisprudence of his district, receive the quarterly reports of the general practitioners, and make an annual report. Besides these state duties, the kreisphysicus has municipal duties, he is to act officially as president of the faculty in his district, to form a book-society, to call meetings of the profession at suitable times and places for the ordinary objects of medical societies in this country, to be the referee and umpire in professional disputes, and a general consultee in cases of difficulty or danger. He is on no account to engage in private practice, is to have his travelling expenses when consulted by a practitioner, but can only receive a fee when called in by desire of the patient. Being thus a consulting physician, it is an essential qualification for office that he have been in practice twenty years. Dr Simeons proposes to fix the salary at from 100*l.* to 125*l.* per annum. Such an officer, but with a much more ample salary, is manifestly suitable to England. The consulting surgeon or public operator is also to have a salary.

As Dr Simeons' plan gives the private practitioner a monopoly of medical practice, it proposes to demand public duties of him in return. The principal of these are, attendance on the poor, vaccination, medical jurisprudence ; for all of which he is to be paid : and the keeping of a daily case-book, or pathological journal, for which he is not to be paid. The proposed mode of keeping this journal is stated by Dr Simeons. An alphabetical index of names and residences and diseases is required to complete the journal, which is to be closed at the end of every year, and transmitted to the kreisphysicus with such notes as the practitioner may think proper to insert. An important duty of the kreisphysicus is to inspect these case-books as he goes his rounds; to see whether due attention is given to important cases, whether the diagnosis of the practitioner is in general good; whether he adopts a clear and definite plan of treatment, or changes it continually as the symptoms change, &c. Dr Simeons adduces numerous arguments in support of this novel mode of supervision. One of these is, that other professional men are subject to a similar discipline, as schoolmasters, clergymen, stipendiary magistrates, apothecaries, &c. And that as practitioners have the care of the *summa bona* of man,—his health and life,— it is proper that they should not handle these without discipline and without control. Disciplinarians ourselves, we acknowledge the propriety of Dr Simeons' views, if not of his arrangements.

On bringing this plan of organization to the test of fitness already laid down (we shall notice the medical relief of the poor subsequently) we find in it much to approve. It provides for many acknowledged wants. The statesman's object in organizing the profession is at least kept in view. Medical science in all its branches is made a part of political economy; the duties of the health officer are well defined. Nor are the objects sought after by the practitioner omitted. The unity of the profession is fully established. The classes of pure surgeons and forensic surgeons are viewed as altogether absurd, and the division of the profession into those who treat external, and those who treat internal diseases considered as belonging to the infancy of science. A consulting physician and an operating physician are alone requisite, and these are strictly limited to their proper sphere. A fixed provision is made for every member of the profession, so that at least none shall starve. The local convocation of the practitioners in a district is established for the purposes of mutual improvement and support; and above all, by the compulsory system of case-books,—(the registrar-general's books are slightly analogous), the best possible foundations for the statistics of pathology are laid, and the idea is attempted to be realised of a whole profession combining not only to practise medical art, but to advance medical science.

Several objections might easily be urged; the greatest is this: the leading principle of the plan of organization is ecclesiastical. It considers the practitioner in his *moral* relations too exclusively. Such a principle may be worked out by the " paternal " governments of the German States, but an *industrial* profession cannot be so trammelled in England. It is further defective in another important point, namely, in restricting the choice by the people at large of a professional man. Medicine is like to theology ; it has its dogmatists and its enthusiasts. A uniformity of medicinal belief and trust is just as impossible as a uniformity of faith and doctrine, or of taste as to a preacher.

ELEEMOSYNARY MEDICINE.—The observation we have just made is applicable also to the systems of eleemosynary medicine adopted by modern governments. The compulsory adoption of a medical attendant is less grievously felt in England by those who apply to medical charities than by the applicants for poor-law medical relief, because the officers of the former are generally more or less eminent in the profession, and if not eminent, the composition of the staff leaves a certain latitude of choice. With the poor-law medical relief, matters are different. The officer is usually more remarkable for his youth, poverty, and inexperience, than for his skill, and is without even a colleague. The poor have, in fact, no choice whatever. Those physicians who have had much practice amongst the poor will bear us out in the opinion that the surgeon of the union has not fair play with his pauper patients, from the circumstance only that he is forced upon them. The love of existence, and of a painless existence, is as fervent in the breast of the pauper as of the peer. Both have alike their opinions as to the individuals most likely to prolong life or relieve pain. The pauper feels it a grievous hardship (as it is) that he cannot have the advice of him in whom he places his confidence. These remarks are also applicable, although in a less degree, to the system of "*sick* clubs."

Dr Simeons has a novel method for the relief of the sick poor; but previously to detailing this, we will note the present methods adopted in certain continental states.   In Denmark, the clergyman of the parish gives the sick pauper a note to the district physician, which the pauper must take himself, if he be able; if not, the clergyman sends an account of the case to the physician. If the latter thinks a visit necessary, he visits, but lets the clergyman know what time will be convenient, and conveyance backwards and forwards is provided for him in rotation by such of the parishioners as keep horses and carriages employed for farm use.

The clergyman, or if he is prevented, the member of the parish committee (a sort of select vestry) nearest the sick person, must see that the prescribed mode of treatment is duly observed. In Berlin, all persons who are too poor to pay for medical attendance, or for medicine, are entitled to medical attendance and medicine, either at home or in a hospital, at the cost of the public fund, which is under the management of a commission. There is a poor's surgeon, or district surgeon, who, on receiving a " certificate" or order from the poor commission, attends the sick, and has power to send them into hospital. The address of an apothecary (who may be named by the patient), is given on the order, at whose shop the medicines prescribed by the surgeon are to be made up. In some instances, however, the individual only receives an order for free attendance, in which case he must pay for his medicine. Paupers, or persons actually receiving relief, are, *ipso facto*, entitled to free medicines and attendance. An order is good for one month only, as the apothecaries' bills are discharged monthly. In Saxony, the system is very similar. Those of the sick that have no comforts at home, are removed to the hospital. The apothecaries compound the medicines at a discount of 25 per cent. from the established or tariff charges. The poor's surgeon may order soup, broth, wine, clothing, bed, fire, baths, &c., if he think them necessary. In Wurtemberg there is a poor's physician and surgeon in every bailiwick, and also a hospital, and apothecary. The regulations are those of Saxony. An apothecary cannot refuse to make up a prescription when the physician signifies its urgency, even if for the poorest person. In case the patient cannot pay, the poor's fund is liable. The arrangements for the relief of the sick poor of a city necessarily differ from those of rural districts. Hamburgh and Berlin are two good examples of the former. Hamburgh is divided into six medical districts, to each of which are appointed two physicians, one surgeon (in the sixth district two), and six apothecaries. The medical expenses for one year (1832) amounted to nearly 5,000*l.*, of which upwards of 3,000*l.* went to the apothecaries for medicines, 285*l.* to the physicians, and 110*l.* to the surgeons. The cost, per head, averages from five to six shillings. A " deputation" of five overseers of the poor is conjoined with the medical staff, who act in the capacity of our English relieving officers.

Dr Simeons proposes that the practitioner of a district, or circuit, shall be the physician of the poor,—in this way. The parishes in his circuit are to raise a rate in the proportion of so many guineas per 1,000 persons, amounting to a fixed annual payment of forty guineas to the physician. For this sum it is proposed that he shall appear in each parish two or three times a week, prescribe for the poor gratuitously, and for other parishioners at a fee minus the ordinary charge for travelling expenses. In cases, however, in which he would be sent for expressly, this charge would be recoverable, and from the public purse in case of paupers. Dr Simeons urges that all classes having ready and cheap access to medical advice, would more frequently consult the physician, and thus many serious illnesses would be prevented. We believe that in many rural districts of England, a system is practised not widely dissimilar from this proposed by Dr Simeons. The surgeon of a district having rural patients in one village, charges them in rotation with the cost of a journey, and makes, at the same time, his visits to the poor.

In marking out a system of eleemosynary medical relief, it is certainly necessary to make a discrimination as to the degrees of poverty analogous to that made in Berlin. There are several such degrees considered with reference to medical relief. At the lowest point is the absolute pauper, entirely dependent on the public for the necessaries of life. Above him is the poor labourer, just able to provide himself and his family with ordinary necessaries, but unable to provide against sickness. A third class comprises mechanics who have a small surplus, out of which they can afford a few shillings for a " doctor " of low charges, or for the druggist. These three classes almost invariably seek eleemosynary medical relief; the first from the union exclusively; the second from the union and the public medical charities indiscriminately; and the third from the public charities exclusively, or from private medical practitioners. It is worthy observation, that the druggist derives from this class the greater number of his patients, and consequently a system which could provide medical relief for this class would effectually put down counter-quackery.

What are the requisites essential to the success of a system of eleemosynary medical relief? Firstly, the sick person must have an opportunity to choose his medical attendant: secondly, attendance on him must be prompt: thirdly, he must contribute so much as his means will permit. A public fund should be formed expressly for the purpose of medical charity. It should comprise, in its objects, a hospital, dispensary, and polyclinic: and should be made up by charitable donations, payments from the union, and payments from the poor (not paupers) on a graduated scale, according to their incomes. In short, the machinery of a self-supporting dispensary should be established, but under the joint control and supervision of the state and the profession.

We do not mean to contend that such a system would not have its defects and difficulties; but we contend that it would counterbalance many defects and difficulties in the existing methods. It would sweep away the whole system of canvassing for poor-law appointments, and public medical charities; a monstrous evil, full of disgrace to the profession and danger to society. It would encourage the young practitioner in a course of kind and diligent attention to the poor, because it would hold out to him a tangible and specific reward. It would throw open the public medical charities to those of the greatest diligence and skill. It would effectually check counter-quackery.

WHAT SHARE OUGHT LAYMEN TO TAKE IN THE ORGANIZA-TION AND THE BUSINESS OF THE PROFESSION?—There can be no doubt the layman has a right to prescribe for himself or for his friend, if the latter request his assistance ; this is essential to civil liberty. There can equally be no doubt that the layman is not justified in assuming for himself the education and title of the regular practitioner. This would be swindling. The lay-man practising medicine ought to do so under the designation of an amateur, and be legally responsible for damages done to health or life by him in his capacity of amateur. The representatives of the patient, if killed, or himself, if he escape, should be the recipients of the sum awarded by a jury.

The profession has always been jealous of any lay interference in its organization. This has been a great mistake. It has cut off a great source of pecuniary sympathy on the part of the public towards the profession. If laymen of rank and wealth had been honoured within it, there would have been a greater number of Warnefords to appreciate its utility, and the funds established for the relief of the destitute practitioner, the education of his children, the establishment of libraries, and other matters of internal economy, would have acquired a proportionate increase. The profession would, in fact, have shared in the provisions made by laymen for the hospitals and dispensaries, in which they have to sue humbly for permission to assist. We think laymen of rank or literary eminence should preside over *local* medical faculties.

We would here close our remarks with a summary of our views on the questions mooted in the legislature. We think,— 1. That the formation of medical municipalities throughout the country would more effectually meet the wishes of the profession than any other system of organization, and more effectually introduce the necessary discipline. 2. That these munici-palities should have a central body acting as the link between the profession and the government. 3. That laymen of rank, wealth, and education, should enter into their composition. 4. That a system of public hygiène should be adopted, and that a staff of officers of health, appointed after examination, sufficiently salaried, and independent of practice, be organized. 5. That there should be a supervision of all medical charities. 6. That the practice of eleemosynary medicine should be thrown open to the whole profession, remunerated by the public, and be developed by a system applicable to every form of eleemosynary medical relief, whether private, public, or pauperal.

If we were called upon to indicate the means by which this scheme might be carried out, we would recommend a Commission of Inquiry as preliminary to any legislation. The results of the inquiry instituted by the Health of Towns' Commission, although but just beginning to appear, are, and will be, so important as to indicate this method as the best. We are certain the interests of the profession, and of society, will appear of greater and greater magnitude as the subject is developed. It is a subject which would reward the statesman for any amount of thought and labour he might bestow upon it. The relations of medical science to political economy are at least as important as the relations of mechanics and physics. With towns rivalling the metropolitan cities of other nations in wealth and population, and with a people teeming and multiplying in a manner scarcely before heard of, public hygiène must become of vital importance, and the medical practitioner will jostle the priest in his influence on society. So fair an opportunity for the exercise of legislative skill rarely happens to a statesman ; and he who succeeds in organizing the medical profession on a wide and enduring basis, will rank with the wisest legislators and greatest benefactors of mankind.   L.

THE
WESTMINSTER

AND

FOREIGN QUARTERLY

Review.

ART. I.—*Epidemics of the Middle Ages,* from the German of
J. F. C. Hecker, M.D. Translated by B. C. Babington, M.D.

2.—*The Remote Causes of Epidemic Diseases.* By John Parkin.
Hatchard and Son.

3.—*Report on Quarantine,* from the General Board of Health.
Hansard.

4.—*Experimental Researches on the Food of Animals.* By Robert
Dundas Thomson, M.D. Longman.

5.—*The Domestic Practice of Hydropathy.* By Edward Johnson,
M.D. Simpkin, Marshall & Co.

THE late epidemic has revealed the existence, and fearfully
illustrated the destructive power, of some unknown agents
of mortality, the precise nature and cause of which, in their
connection with known and more familiar morbific influences,
have hitherto been suffered to remain involved in the deepest
obscurity. It leaves us with the unpleasant conviction that the
accounts handed down to us of the ravages of pestilence in ancient
times, were not historical exaggerations, as they have generally
been considered, and that we have been labouring under a mistake
in supposing that modern civilization had attained an immunity
from similar desolating and wide-spread calamities. The work of
Dr. Hecker on the epidemics of the middle ages, recently translated by Dr. Babington, has now become one of serious interest,
as belonging, not to the past alone, but connecting the past with

the present, and relating to physical phenomena which there is now reason to believe to be constantly latent, and the manifestation of which may be expected at frequently recurring intervals. With a view to the practical conclusions which may perhaps be drawn from this volume, and from other sources, we propose to give some account of its contents.

The work, which we owe to the Sydenham Society, by whom it is published, commences with a treatise upon the pestilence of the fourteenth century, called the ' Black Death,' by which it is computed twenty-five millions of people—one-fourth of the then population of Europe, were destroyed. This pestilence broke out in the reign of Edward the Third, and was undoubtedly the most marked event of that reign; but it is passed over by Hume, in his life of that monarch, in a paragraph of a dozen lines, with a note of reference to Stow—a striking instance of the haste and superficial carelessness with which history is sometimes written. Stow mentions it, in his ' Survey of London,' in explanation of the appropriation of a large plot of ground, without the walls, to the purposes of a cemetery, situate at the back of what is now Charter-house-square, and bounded on the north by Wilderness-row, St. John-street.

His account is the following:—

" A great pestilence entering this island, which began first in Dorsetshire, then proceeded into Devonshire, Somersetshire, Gloucestershire, and Oxfordshire, and at length came to London, and overspread all England, so wasting the people, that scarce the tenth person of all sorts was left alive ; and churchyards were not sufficient to receive the dead, but men were forced to choose out certain fields for burials ; whereupon, Ralph Stratford, Bishop of London, in the year 1348, bought a piece of ground called ' No Man's Land,' which he inclosed with a wall of brick, and dedicated for burial of the dead, building thereupon a proper chapel, which is now enlarged and made a dwelling-house ; and this burying-plot is become a fair garden, retaining the old name of Pardon churchyard. About this, in the year 1349, the said Sir Walter Manny, in respect of danger that might befall in this time of so great a plague and infection, purchased thirteen acres and a rod of ground adjoining to the said No Man's Land, and lying in a place called ' Spittle Cross,' because it belonged to St. Bartilmewe's Hospital, since that called the new church-haw, and caused it to be consecrated by the said Bishop of London to the use of burials.

" In this plot of ground there were in that year more than fifty thousand persons buried, as I have read in the charters of Edward III. ; also, I have seen and read an inscription fixed on a stone cross, some time standing in the same churchyard, and having these words :—
' *Anno Domini* 1349, *regnante magna pestilentia consecratum fuit hoc cœmiterium, in quo et infra septa presentis monasterii, sepulta fuerunt*

mortuorum corpora plusquam quinquaginta millia, præter alia multa abhinc usque ad presens, quorum animabus propitietur Deus. Amen.'" *

This ancient cemetery, or the greater part of it, is now used as a play-ground and garden by the boys of the Charter-house, and few persons in London are aware of the original destination of the large enclosure of this neighbourhood, the interior of which is hidden by high walls from surrounding observation.

The disease which led to its appropriation as a burial ground, is described by Hecker as a species of oriental plague, exhibiting itself in inflammatory boils and tumours of the glands, accompanied with burning thirst; sometimes, also, with inflammation of the lungs, and expectoration of blood; in other cases, with vomitings of blood and fluxes of the bowels, terminating, like malignant cholera, with a discoloration of the skin, and black spots indicating putrid decomposition, from which it was called, in the north of Europe, the "Black Death." In Italy it obtained the name of "*La mortalega granda,*"—the great mortality. The attacks were usually fatal within two or three days of the first symptoms appearing, but in many cases were even more sudden, some falling as if struck by lightning. Its effects were not confined to man; in some countries affecting dogs, cats, fowls, and other animals, which died in great numbers; and in England the disease was followed by a murrain among the cattle, occasioning a great rise in the price of food.†

The Black Death was supposed to have commenced in the kingdom of Cathay, to the north of China, in the year 1333, and thence to have spread in a westerly direction across the continent

---

* Stow's Survey of London, p. 160.

† At the commencement, there was in England a superabundance of all the necessaries of life; but the plague, which seemed then to be the sole disease, was soon accompanied by a fatal murrain among the cattle. Wandering about without herdsmen they fell by thousands; and, as has likewise been observed in Africa, the birds and beasts of prey are said not to have touched them. Of what nature this murrain may have been, can no more be determined, than whether it originated from communication with plague patients, or from other causes; but thus much is certain, that it did not break out until after the commencement of the Black Death. In consequence of this murrain, and the impossibility of removing the corn from the fields, there was everywhere a great rise in the price of food which to many was inexplicable, because the harvest had been plentiful; by others it was attributed to the wicked designs of the labourers and dealers; but it really had its foundation in the actual deficiency arising from circumstances by which individual classes at all times endeavour to profit. For a whole year, until it terminated in August, 1349, the Black Plague prevailed in this beautiful island, and everywhere poisoned the springs of comfort and prosperity.—*Hecker's 'Epidemics of the Middle Ages.'*

Y 2

of Asia to Constantinople, where it made its appearance in the year 1347. In 1348 it visited Avignon, and other cities in the south of France and north of Italy and Spain. The following year it ravaged England, appearing first in Dorsetshire, attacking Bristol, Gloucester, Oxford, and London, and thence proceeding north-ward to Norwich, Yarmouth, Leicester, and York, which suffered immense losses; some of these cities losing nine-tenths of their inhabitants. The pestilence next visited Scotland, Norway, Russia, and Poland, which latter country, however, it did not reach until two years after its first appearance in the south of Europe. In Poland, it is stated, three-fourths of the entire population perished, and in Norway two-thirds. In Russia, also, the mortality is said to have been equally great. The total mortality of this period is thus summed up by Dr. Hecker:—

" Kairo lost daily, when the plague was raging with its greatest violence, from 10,000 to 15,000 ; being as many as, in modern times, great plagues have carried off during their whole course. In China, more than thirteen millions are said to have died ; and this is in cor-respondence with the certainly exaggerated accounts from the rest of Asia. India was depopulated. Tartary, the Tartar kingdom of Kaptschaka, Mesopotamia, Syria, Armenia, were covered with dead bodies : the Koords fled in vain to the mountains. In Caramania and Cæsarea none were left alive. On the roads, in the camps, in the caravansaries, unburied bodies alone were seen ; and a few cities only (Arabian historians name Maara-el-nooman, Schiesur, and Harem) remained in an unaccountable manner free. In Aleppo 500 died daily ; 22,000 people, and most of the animals, were carried off in Gaza within six weeks. Cyprus lost almost all its inhabitants ; and ships without crews were often seen in the Mediterranean, or afterwards in the North Sea, driving about, and spreading the plague wherever they went on shore. It was reported to Pope Clement, at Avignon, that throughout the East, probably with the exception of China, 23,840,000 people had fallen victims to the plague. Considering the occurrences of the 14th and 15th centuries, we might, on first view, suspect the accuracy of this statement. How, it might be asked, could such great wars have been carried on—such powerful efforts have been made ? how could the Greek empire, only a hundred years later, have been overthrown, if the people really had been so utterly destroyed ?

" This account is nevertheless rendered credible by the ascertained fact, that the palaces of princes are less accessible to contagious dis-eases than the dwellings of the multitude ; and that in places of im-portance, the influx from those districts which have suffered least soon repairs even the heaviest losses. We must remember, also, that we do not gather much from mere numbers, without an intimate know-ledge of the state of society. We will, therefore, confine ourselves to exhibiting some of the more credible accounts relative to European cities.

In Florence there died of the Black Plague	60,000
In Venice	100,000
In Marseilles, in one month	16,000
In Siena	70,000
In Paris	50,000
In St. Denis	14,000
In Avignon	60,000
In Strasburg	16,000
In Lübeck	9,000
In Basle	14,000
In Erfurt, at least	16,000
In Weimar	5,000
In Luisburg	2,000
In London, at least	100,000
In Norwich	51,000
To which may be added	
Franciscan Friars in Germany	124,434
Minorites in Italy	30,000

" This short catalogue might, by a laborious and uncertain calculation, deduced from other sources, be easily further multiplied, but would still fail to give a true picture of the depopulation which took place. Lübeck, at that time the Venice of the North, which could no longer contain the multitudes that flocked to it, was thrown into such consternation on the eruption of the plague, that the citizens destroyed themselves as if in frenzy."

The consternation which seized the inhabitants of every country through which the plague passed was such, that in a multitude of instances the effects of fear alone were probably as fatal as the pestilence. Everywhere a feeling of torpor and a depression of spirits, almost amounting to despair, became universal; and this frequently taking a religious form, the wealthy, we are told, abandoned their treasures, and gave their villages and estates to the churches and monasteries, as the surest way, according to the notions of the age, of securing the forgiveness of their past sins. Thus was the first impulse given to the erection of those magnificent cathedrals, which yet remain to the admirers of what is called Gothic architecture, in the northern parts of Europe; buildings, commenced for the most part in the fourteenth century, and which were completed by the piety of the succeeding age.

The same spirit was manifested in a more superstitious shape in a zeal for fasting and penance, which revived and extended a new order of religionists, said to have been founded by St. Anthony in the preceding century, styling themselves Brothers of the Cross, or Cross-bearers, but called by the people flagellants, from their rule of submitting to a severe public flogging as a means of averting the anger of Heaven. This order was at first confined to the poorer classes, but ultimately many nobles and ecclesiastics enrolled themselves in the order. Their practice was to march through cities in well-organized processions, clothed in sombre garments, their faces covered up to the forehead, knotted scourges in their hands, and singing hymns with their eyes fixed upon the ground. Tapers and magnificent banners of velvet and cloth of gold were carried before them, and wherever they made their appearance the bells were set ringing, and the people flocked to welcome them as a holy band, by whose intercession the pestilence might be diverted from its course.

" Whoever was desirous of joining the brotherhood, was bound to remain in it thirty-four days, and to have four-pence per day at his own disposal, so that he might not be burthensome to any one; if married, he was obliged to have the sanction of his wife, and give the assurance that he was reconciled to all men. The Brothers of the Cross were not permitted to seek for free quarters, or even to enter a house without having been invited; they were forbidden to converse with females; and if they transgressed these rules, or acted without discretion, they were obliged to confess to the superior, who sentenced them to several lashes of the scourge, by way of penance. Ecclesiastics had not, as such, any pre-eminence among them; according to their original law, which, however, was often transgressed, they could not become masters, or take part in the *secret councils*. Penance was performed twice every day; in the morning and evening, they went abroad in pairs, singing psalms, amid the ringing of the bells; and when they arrived at the place of flagellation, they stripped the upper part of their bodies, and put off their shoes, keeping on only a linen dress, reaching from the waist to the ankles. They then lay down in a large circle, in different positions, according to the nature of their crime—the adulterer with his face to the ground; the perjurer on one side, holding up three of his fingers, &c., and were then castigated, some more and some less, by the master, who ordered them to rise in the words of a prescribed form. Upon this they scourged themselves, amid the singing of psalms and loud supplications for the averting of the plague, with genuflexions and other ceremonies, of which cotemporary writers give various accounts; and at the same time constantly boasted of their penance, that the blood of their wounds was mingled with that of the Saviour. One of them, in conclusion, stood up to read a letter which it was pretended an angel had brought from Heaven, to St. Peter's church, at Jerusalem, stating that Christ, who was sore displeased at the sins of man, had granted, at the intercession of the Holy Virgin and of the angels, that all who should wander about for thirty-four days, and scourge themselves, should be partakers of the Divine grace. This scene caused as great a commotion among the believers as the finding of the holy spear once did at Antioch; and if any among the clergy inquired who had sealed the letter? he was boldly answered, the same who had sealed the Gospel!

" All this had so powerful an effect, that the church was in considerable danger; for the flagellants gained more credit than the priests,
from whom they so entirely withdrew themselves, that they even
absolved each other. Besides, they everywhere took possession of
the churches; and their new songs, which went from mouth to mouth,
operated strongly on the minds of the people."

Two hundred flagellants, who entered Strasburg in 1349, were
speedily augmented to a thousand; when they divided into two
bodies, and separated, travelling to the north and south. Similar
bodies were found in other towns, and in this manner all Germany
became overrun with wandering tribes of fanatics, expecting everywhere to be received with hospitality, and the mania of joining
them threatened to become as formidable as that of the Crusades.
But at last the public closed their doors against them; partly from
suspicion that instead of diverting the plague, they were the
means of spreading it over the country; and the Pope interdicting
their processions, and public penances, the brotherhood melted
away, and gradually disappeared.

The superstitious fears of the age appeared again, but in a
more horrible form—in a persecution of the Jews, who were
everywhere accused of being the authors of the calamity. It is
to be remarked, in the history of all destructive epidemics, that
their effects are so analogous to those of poison, that an opinion
has always prevailed, on the outbreak of the pestilence, that the
food or water of the first victims had been tampered with. We
have seen this notion obtain very general credence in modern
times, especially in Paris and St. Petersburg, in 1832, when many
persons nearly lost their lives in popular commotions, occasioned
by the belief, that the persons who had first died of malignant
cholera had been made to drink of poisoned water. It was so in
Germany on the appearance of the Black Death, but with this
difference, that the suspicion of the people lighted not upon
individuals, but upon a whole class of persons obnoxious to the
religious prejudices of the day, and who were supposed to have
entered into a general conspiracy to destroy the Christian population of every city. The consequences of this monstrous charge,
and the credulity of the people by whom it was entertained, form,
as detailed by Dr. Hecker, one of the most painful episodes of
history.

" Already, in the autumn of 1348, a dreadful panic, caused by this
supposed empoisonment, seized all nations; in Germany especially,
the springs and wells were built over, that nobody might drink of
them, or empty their contents for culinary purposes; and for a long
time, the inhabitants of numerous towns and villages used only river

and rain water. The city gates were also guarded with the greatest
caution : only confidential persons were admitted; and if medicine, or
any other article which might be supposed to be poisonous, was found
in the possession of a stranger,—and it was natural that some should
have these things by them for their private use,—they were forced to
swallow a portion of it. By this trying state of privation, distrust
and suspicion, the hatred against the supposed poisoners became
greatly increased, and often broke out in popular commotions, which
only served still further to infuriate the wildest passions. The
noble and the mean fearlessly bound themselves by an oath, to
extirpate the Jews by fire and sword, and to snatch them from
their protectors, of whom the number was so small, that throughout all Germany, but few places can be mentioned where these
unfortunate people were not regarded as outlaws, and martyred and
burnt. Solemn summonses were issued from Berne to the towns of
Basle, Freyburg in the Breisgau, and Strasburg, to pursue the Jews
as poisoners. The burgomasters and senators, indeed, opposed this
requisition ; but in Basle the populace obliged them to bind themselves
by an oath, to burn the Jews, and to forbid persons of that community
from entering their city, for the space of two hundred years. Upon
this, all the Jews in Basle, whose number could not have been incon-
siderable, were enclosed in a wooden building, constructed for the
purpose, and burnt together with it, upon the mere outcry of the
people, without sentence or trial ; which indeed would have availed
them nothing. Soon after, the same thing took place at Freyburg.
A regular diet was held at Bennefeld, in Alsace, where the bishops,
lords and barons, as also deputies of the counties and towns, consulted
how they should proceed with regard to the Jews ; and when the
deputies of Strasburg—not, indeed, the bishop of this town, who proved
himself a violent fanatic—spoke in favour of the persecuted, as nothing
criminal was substantiated against them, a great outcry was raised,
and it was vehemently asked, why, if so, they had covered their wells
and removed their buckets? A sanguinary decree was resolved upon,
of which the populace, who obeyed the call of the nobles and superior
clergy, became but the too willing executioners. Wherever the Jews
were not burnt, they were at least banished ; and so being compelled
to wander about, they fell into the hands of the country people, who
without humanity, and regardless of all laws, persecuted them with
fire and sword. At Spires, the Jews, driven to despair, assembled in
their own habitations, which they set on fire, and thus consumed
themselves with their families. The few that remained were forced
to submit to baptism ; while the dead bodies of the murdered, which
lay about the streets, were put into empty wine casks, and rolled into
the Rhine, lest they should infect the air. The mob were forbidden
to enter the ruins of the habitations that were burnt in the Jewish
quarter; for the senate itself caused search to be made for the treasure,
which is said to have been very considerable. At Strasburg, two
thousand Jews were burnt alive in their own burial-ground, where

a large scaffold had been erected : a few who promised to embrace Christianity, were spared, and their children taken from the pile. The youth and beauty of several females also excited some commiseration, and they were snatched from death against their will : many, however, who forcibly made their escape from the flames, were murdered in the streets."

Dr. Hecker proceeds to relate that the effects of the Black Death had scarcely subsided, before a new epidemic appeared in Europe, of an extraordinary character, showing itself in an involuntary motion of the muscles, of which examples are still occasionally met with in the practice of physicians, but in a mild form,* and which continues to be known by its ancient name of St. John or St. Vitus's Dance—so called from the names of the two patron saints supposed to possess the power of curing the disease by their miraculous interposition. It would appear that the disease having first shown itself in violent and involuntary contractions of the muscles of the legs, the physicians of the time formed the idea, that if the patients were encouraged to dance until they fell down exhausted with the fatigue of the exertion, a reaction would commence, by which a cure might be promoted. Bands of music were therefore provided for the use of the afflicted, and airs, somewhat of the polka character, were composed, to suit the wild kind of Bacchanalian leaps which their dancing resembled. The public exhibition, however, of

---

* Instances, indeed, are not altogether uncommon of the disease showing itself in all the violence by which it was marked in the middle ages. Dr. Babington remarks that—

"In the third volume of the 'Edinburgh Medical and Surgical Journal,' p. 434, there is an account of ' some convulsive diseases in certain parts of Scotland,' which is taken from Sir J. Sinclair's statistical account, and from which I have thought it illustrative of our author's subject to make some extracts ; the first that is noticed is peculiar to a part of Forfarshire, and is called the leaping ague, which bears so close an analogy to the original St. Vitus's Dance, or to Tarantism, that it seems to want only the ' foul fiend,' or the dreaded bite, as a cause, and a Scotch reel or strathspey as a cure, to render the resemblance quite complete. ' Those affected with it first complain of a pain in the head, or lower part of the back, to which succeed convulsive fits, or *fits of dancing*, at certain periods. During the paroxysm they have all the appearance of madness, distorting their bodies in various ways, and leaping and springing in a surprising manner, whence the disease has derived its vulgar name. Sometimes they run with astonishing velocity, and often over dangerous passes, to some place out of doors which they have fixed on in their own minds, or, perhaps, even mentioned to those in company with them, and then *drop down quite exhausted*. At other times, especially when confined to the house, they climb in the most singular manner. In cottages, for example, they leap from the floor to what is called the baulks, or those beams by which the rafters are joined together, springing from one to another with the agility of a cat, or whirling round one of them with a motion resembling the fly of a jack. Cold bathing is found to be the most effectual remedy ; but when the fit of dancing, leaping or running comes on, *nothing tends so much to abate the violence of the disease, as allowing them free scope to exercise themselves till nature be exhausted.*'"

these dances seems to have had the effect of propagating the
disorder over the whole of Germany, doubtless through the
power of that sympathetic action of the nervous system which,
in the familiar instances of laughing and yawning, will impel a
large company to imitate the example of a single individual.

" So early as the year 1374, assemblages of men and women were
seen at Aix-la-Chapelle, who had come out of Germany, and who,
united by one common delusion, exhibited to the public, both in the
streets and in the churches, the following strange spectacle. They
formed circles hand in hand, and, appearing to have lost all control
over their senses, continued dancing, regardless of the bystanders, for
hours together, in wild delirium, until at length they fell to the ground
in a state of exhaustion. They then complained of extreme oppression,
and groaned as if in the agonies of death, until they were swathed in
cloths bound tightly round their waists, upon which they recovered, and
remained free from the complaint until the next attack. This practice of swathing was resorted to on account of the tympany which followed these spasmodic ravings; but the bystanders frequently relieved
patients in a less artificial manner, by thumping and trampling upon
the parts affected. While dancing they neither saw nor heard, being
insensible to external impressions through the senses, but were
haunted by visions, their fancies conjuring up spirits, whose names
they shrieked out. And some of them afterwards asserted that they
felt as if they had been immersed in a stream of blood, which obliged
them to leap so high ; others, during their paroxysms, saw the heavens
open, and the Saviour enthroned with the Virgin Mary, according as
the religious notions of the age were strangely and variously reflected
in their imaginations."

The symptoms varied with the character of the patients. The
visions might be occasioned by a morbid action of the visual
organs producing optical delusions, or by a predisposition to
fanaticism. The common notion of the time, countenanced by
the clergy, was, that the persons afflicted were possessed, and the
patients themselves generally fell into the same belief, and acted
accordingly.

" It was but a few months ere this demoniacal disease had spread
from Aix-la-Chapelle, where it appeared in July, over the neighbouring
Netherlands. In Liege, Utrecht, Tangier, and many other towns of
Belgium, the dancers appeared with garlands in their hair, and their
waists girt with cloths, that they might, as soon as the paroxysm was
over, receive immediate relief on the attack of the tympany. This
bandage was, on the insertion of a stick, easily twisted tight. Many,
however, obtained more relief from kicks and blows, which they found
numbers of persons ready to administer, for wherever the dancers
appeared, the people assembled in crowds to gratify their curiosity
with the frightful spectacle. At length the increasing numbers of the

affected, excited no less anxiety than the attention that was paid to them. In towns and villages, they took possession of the religious houses ; processions were everywhere instituted on their account, and masses were said, and hymns were sung, while the disease itself, of the demoniacal origin of which no one entertained the least doubt, excited everywhere astonishment and horror. In Liege the priests had recourse to exorcisms, and endeavoured by every means in their power to allay an evil which threatened so much danger to themselves; for the possessed assembling in multitudes, frequently poured forth imprecations against them, and menaced their destruction. They intimidated also the people to such a degree, that there was an express ordinance issued that no one should make any but square-toed shoes, because these fanatics had manifested a morbid dislike to the pointed shoes which had come into fashion immediately after the great mortality of 1350. They were still more irritated at the sight of red colours, the influence of which on the disordered nerves, might lead us to imagine an extraordinary accordance between this spasmodic malady, and the condition of infuriated animals."

At Cologne five hundred persons became affected by this dancing plague, and at Metz eleven hundred. Peasants left their ploughs, mechanics their workshops, housewives their domestic duties to join the wild revels, and the most ruinous disorder prevailed in the city. The epidemic extended to Italy, where it was attributed to the bite of a ground spider, common in Apulia, called the *tarantula;* whence the disease was known under the name of *Tarantism.*

" At the close of the fifteenth century, we find that Tarantism had spread beyond the boundaries of Apulia, and that the fear of being bitten by venomous spiders had increased. Nothing short of death itself was expected from the wound which these insects inflicted, and if those who were bitten escaped with their lives, they were said to be seen pining away in a desponding state of lassitude. Many became weak-sighted, or hard of hearing ; some lost the power of speech, and all were insensible to ordinary causes of excitement. Nothing but the flute or the cithern afforded them relief. At the sound of these instruments they awoke as if by enchantment, opened their eyes, and moving slowly at first according to the measure of the music, were, as the tune quickened, gradually hurried on to the most passionate dance. Cities and villages alike resounded throughout the summer season with the notes of fifes, clarionets and Turkish drums ; and patients were everywhere to be met with who looked to dancing as their only remedy. Alexander ab Alexandro, who gives this account, saw a young man in a remote village who was seized with a violent attack of Tarantism. He listened with eagerness and a fixed stare to the sound of a drum, and his graceful movements gradually became more and more violent, until his dancing was converted into a succession of frantic leaps, which required the utmost exertion of his whole strength. In the midst of this overstrained exertion of mind and body the music suddenly ceased, and he immediately fell powerless to the ground, where he lay senseless and motionless, until its magical effect again aroused him to a renewal of his impassioned performances.*

"At the period of which we are treating there was a general conviction that by music and dancing the poison of the *tarantula* was dis-

* A modern instance of the power of music in this disorder is narrated by Mr. Kinder Wood, in the seventh volume of the ' Medico Chirurgical Transactions,' The patient was a young married woman, who was attacked by headache, sickness, followed by an involuntary motion of the eyelids, and extraordinary contortions of the trunk and extremities, and who finally exhibited all the symptoms, in the most marked manner, of the dancing mania of the middle ages.

The following are extracts :

"Feb. 27th.—The attack commenced in bed, and was violent, but of short duration. When she arose, about ten, she had a second attack, continuing an hour, except an interval of five minutes. She now struck the furniture more violently and more repeatedly. Kneeling on one knee, with the hands upon the back, she often sprang up suddenly, and struck the top of the room with the palm of the hand. To do this she rose fifteen inches from the floor, so that the family were under the necessity of drawing all the nails and hooks from the ceiling. She frequently danced upon one leg, holding the other with the hand, and occasionally changing the legs. In the evening, the family observed the blows upon the furniture to be more continuous, and to assume the regular time and measure of a musical air. As a strain or series of strokes was concluded, she ended with a more violent stroke, or a more violent spring or jump.   *   *   *

"In the afternoon of the 28th the motions returned. At this time a person present, surprised at the manner in which she beat upon the doors, &c., and thinking he recognised the air, without further ceremony began to sing the tune; the moment this struck her ears, she turned suddenly to the man, and dancing directly up to him, continued doing so till he was out of breath. The man now ceased a short time, when, commencing again, he continued till the attack stopped. The night before this her father had mentioned his wish to procure a drum, associating this dance of his daughter with some ideas of music. The avidity with which she danced to the tune when sung, as above stated, confirmed this wish, and accordingly a drum and fife were procured in the evening. After two hours of rest the motions again reappeared, when the drum and fife began to play the tune to which she had danced before, viz., the 'Protestant Boys,' a favourite popular air in this neighbourhood. In whatever part of the room she happened to be, she immediately turned and danced up to the drum, and as close as possible to it, and there she danced till she missed the step, when the involuntary motion instantly ceased. The first time she missed the step in five minutes, but again rose and danced to the drum two minutes and a half by her father's watch, when, missing the step, the motions instantly ceased. She rose a third time, and missing the step in half a minute, the motions immediately ceased. After this, the drum and fife commenced as the involuntary actions were coming on, and before she rose from her seat; and four times they completely checked the progress of the attack, so that she did not rise upon the floor to dance."

By acting upon this hint a cure was effected. A roll of the drum at the commencement of every attack interrupted the current of associations in the patient's mind, and acting perhaps as a counter-irritant to the nerves, neutralised their action. On the 2nd of March an irruption appeared on the skin, after which the patient became rapidly convalescent.

tributed over the surface of the whole body, and expelled through the skin, but that if there remained the slightest vestige of it in the vessels this became a permanent germ of the disorder, so that the dancing fits might again and again be excited *ad infinitum* by music."

The belief that the disorder was occasioned by the bites of spiders was of course a delusion, but one which had taken such firm hold of the mind, that no one in Italy seems to have questioned the fact; and it appears that a dread of venomous spiders prevailed about the same time in distant countries of Asia, where insects being a greater pest than in Europe, the idea probably originated. While the delusion lasted, and it appears not to have been dispelled for several centuries, every kind of insect bite was set down to the account of the tarantula; and if the person bitten had a constitution already predisposed to nervous affections, an attack would frequently follow from the power of the imagination. The celebrated Fracastoro found the robust bailiff of his landed estate groaning, and with the aspect of a person in the extremity of despair, and suffering the agonies of death from a sting in the neck inflicted by some unknown insect, which was believed to be a tarantula. A little vinegar and Armenian bole reduced the inflammation, and hope returning as the pain subsided, the dying man was, as if by a miracle, restored to life and the power of speech.

The world is not so much wiser in our own day that we can at all afford to smile at this chimera of public credulity. The belief continues unabated, even among the majority of medical men, of the connexion of hydrophobia in human beings with the bite of a mad dog, and every year hundreds of persons bitten by dogs allow their wounds to be cruelly cauterized with a view of extirpating the poison supposed to be communicated by the saliva of a dog—a poison abundantly proved by chemical analysis and experiment to have no existence.* An injury to a nerve, when

---

* We regret to see this popular error countenanced by so high an authority as that of the Registrar-General. In his report for the third quarter of the present year it is stated, after alluding to the decrease of nervous affections, and to the fact that there had been no death by hydrophobia recorded in London during the last five summers, that

"Hydrophobia disappears when the dogs which are liable to become mad, or to be bitten every summer, are removed by police regulations."

This statement it would be very difficult to support by any evidence entitled to credit. 1. There has been no such extraordinary vigilance of the police but that unmuzzled dogs have been seen running about the streets in summer time; and especially on Mondays, in Smithfield-market; whatever formal instructions may have been issued respecting them. 2. In the cities of the East, as in Constantinople, where the heat of summer is greatest, and where dogs and pigs are the only scavengers, the inhabitants do not suffer more from hydrophobia

of such a character as to be difficult of healing, whether occasioned by a bite, a scratch, or even the prick of a pin, may so
affect the system, as to bring on, in some cases, tetanus, and
in others death by convulsions; but beyond this the only poisonous influence to be feared is that of a morbid fancy; the
effects of which may, however, be sufficiently serious. Many
have undoubtedly gone mad from the belief that madness was
inevitable. Zimmerman narrates a case of an epidemic of the
fifteenth century, contemporaneous with the dancing plague,
which began with a nun in a German nunnery showing a propensity to bite her companions. Soon after, all the nuns of the
convent began biting each other. The news of this infatuation
reached other convents, and the biting mania spread from nunnery to nunnery throughout the greater part of Germany and
Holland, and extended even as far as Rome. He mentions
another case of a sick nun in a convent of France, who began
mewing like a cat; when the example became equally infectious.
All the nuns in the convent commenced mewing at a certain
time in the day for several hours together, to the great scandal of
the neighbourhood, and this daily cat-like concert did not cease
until soldiers were sent to the convent with rods to flog, or
threaten to do so, those in whom this strange propensity might
be incurable.

Nervous affections appear to have been unusually prevalent
in Europe during the fifteenth and sixteenth centuries; and the
dancing mania, or Tarantisnt, continued in Italy during the
seventeenth century, long after it had disappeared from Germany.
This may perhaps in part be accounted for by the more lively
temperament of the Italians, who were perhaps glad of an excuse for dancing when the physical necessity for it had ceased.
Indeed, the dance of the *Tarantella* is still a favorite popular
pastime; although its origin has been forgotten.

The close of the fifteenth century was marked by a train of
malignant epidemics, chiefly of an inflammatory kind. In 1482

---

than in Europe. 3. It has been proved by M. Trolliet, who published, in a
memoir, the dates of all the cases of hydrophobia of which any account had
appeared, that the greatest number had occurred in January, the coldest month
of the year, and the smallest number in August, which is the hottest. 4. It
has been shown by the records of hospitals, that not more than one person
in twenty-five said to be bitten by mad dogs ever suffers from hydrophobia;
and in that case the influence of fear upon weak nerves may have been as much
a cause as the actual laceration. 5. Although there are few persons who have
not been bitten by dogs or cats, the disease has frequently occurred in human
beings where no possible connexion could be traced between the malady and
any previous bite or scratch.

France was devastated by an inflammatory fever, attended with such intense pain in the head, that many, it is said, destroyed themselves to avoid the endurance of the agony. The king Louis XI., in terror, shut himself up in his castle of Plessis des Tours, and forty men with cross-bows kept guard, to put to death every living thing that might approach and communicate the infection. A fever of a corresponding character raged in Italy and the North of Germany about the same time; and in 1485 a plague called the Sweating Sickness, broke out in England, the fatality of which was nearly as great as that of the Black Death. This disorder was a violent inflammatory fever, which prostrated the powers as if by a blow; and amidst painful oppression at the stomach, headache, and lethargic stupor, suffused the whole body with a fetid perspiration. The disease arrived at a crisis in a few hours, its duration seldom extending above a day and a night; and its fatality was so great that not more than one in a hundred of those attacked escaped with life.

The Sweating Sickness principally attacked robust and vigorous men, or persons of a full habit of body from high living; passing over almost entirely children and the aged. In London, two lord-mayors and six aldermen died within one week, with many merchants of high standing, and some numbers of the nobility. No record has been kept of the total mortality it occasioned, but Bacon tells us that "infinite persons" died, and Stow "a wonderful number."

The disorder appeared in England in the beginning of August, about the time of the landing of Henry the Seventh at Milford Haven, and is said to have first broke out in his camp on the banks of the Severn. It would seem, however, to have prevailed generally in the west of England at the same period; for Lord Stanley assigned the prevalence of the new disease as a sufficient excuse for not joining the army of Richard. It reached London about the 21st of September, compelling the postponement of the coronation, and then spread all over England; but did not extend to either Ireland or Scotland.

In 1499, a plague in London, of the oriental character, carried off 30,000 persons, and in 1506 the Sweating Sickness re-appeared in England, but in a curative form, which occasioned comparatively little uneasiness. In 1517 it raged with extreme violence from July to December, and was so rapid in its course that it carried off multitudes of those attacked in two or three hours. Ammonius of Lucca, private secretary to Sir Thomas More, Lords Grey and Clinton, with many knights, officers, and gentlemen of the court, fell victims to the disease; while Oxford and Cambridge lost many of their most distinguished scholars.

Henry VIII., in alarm, retired to a country-seat, where he received message after message from different towns and villages, announcing that in some a third, in others even half the inhabitants were swept away by this pestilence. In this case, the presence of the Sweating Sickness was not marked by the extreme humidity of former seasons. The summer of 1517 was one of the ordinary character, following a cold winter. The disease did not cross the Scottish borders, nor extend south beyond Calais; and Dr. Hecker concludes that the reason it was principally confined to the English was their intemperate habits at that period; it being the practice to drink strong wine immediately after rising in the morning, to eat in excess flesh-meats seasoned with spices, and to indulge frequently in nocturnal carousings. The people of Holland and Switzerland, however, had been visited at a little earlier period by a malignant inflammation of the throat, accompanied by convulsive paroxysms, which proved generally fatal.

In May, 1528, the Sweating Sickness appeared for the fourth time in England, and manifested itself with the same intensity as in the last visitation. Between health and death there lay but a brief interval of six hours. Public business was postponed; the courts were closed; and the king, alarmed at the death of two chamberlains, and numerous other persons of distinction, left London immediately, and endeavoured to avoid the epidemic by rapid travelling,—finally isolating himself at Tytynhanga, and surrounding his lonely residence with fires for the purification of the air.

In this instance the disease was attended, and was doubtless aggravated, by a season of excessive moisture. The winter had been mild and wet, and although March was dry, the rains again set in with April and continued without intermission for eight weeks, entirely destroying the hopes of harvest. Heavy rains and floods prevailed throughout Europe during the summer of this year, and the year following, and inflammatory fevers, in some countries corresponding with the Sweating Sickness of England, were universal.

In France, the epidemic of this period was known under the name of the *trousse-galant,** or short thrift, which is described as attended both with inflammation, fever, and a morbid condition of the bowels, often carrying off the patient in a few hours. In the dictionary of the French Academy the term *trousse-galant,* is explained as the ancient name of *cholera-morbus,* from which the identity of this epidemic with the malignant cholera

---

* From *trousser*, to turn up; the allusion being to the quick work of death made by the hangman.

of modern times may be reasonably surmised; profuse perspirations being sometimes one of its symptoms, and its effects upon the skin or the bowels apparently depending upon the habit of body and constitution of the patient.

The political effects of pestilence in the year 1528 were of unusual significance. It led to the total destruction of the French army before Naples, and changed the destiny of nations. Francis I., in league with England, Switzerland, Rome, Geneva, and Venice, against the Emperor of Germany, led a fine army into Italy, burning to revenge the disgrace of Pavia. The emperor's troops everywhere gave way, and Naples alone, weakly defended by a few German lansquenets and Spaniards, remained to be vanquished. The city was already blockaded by Doria with Genoese galleys; and, on the land side, 30,000 veteran warriors, with a small body of English, sat down before the walls to await, as they imagined, an easy conquest. This expectation was destined never to be realised. Sickness, with diarrhœa, attributed in the first instance to fruit, broke out in the camp in the beginning of June, and rapidly increased;—the measures taken by Lautrec, the commander, to deprive the city of water by cutting off the supplies at Poggio, turning against the besiegers.

" The water, having now no outlet, spread over the plain where the camp was situated, which it converted into a swamp, whence it rose, morning and evening, in the form of thick fogs. From this cause, and while a southerly wind continued to prevail, the sickness soon became general. Those soldiers, who were not already confined to bed in their tents, were seen with pallid visages, swelled legs, and bloated bellies, scarcely able to crawl; so that, weary of nightly watching, they were often plundered by the marauding Neapolitans. The great mortality did not commence until about the 15th of July; but so dreadful was its ravages, that about three weeks were sufficient to complete the almost entire destruction of the army. Around and within the tents, vacated by the death of their inmates, noxious weeds sprang up. Thousands perished without help, either in a state of stupor, or in the raving delirium of fever. In the entrenchments, in the tents, and wherever death had overtaken his victims, there unburied corpses lay; and the dead that were interred, swollen with putridity, burst their shallow graves, and spread a poisonous stench far and wide over the camp. There was no longer any thought of order or military discipline, and many of the commanders and captains were either sick themselves, or had fled to the neighbouring towns, in order to avoid the contagion.

" The glory of the French arms was departed, and her proud banners cowered beneath an unhallowed spectre. Meanwhile the pestilence broke out among the Venetian galleys under Pietro Lundo. Doria had already gone over to the Emperor; and thus was this expedition,

Epidemics.

begun under the most favourable auspices, frustrated on every side by the malignant influences of the season."

On the 29th of August, the army broke up ; and in the midst of a storm of thunder and heavy rain, endeavoured to effect a retreat : but reduced to a mere skeleton of its former strength, and in an enfeebled condition, they were speedily captured by the Imperialists. It is said that 5,000 of the French nobility, including the commander himself, perished with this army. The blow was too heavy to be recovered. It reminds us of the scriptural account of the delivery of Jerusalem by the destruction of the Assyrian host in the days of Hezekiah, doubtless effected by some similar pestilential agency :—

" And it came to pass that night, that the angel of the Lord went out, and smote in the camp of the Assyrians an hundred fourscore and five thousand: and when they arose early in the morning, behold, they were all dead corpses. So Sennacherib king of Assyria departed, and went and returned, and dwelt at Nineveh." *

A fifth visitation of the Sweating Sickness occurred in 1551, said to have been the last appearance of the disease in England ; by which we are merely to understand that it was the last appearance of any epidemic known by that particular name—a name probably dropped by physicians of a later date, as not sufficiently generic, and as belonging to a symptom not found to be invariable in complaints otherwise of a similar character. It broke out this year in the same locality as when it made its first appearance, in the time of Henry the Seventh, on the banks of the Severn ; and on this occasion nearly depopulated the town of Shrewsbury, before it was at all seen in the northern and eastern parts of the kingdom.

" Here, during the spring, there arose impenetrable fogs from the banks of the Severn, which, from their unusually bad odour, led to a fear of their injurious consequences. It was not long before the Sweating Sickness suddenly broke out on the 15th of April. To many it was entirely unknown, or but obscurely recollected ; for, amidst the commotions of Henry's reign, the old malady had long since been forgotten.

" The visitation was so general in Shrewsbury and the places in its neighbourhood, that every one must have believed that the atmosphere was poisoned, for no caution availed—no closing of the doors and windows ; every individual dwelling became an hospital, and the aged and the young, who could contribute nothing towards the cure of their relatives, alone remained unaffected by the pestilence. The disease came as unexpectedly, and as completely without all warning, as it had ever

---

* 2 Kings, xix. 35, 36.

done on former occasions; at table, during sleep, on journeys, in the midst of amusement, and at all times of the day; and so little had it lost of its old malignity, that in a few hours it summoned some of its victims from the ranks of the living, and even destroyed others in less than one. *Four-and-twenty hours,* neither more nor less, *were decisive as to the event;* the disease had thus undergone no change.

" In proportion as the pestilence increased in its baneful violence, the condition of the people became more and more miserable and forlorn: the townspeople fled to the country, the peasants to the towns; some sought lonely places of refuge, others shut themselves up in their houses. Ireland and Scotland received crowds of the fugitives. Others embarked for France or the Netherlands; but security was nowhere to be found, so that people at last resigned themselves to that fate which had so long and heavily oppressed the country. Women ran about negligently clad, as if they had lost their senses, and filled the streets with lamentations and loud prayers; all business was at a stand, no one thought of his daily occupation; and the funeral bells tolled day and night, as if all the living ought to be reminded of their near and inevitable end. There died, within a few days, nine hundred and sixty of the inhabitants of Shrewsbury, the greater part of them robust men and heads of families; from which circumstance we may judge of the profound sorrow that was felt in this city.

" The epidemic spread itself rapidly over all England, as far as the Scottish borders, and on all sides to the sea coasts, under more extraordinary and memorable phenomena than had been observed in almost any other epidemic. In fact, it seemed that *the banks of the Severn* were *the focus of the malady,* and that from hence a true impestation of the atmosphere was diffused in every direction. Whithersoever the winds wafted the stinking mist, the inhabitants became infected with the Sweating Sickness, and, more or less, the same scenes of horror and of affliction which had occurred in Shrewsbury were repeated. These poisonous clouds of mist were observed moving from place to place, with the disease in their train, affecting one town after another, and, morning and evening, spreading their nauseating insufferable stench. At greater distances, these clouds being dispersed by the wind, became gradually attenuated; yet their dispersion set no bounds to the pestilence, and it was as if they had imparted to the lower strata of the atmosphere a kind of ferment, which went on engendering itself even without the presence of the thick misty vapour, and being received into men's lungs, produced the frightful disease everywhere. Noxious exhalations from dung-pits, stagnant waters, swamps, impure canals, and the odour of foul rushes which were in general use in the dwellings in England, together with all kinds of offensive rubbish, seemed not a little to contribute to it; and it was remarked universally, that wherever such offensive odours prevailed, the Sweating Sickness appeared more malignant. It is a known fact, that in a certain state of the atmosphere, which is perhaps principally dependent on electrical conditions and the degree of heat, mephitic odours exhale more easily and powerfully. To the quality of the air at that time prevalent in England, this peculiarity may certainly be attributed, although it must be confessed that upon this point there are no accurate data to be discovered."

The disease remained in the country, on the whole, about half a year, namely from the 15th of April to the 30th of September, and was attended, as usual, with a train of inflammatory epidemics breaking out in different parts of Europe about the same period. It is further traced by Dr. Hecker as appearing in Saxony in 1652, in France and Piedmont in 1715, at Rottingen in Germany in 1802; and he concludes by showing its connexion, although not absolute identity, with the present miliary fevers on the continent.

The work of Dr. Hecker closes here, as far as it relates to England; but we learn from other writers that fatal epidemics, popularly known as plagues, continued, after the year 1551, to be of frequent occurrence; and it is remarked by Sir William Petty that "a plague happeneth in London every twenty years, or thereabouts, and do commonly kill one-fifth of the inhabitants." There was a plague in London in 1592, the year when a first attempt at a general registration of deaths was made by an association of parish clerks, in the publication of " bills of mortality." In the succeeding century there were four visitations of plague, including that of the great plague of 1665, immediately preceding the fire of London. The number of persons carried off by these epidemics was as under:—

Date.	Died of plague in London.	Total deaths in London.
1603	30,561	37,294
1625	35,417	51,758
1636	10,400	23,357
1665	68,596	97,306

The plague had appeared in Amsterdam in 1664, and ships from Holland were ordered into a quarantine of thirty days, but without effect. Isolated cases of plague appeared in London during the winter; and as the following summer advanced, which was exceedingly hot, it began to rage with extreme virulence. For the week ending Sept. 19, the deaths were 7,165, of which 4,000 are stated by Dr. Hodges to have occurred in one night; but from this time the disease began to decline. The following week the deaths were 5,533; the next 4,929; and in the first week of December they declined to 210. The disease is described as commencing with shivering, nausea, headache, and delirium, followed by sudden faintness, total prostration of strength, and sometimes paroxysms of frenzy. If the patient survived these to the third day, buboes commonly appeared, and when these could be made to suppurate, there was hope of recovery.

The buboes, like the profuse perspiration of the Sweating Sickness, the purgings and vomitings of epidemic cholera, and the eruptions of small-pox, were doubtless the result of an effort of nature to throw off from the system some morbific agent; and there is reason to believe that in all cases of plague the whole of these symptoms have been more frequently manifested than has been generally supposed. In the middle ages every disease was plague that produced a sudden and great mortality: and the malady only obtained a more specific name when some one of its various symptoms exhibited itself more generally than another; and this would obviously depend more upon diet, temperature, and the state of the patient's constitution, than upon the action and insidious cause of the disease itself, whatever its origin.

In a table of London casualties given by Graunt, there is set down among eighty different causes of death, a disease called "the plague of the guts," which carried off 253 persons in 1659, and 402 in 1660, beyond which the tables were not continued. There can be little doubt but this disease was cholera in its malignant form ; common dysentery being separately mentioned under the heads of " bloody flux " and " scouring," and that it exhibited itself in 1665, when the deaths occurred with too great rapidity for the clerks who framed the bills of mortality to make nice distinctions between one kind of plague and another. We hear of it again as occasioning great devastation in 1670 and 1699, from Dr. Tralles in his ' Historia Choleræ Atrocissimæ,' a work published in 1753, the minute descriptions of which identify the disease with the epidemic of the last summer and autumn.

The work of Dr. Tralles must completely set at rest the controversy about the modern Asiatic origin of malignant cholera. The received opinion of the medical profession, with few exceptions (Mr. Thackeray and Dr. Chambers among the chief), has been that malignant cholera is altogether a new disease, first appearing in August 1817, in the delta of the Ganges, at Jessore, after the annual inundation of the marsh lands by which it is surrounded, and there carrying off 10,000 persons (a sixth of the population) in a few weeks ; thence proceeding to Calcutta, and devastating every town and village within an area of several thousand square miles. It is admitted, however, that Brahminical records notice vaguely a disease of a somewhat similar character to have prevailed among the Hindoos of remote anti-quity, and our own occupation of India is not so recent, but that a little research has now established the fact that it appeared in 1781 at Ganjam, 500 miles to the north-east of Madras, where 500 men sunk beyond recovery within an hour; at Madras, the following year, when it attacked the army of Sir John Burgoyne; and the next year at Hurdwar, where it swept off 20,000 pilgrims. It was then called by the Moslems *mordechim*, or bowel-death, corrupted by the Europeans into *mort-de-chien;* and it was remarked that at the same period a severe epidemic influenza, or catarrhal fever, visited Russia, England, Germany and France, and occasioned a great mortality.

The doctrine, therefore, that malignant cholera is new in India, rests entirely upon assumption; and that it is new in Europe, can hardly be maintained as in the slightest degree pro-bable by any one who has attentively considered the analogous effects of several of the epidemics of the middle ages, as de-scribed by Dr. Hecker. The testimony, however, of Dr. Tralles is decisive of the fact that epidemic cholera was known in Eng-land in the seventeenth and eighteenth centuries. Those who hold the contrary opinion have generally maintained that the cholera morbus of antiquity was a violent dysentery, charac-terised by the presence of bile; but Dr. Tralles shows that in his time the absence of bile had not only been noticed, but various theo-ries formed to account for the want of this secretion. He notices the serous and aqueous discharges by vomitings and purging; the draining of the body of all its fluids; the thickening of the blood by the loss of its serous portion, and consequent arrest of circulation; the icy coldness; the consecutive fever; the rapid death in a few hours, with cramps and spasms in severe cases, and their frequent sudden occurrence in the middle of the night; all of which have been marked features of the epidemic recently prevailing among us. Commenting upon this evidence, the editor of the ' London Medical Gazette' observes—

" We began the investigation already prejudiced in favour of the view entertained by Dr. Copland and other reputable authorities, namely, that before the year 1817 it was altogether unknown either in India or Europe, and that the *materies morbi* first sprang from the jungles of Jessore in that year. We must admit, however, that the description given by Dr. Trotter of cholera, as it was known to medical writers in 1753, has satisfied us that a much older date must be assigned to the first outbreak of this pestilence. His description is, perhaps, as complete as the state of pathology at that time would admit, and if we except the want of reference to any account of the state of the renal secretion, all the marked peculiarities of the present disease are clearly indicated *

Celsus, the Hippocrates of Rome, is quoted by Dr. Chambers to prove the existence of cholera, with serous discharges, in the first century; and in looking attentively at Dr. Hecker's summary of the statements of ancient medical writers, respecting the *cardiac,* or heart disease, referred to as early as the time of Alexander the Great, 300 years before Christ, it is impossible to resist the conclusion that they were describing, under another name, the last stage of malignant cholera. The disease was called *morbus cardiacus,* not by medical writers, but by the people, who concluded the heart to be the seat of the malady from the irregular beatings and violent palpitations which were one of its symptoms. Other symptoms were "cold numbness of the limbs" (*torpor frigidus;*) "profuse and clammy perspirations;" "a feeble and almost extinct pulse;" "a thin and trembling voice;" "a countenance pale as death;" "an insufferable oppression on the left side, or even over the whole chest;" "eyes sunk in the sockets, and, in fatal cases, the hands and feet turning blue;" "and while the heart, notwithstanding the universal coldness of the body, still beat violently, they, for the most part, retained possession of their senses." Finally, "the nails became curved on their cold hands, and the skin wrinkled."† These are nearly the very expressions used by Dr. Adair Crawford, in describing the last stage of malignant cholera, as it occurred in St. Petersburgh in 1848.

"The whole surface of the body became as cold as marble, and covered sometimes with a clammy moisture; the pulse extremely feeble, and often imperceptible; the face sunk, and the features contracted to, sometimes nearly half their usual size; the eyes sunk deep in their sockets, and surrounded by a dark circle, and the pupils generally dilated. The cheeks, hands, feet, and nails assumed a leaden-blue or purplish colour, and likewise, though in a less degree, the entire surface of the skin, whose functions seemed completely paralysed. One remarkable phenomenon was the sudden collapse of the soft parts of the body, the effect necessarily of all the vessels being nearly emptied of their fluids, and of the rapid absorption of the adipose substance; so that patients were reduced, sometimes in twenty-four hours, perhaps one-third or more of their previous size. The skin of the hands and feet was shrivelled up; the violence of the cramps usually diminished, though not always, and they were limited chiefly to the hands and feet, which often remained contracted after

---

* See the numbers of the 'London Medical Gazette' for September 28th and October 5th, 1849, in which numerous extracts from the work of Dr. Tralles are given at length.

† Hecker's 'Epidemics of the Middle Ages,' page 308.

death. The vomiting and diarrhœa were also less urgent; the tongue
was moist, flabby, and cold; the respiration hurried, or else slow, and
much oppressed with frequent deep sighing; the breath cold, the
voice plaintive and reduced almost to a whisper. There was great
heat, oppression, and anguish in the epigastrium and about the heart,
to which regions all the suffering was referred."*

These facts are important, for they help to dispel much of that
mystery about cholera which has made it the object of superstitious terrór, and point out the path to be followed by those
who would learn the cause of epidemics and the means of obviating their effects. It is a great step towards a true knowledge of
the evil to discover\that epidemics are not caprices of nature, to
be regarded as original marvels, but *periodical* visitants, obeying
therefore fixed laws which it may be possible to trace out by
closely watching the recurrence of their operation.

It is of vast moment, also, to the interests of humanity, in a
moral as well as in a commercial view, to be thus enabled to get
rid of that most mischievous of medical errors—the doctrine that
epidemics, like the cholera, are propagated by contagion. We would
guard this observation by an admission that in all cases of disease
the air of an unventilated room may be rendered poisonous to the
healthy by the sick, and that the sick may otherwise predispose
the healthy to attack, by the influence upon the nervous system
of fear and sympathy; but that the casual contact of strangers with
the person or the clothes of a sick man has ever been a cause of
the spread of cholera, or of any other epidemic, is a notion at
variance alike with probability and fact. In a paper presented
by Dr. Strong, of the Bengal army, to the Statistical Society, he
states, that during the twenty years ending with 1847, there were
deaths annually from cholera in the gaols under his superintendance, but that it did not spread ; never attacking more than one
in nine of the inmates. But the sudden cessation of cholera in
London at the close of the last autumn, and its equally sudden
disappearance from other cities, after raging for an average interval of eight or ten weeks, demonstrates the fact that its propagation depends upon atmospherical conditions, and not upon
human intercourse. Even in the height of an epidemic season,
the nurses and physicians in constant attendance on cholera
patients, have not suffered more than the rest of the community,
from the supposed danger of their exposed position, and have
enjoyed comparative immunity where the arrangements of ventilation and drainage have been perfect. In the general hospital
of Hamburgh, no case of cholera occurred among its 1,600 in-

* ' Official Circular,' for Oct. 10, 1848.

mates, although 117 cholera cases were admitted between the 7th and 22nd of September ;* and in London, at St. Bartholomew's hospital, where 478 cholera patients were admitted during the past summer, of whom 199 died, the disease proved fatal to one only of the nurses of that institution. The attacks in other cases being confined to premonitory diarrhœa, which, by prompt attention, were speedily subdued.

If it be said that its appearance in different countries has not been exactly simultaneous—that it is in India one year and in Europe the next—in France in the summer, and in England in the autumn, showing a march or progress like that attributed to contagion—the answer is, that neither do corresponding seasons always occur in different countries in precisely the same years or months. The weather is often wet in England when it is dry in Germany; cold and dry in England when it is hot and damp in Russia; winds blow from different points of the compass, even within the same country—moving in eddies or circles ;† electrical phenomena equally vary, and the course of epidemics must obviously vary with them.

Little, however, remains to be said on this subject, after the able and conclusive reports of the Board of Health on the uselessness of quarantine establishments as a means of prevention, in which the fallacy of popular ideas, on the supposed contagious character of epidemics, is fully exposed. For the interests of civilization, we trust that translated copies of this valuable report will be forwarded to every government of Europe and Asia with which we maintain friendly relations; and we think that the present cabinet will be wanting in its duty to the country, if they do not promptly act upon its recommendations, in abolishing during the next session, as an example to other nations, English quarantine regulations, and in otherwise exerting themselves to cause the example to be followed. Wherever the principle of quarantine is maintained, a standing lesson of inhumanity is inculcated. It is a practical mode of teaching the people the wisdom of abandoning the sick and leaving them to perish, as a cruel necessity; while, at the same time, it diverts the mind from an investigation of the true causes upon which the propagation of epidemics chiefly depend. Upon the disastrous effects of quarantine in paralysing the trade and industry of commercial countries, we need offer no observation. They are now too well known to require comment.

Quarantine regulations are a relic of the ignorance and super-

---

* Report on Quarantine, page 23.

† A fact established by the very useful meteorological tables published in the *Daily News;* a further elucidation of Captain Reid's theory of the law of storms.

stition of the middle ages. They were first established at Venice and in Italy about the close of the fifteenth century, in the vain but abortive hope of opposing a barrier to the eruption of the plague; and bills of health were introduced about the period of the destruction of the French army, before Naples, by an epidemic in 1528. The notion of the importance of a forty days' detention was founded upon the religious ideas of the period, of some magical virtue residing in forty-day epochs. Christ had fasted forty days in the wilderness; forty days were asserted to be the limit of separation between acute and chronic diseases; forty days were assigned for the perfect recovery of lying-in women; forty days were supposed to be necessary for every change in the growth of a fœtus; and forty days composed the philosophical month of the alchymists. Let us hope that we are not far from the time when, instead of lazarettos of imprisonment founded upon such puerile theories, marine hospitals will be established in every port for the immediate but voluntary occupation of all sick persons landing after a voyage, and that the principle of the forcible detention of a ship's crew or passengers will be utterly abandoned.

It may be observed here, that very little faith ought to be placed in the correctness of any of the numerous statements that have appeared of the precise course of the cholera in its march from Asia to Europe, from the date of its appearance at Jessore in 1817. We know of course the year and month when it broke out at Newcastle-upon-Tyne, in London, Paris, St. Petersburg, and other European cities; and we assume it to be true, that it had appeared as we are told, previously at Teflis, Astrachan, Saratoff, and other places of which we know little; but all these statements amount to nothing more than industrious collections of newspaper paragraphs; and it will be obvious, on a moment's reflection, that cholera may, and doubtless has appeared in a thousand places where there has been no newspaper reporter to testify of its existence. Who will prove to us that it was not raging last September in the interior of Thibet, or at the sources of the Niger, or on the banks of the Amazon? Even its existence last summer in the United States has been but little noticed in England; and although the mortality in many towns of the Union has been excessive, the contagionists have failed to explain to us when and by what mode it crossed the Atlantic ocean, and appeared, without local spontaneity of origin, at New York.

We shall not, therefore, attempt to follow the narrative of any so-called history of the progress of cholera that has yet been written; and not to extend this paper to a length too great for the patience of the reader, we shall now confine ourselves to the statistics of the disease as it manifested itself in Paris and London.

The following is an analysis of the principal facts connected with the appearance of cholera in Paris in 1832, drawn up by M. de Watteville.*

" Cholera showed itself in Paris on the 26th of March, 1832 ; four persons were suddenly attacked, and died in a few hours.

" The next day, March 27, six other individuals were attacked ; on the 28th, those attacked were 22 in number ; on the 31st, there were 300 ; and the cholera had already invaded 35 out of the 48 quarters of Paris.

" Out of the 300 cholera patients on the 31st of March, 86 had ceased to exist before the end of that day. On the 2nd of April, the number of deaths amounted to more than 100 ; on the 3rd, to 200 ; the 5th, to 300. On the 9th, more than 1,200 individuals were attacked, and 814 died. In short, eighteen days after the breaking out of the malady, namely, on the 14th of April, the number of attacks was 13,000, with 7,000 deaths.

" At length the virulence of the epidemic began to abate ; on the 15th of April, the number of deaths fell from 756 to 631 ; on the 30th they were but 114 ; and from the 17th of May to the 17th of June, no more than from 15 to 20 per diem occurred. All at once, this limit was exceeded ; on the 9th of July, 71 persons succumbed to the malady ; on the 13th, 88 died ; the next day, 107 ; the 15th, 128 ; the 16th, 170 ; and the 18th, 225. But, on the 19th, the number of deaths decreased to 130, and this rapid diminution continuing daily, the alarm of the public began to subside. The epidemic went on decreasing up to the end of September, and on the 1st of October, the cholera was regarded as extinct.

" The total duration of this epidemic, in Paris, was 129 days, or 27 weeks, from the 26th of March to the 30th of September, or from the vernal to the autumnal equinox.

" The period of augmentation or increase was 15 days, and that of diminution 62. Thus the second period lasted four times as long as the first.

" The cholera carried off 18,402 individuals in the French capital, viz. :—

March (from the 26th only)	90 deaths.
April	12,733
May	812
June (from the 15th to the 30th, second increase, *recrudescence*)	602
July	2,573
August	969
September	357
General total	18,402

* See the *Journal des Economistes* for April, 1849, a periodical of great merit, but too little known in this country. It is published by Guillaumin in Paris, and may be had of G. Luxford, Whitefriars-street, London.

" This total of 18,402 comprised 9,170 men and 9,232 women ; and bears a proportion to the general population of 1 to 4,270.

" Of these 18,402 deaths, there were,—

Under 5 years of age	.. 1,311	From 55 to	60 years	..	1,440
From 5 to 10	 392	„ 60 to	65 „	..	1,527
„ 10 to 15	 202	„ 65 to	70 „	..	1,594
„ 15 to 20	 377	„ 75 to	80 „	..	756
„ 20 to 25	 959	„ 80 to	85 „	..	307
„ 25 to 30	 1,206	„ 85 to	90 „	..	58
„ 30 to 35	 1,423	„ 90 to	95 „	..	13
„ 35 to 40	 1,348	„ 95 to 100 „		..	1
„ 40 to 45	 1,311				
„ 45 to 50	 1,416	Total		..	.. 18,402
„ 50 to 55	 1,473				

" We may add, as a curious piece of information, the number of deaths which occurred in the different parts of houses, during the six months of the prevalence of the epidemic :—

Ground floor	..	..	..	..	..	1,506
First floor	..	..	..	..	..	2,868
Second floor	..	..	..	..	..	2,264
Third floor	..	..	..	..	..	2,023
Fourth floor	..	..	..	..	..	1,375
Fifth, sixth, and seventh floors	..		..	..	..	962
Not indicated	..	..	..	..	..	170
	Total	..	..	..	..	11,168 "

The last table, which M. de Watteville introduces as a curious piece of information, is the most important part of the whole. It establishes two facts upon which our attention cannot be too strongly fixed, and which there is abundant additional evidence to confirm—first, that the cholera does not attack the poor in preference to the rich, where the poor are not unhealthfully lodged; second, that the mortality is greatest where the air is the densest, namely, at its lowest level. In Paris, the reader is probably aware that few persons rent private houses as in England. The different classes of society occupy separate suites on the different floors of houses, built somewhat upon the plan of the chambers of our inns-of-law. The only persons who sleep on the ground-floor are the porters and their families, who suffered largely, although the number does not appear so great as on the next floor, because the ground is principally devoted to shops and warehouses. The *première* and *seconde*, or first and second floors, are exclusively occupied by classes in easy circumstances, and it will be noticed that it was among them that the greatest number of deaths occurred. Higher up live the families of the poorer class, and it will be seen that there were fewer deaths on the third floors than on the second, fewer still on the fourth, and that the inmates of the attics or *mansardes* (always the very poorest of the poor), nearly escaped altogether.

In noticing the return of the aggregate deaths in each of the different arrondissements of Paris, the same rule may be observed. The cholera made no distinction between rich and poor, nor between crowded and thinly inhabited districts. The mortality was greatest in proportion to the number of residents, where the houses were built on the lowest land. Thus it was greatest in the tenth arrondissement, which includes the fashionable Faubourg of St. Germain, where many of the houses are isolated and surrounded by gardens, but the level of which is low, corresponding with that of Lambeth in respect to London; and it was in Lambeth where the ravages of cholera in the British Metropolis were the most severe during the late autumn. The smallest number of deaths occurred in the third arrondissement, which embraces part of the Faubourg Poissonnière and Montmartre, inhabited by a poor population, *but situated upon high ground.*

Next to the tenth arrondissement, the mortality was greatest in the eighth and ninth arrondissements; the districts including the canals and ditches of the *Marais* and the *Cité*, which is an island, or collection of sand-banks in the middle of the Seine.* Here the cholera made considerable havoc, which is strangely enough attributed, by M. de Watteville, to the population being "poor and miserable," although he had just before admitted that "it more especially attacked those whose professions commanded competent means."

The returns explain another of the difficulties of this writer, who says that "the disease was not more formidable in places known to be infected by putrid emanations than in other localities," forgetting the *Marais*, and alluding to the open reservoirs of night-soil then existing (but since removed) at Montfaucon, near Montmartre, the highest ground in Paris. It would not be there on the hill top that there would be any great concen-

---

* The number of deaths in the various arrondissements of Paris, exclusive of those who died in the hospitals, were as follows :—

1st arrondissement	..	600	8th arrondissement	..	1,306
2nd	,,	.. 535	9th	,,	.. 1,239
3rd	,,	.. 403	10th	,,	.. 1,685
4th	,,	.. 528	11th	,,	.. 1,051
5th	,,	.. 619	12th	,,	.. 1,194
6th	,,	.. 817			
7th	,,	.. 1,201	Total	..	11,178

tration of malignant vapour; and we have to remember that, as gases follow the same law as fluids, the exhalations from Montfaucon on cooling at night, would descend, not on the spot whence they rose, but mixing with other vapours would seek the lowest level, as naturally as a running stream.

This is suggestive of the reason of the frequency of night attacks during severe epidemics, as remarked in the epidemics of the middle ages, as also during the late visitation, and in ordinary cases of marsh fever. It was in one *night* that 4,000 perished in the plague of London of 1665. It was at *night* that the army of Sennacherib was destroyed. Both in England and on the continent a large proportion of the cholera cases, in its several forms, have been observed to have occurred between one and two o'clock in the morning. The " danger of exposure to *night* air " has been a theme of physicians from time immemorial; but it is remarkable that they have never yet called in the aid of chemistry to account for the fact.*

It is at night that the stratum of air nearest the ground must always be the most charged with the particles of animalized matter given out from the skin, and deleterious gases, such as carbonic acid gas, the product of respiration, and sulphuretted hydrogen, the product of the sewers. In the day, gases and vapourous substances of all kinds rise in the air by the rarefaction of heat; at night when this rarefaction leaves them, they fall by an increase of gravity, if imperfectly mixed with the atmosphere, while the gases evolved during the night, instead of ascending, remain at nearly the same level. It is known that carbonic acid gas at a low temperature partakes so nearly of the nature of a fluid, that it may be poured out of one vessel into another: it rises at the temperature at which it is exhaled from the lungs, but its tendency is towards the floor, or the bed of the sleeper, in cold and unventilated rooms.

At Hamburg, the alarm of cholera at night in some parts of the city, was so great, that on some occasions many refused to go to bed, lest they should be attacked unawares in their sleep. Sitting up, they probably kept their stoves or open fires burning for the sake of warmth, and that warmth giving the expansion to any deleterious gases present, which would best promote their escape, and promote their dilution in the atmosphere, the means of safety were thus unconsciously assured. At Sierra Leone, the natives have a practice in the sickly season of keeping fires constantly burning in their huts at night, assigning that the fires

---

* Formerly it was ascribed to lunar influences; whence the phrase " moonstruck," and the scripture, " the moon shall not smite thee by night."

kept away the evil spirits, to which, in their ignorance, they attribute fever and ague. Latterly, Europeans have begun to adopt the same practice; and those who have tried it, assert that they have now entire immunity from the tropical fevers to which they were formerly subject.

In the epidemics of the middle ages, fires used to be lighted in the streets for the purification of the air; and in the plague of London, of 1665, fires in the streets were at one time kept burning incessantly, till extinguished by a violent storm of rain. Latterly, trains of gunpowder have been fired, and cannon discharged, for the same object; but it is obvious that these measures, although sound in principle, must necessarily, *out of doors*, be on too small a scale, as measured against an ocean of atmospheric air, to produce any sensible effect. Within doors, however, the case is different. It is quite possible to heat a room sufficiently to produce a rarefaction and consequent dilution of any malignant gases it may contain; and it is of course the air of the room, and that alone at night, which comes into immediate contact with the lungs of a person sleeping.

The mortality occasioned by cholera in Paris in 1849, appears to have very nearly corresponded with that of 1831-2, but there was this remarkable difference: in 1832, two-thirds of the deaths, 12,733, of the whole number occurred in the month of *April*, while, in the recent instance, the deaths in April were but 694, and the greatest mortality was in June.* In England, the disease reached its greatest height in August and September, and has been much more violent than on its former visitation. In 1831-2, the deaths from cholera in the metropolis were 5,275. In 1849, 13,631, exclusive of 2,981 deaths by diarrhœa;† and

---

* The deaths in Paris from cholera, of persons who died at their own residences in 1849, were as follows :—

March	...	...	130	July	...	...	419
April	...	...	694	August	...	...	810
May	..	...	2,426	September		...	670
June	...	...	5,769	October	...	...	32

To this must be added the deaths in the hospitals. The greatest mortality was in the neighbourhood of the Jardin des Plantes.

† Deaths in London from Cholera, 1849.

Quarter ending March	31	...	...	...	516
„ June	30	...	...	...	268
„ September	30	...	...	...	12,847

13,631

Deaths in London from Diarrhœa, 1849 :—

Quarter ending March	31	...	...	...	284
„ June	30	...	...	...	240
„ September	30	...	...	...	2,457

2,981

the registrar-general's reports for the whole of England and Wales show an excess of 60,492 deaths for the last summer quarter over the summer quarter of 1845—an excess principally to be attributed to the epidemic, the mortality of the quarter exceeding the average by 53 per cent. The effects of the epidemic may also be traced in a falling off in the number of births, which had been 140,361 for the summer quarter of 1848, but only 135,200 in 1849, exceeding the number of deaths by only 164; so that, if there be truth in the common estimate, that nearly 300,000 persons have left the shores of the United Kingdom within the last twelvemonth, we have now a rapidly decreasing population. It may be noted also as probable, that population has remained stationary, or been turned back in its course throughout the world during the past year, for no part of the globe appears to have wholly escaped the ravages of the disease, and we hear of it as appearing at about one and the same time in Russia and Spain,* in Paris and New York, on the shores of the Medi-

---

* " From Bangkok, the metropolis of the kingdom of Siam, we have received accounts to the 26th July. These communications give fearful details of the havoc wrought by the scourge cholera. At Quedah, thousands were carried off by cholera at the beginning of the year; and passing from thence along the eastern coast of the Malayan peninsula, the scourge visited Tringanu, Pahang, and Calantan, where it still rages with much virulence. Passing eastward, at the commencement of June, it visited the provinces of Siam, and on June 7th broke out in the capital, Bangkok. So few cases occurred at this latter place that no alarm was excited; but on the 9th its ravages had increased to the extent of two or three hundred; and 80 persons within the city were carried to one wat, or burning-place. On June 11, and two succeeding days, the cholera raged with frightful virulence, carrying off rich and poor. An eye-witness, an American missionary, remarks that its horrors were beyond all description. The streets were thronged with the dead and dying; it was impossible to walk even a short distance without witnessing the dead bodies lying in all directions, exposed to a tropical sun, and persons were attacked whilst walking from one place to another. The inhabitants became panic-struck. The deaths were so numerous that to burn the corpses was impossible, and multitudes were thrown into the river just as they had died. In many of the wats four hundred bodies were burned each day, without parade or mourners; they were placed like logs and left to the flames, or putrified on the ground. From correct returns it was ascertained that nearly three thousand perished daily in the city alone, whilst in the suburbs and provinces, the number is untold. From the government census it was ascertained at the end of twelve days that more than twenty thousand souls were swept from Bangkok, and within a radius of from twenty to thirty miles the deaths are estimated at thirty thousand. Amongst the early victims was Chau Khun Bodin, a noble of high rank, who commanded the Siamese troops against the Cochin-Chinese for possession of Cambodia, and who had returned to Bangkok but a few months previously, after an absence of ten years in the border war. In the sugar districts the fatality was also frightful, carrying off the Siamese by thousands, but being less fatal among the Chinese population."—*Daily News,* October 29, 1849.

terranean and the banks of the Mississippi, the mortality in some places extending to the lower animals.*

In all cases, however, we find the mortality has been greatest in *low-lying districts.* On high and naturally salubrious situations, comparatively few deaths by cholera have occurred, and the mortality has even been less than usual. In London it was almost wholly confined to the banks of the river, the district between Waterloo Bridge and Battersea, which in the time of the Romans was an unreclaimed marsh ; and the low, but slightly more elevated, levels of Whitechapel, Bethnal Green, and Shoreditch. In the large parishes of Marylebone and St. George's, Hanover-square, the greater part of which lie between 50 and 100 feet above high water mark, deaths were scarcely above the average, and nowhere exceeded the births. Although most destructive on the Surrey side of the river, the cholera did not touch the Surrey Hills.†

The returns to the registrar-general from parts of the country where the towns are situated on elevated lands, as in central and North Devon, Leicestershire, and the West Riding of Yorkshire, state the population to have been unusually healthy, and the deaths below the average. The exceptions have everywhere been of the kind that prove the rule. Cholera was fatal at Huddersfield among some labourers' cottages, which although situated on a hill side, were without drainage, surrounded by filth and refuse, and exposed to the malaria of an uncleansed fish-pond.

At Leeds, the deputy-registrar remarks, that although the ravages of cholera had been truly awful, it had been confined, in his district, almost exclusively to that part of the population that

---

* It was publicly announced from the pulpit in St. Louis, on the Mississippi, a few days since, that there had been 8,000 victims to the pestilence in that city alone. So shocking were the ravages of cholera in Landusky, Ohio, that even after the population had been reduced from 300 to 600 by death, and by flight inspired by terror, the deaths averaged from 30 to 40 per day, for several days together. The physicians, a rare instance, deserted the town, but several other physicians very nobly repaired to the afflicted place from Cleveland, Cincinnati, and even from Philadelphia. A few of the most distinguished men of Landusky, who resisted the panic and remained at home, perished by the epidemic, while many of those who fled also became victims. It is singular, that in Cincinnati *both fowls and hogs have died in immense numbers, as if by an epidemic somewhat resembling the cholera ; while at Wheeling, nearly all the cats have been carried off in a similar manner.—Correspondent of the Morning Chronicle.*

† Nor the chalk hills of Kent. At Fairscat, situated on the Wrotham range, about 800 feet above the level of the sea, there is, near the residence of the Editor, a boarding school establishment for young ladies, containing forty-four pupils, amongst whom not a single case of sickness of the most ordinary kind, has occurred during the whole of the half-year ending with December, 1849.

dwell in cellars, although sometimes better drained than the unoccupied cellars of other streets,—a circumstance which makes the deputy-registrar undervalue the importance of drainage, he not perceiving that malignant vapours are not necessarily confined to the spot where they rise, but may flow from their own gravitation, or be drifted by the wind, into cellars a mile distant.

The following is the proportion of deaths to the population in some of the towns where the mortality was greatest:—

Deaths from Cholera during the summer quarter of 1849 :—

	Males.		Females.	
Hull	1 in	28	1 in	28
Plymouth	1 „	38	1 „	46
Merthyr Tydvil	1 „	39	1 „	39
Portsea Island	1 „	44	1 „	50
Liverpool	1 „	47	1 „	43
Tynemouth	1 „	61	1 „	64
Bristol	1 „	66	1 „	78

Of the numerous communications published by the Board of Health to throw light upon the causes of the epidemic, perhaps the following, addressed to Lord Carlisle by Mr. K. B. Martin, harbour-master of Ramsgate, is one of the most important.

" During the heats of the last days of August, having a considerable body of officers and men under my surveillance, I watched their state and habits with great care and anxiety. I knew they were exposed in no common degree to all the admitted predisposing causes. Some were occasionally at work in a sewer in progress ; others in a coffer-dam, surrounded by a fetid blue mud, and offensive sullage. All were employed in a harbour partially dry at low-water, and with a hot sun, liable to exhalations from decomposed marine exuviæ; yet, to my great consolation, all these poor men, *thus employed*, continued well. The exception is extraordinary. The crew of my steam towing-vessel *Samson*, continually employed in the fresh sea-breeze, when at home living in well-ventilated comfortable houses, temperate in their habits, hále and young ; and yet they were attacked, under the following curious and interesting circumstances. At midnight of the 31st of August, the *Samson* proceeded to the Goodwin Sands, where they were employed under the Trinity agent, assisting in work carried on there by that corporation. While there, at 3, *a. m.* on the 1st of September, a hot humid haze, with a bog-like smell, passed over them ; and the greater number of the men there employed instantly felt a nausea. They were in two parties. One man at work on the sand was obliged to be carried to the boat ; and before they reached the steam-vessel at anchor, the cramps and spasm had supervened upon the vomitings : but here they found two of the party on board similarly affected, and after heaving up the anchor they returned with all the despatch they could to Ramsgate. Hot baths were immediately put in requisition, and by proper medical treatment they were convalescent in a few days. Here, then, is a very marked case, without one known predisposing local cause; while our labourers escaped, surrounded by local and continual disadvantages. Doubtless it was atmospheric, and in the hot blast of pestilence which passed over them. * * * * * * * *

"My men were carried home, where every comfort awaited them, and not a member of their families was infected."

The facts to be noticed here are—first, the connexion of cholera with "a humid haze with bog-like smell," corresponding with the "stinking mists" remarked during the progress of the epidemics of the middle ages; and, second, the circumstance that it was soon after *midnight*, or at 3, *a. m.*, when the crew of the *Samson* were attacked; while fourteen men who had been employed in the daytime in the docks, amid fetid exhalations, under a hot sun, continued well. Here we have again the most decisive evidence, not that fetid exhalations are harmless, as Mr. Martin would seem to infer, but that they are least hurtful when most rapidly disengaged and expanded by the action of heat; and that in their effects upon human beings, their malignity depends upon the accidents of temperature and winds that may cause them to sweep along the surface of the ground in a concentrated form. For aught that can be shown to the contrary, the "humid haze" seen by Mr. Martin may have been impregnated with the sulphuretted hydrogen exhaled the day before from the very dock he has described.

The presence of aqueous vapour appears to be one of the essential conditions of all epidemics; but the effect is not produced by aqueous vapour alone, for an ordinary Scotch mist will hurt nobody; the vapour must be impregnated with poisonous gases. It, then, naturally produces the same effect upon the lungs as poisoned water upon the stomach; and here it may be observed, that in numerous cases, quoted by the registrars and the Board of Health—as for example, the deaths in Wandsworth-terrace—cholera has been directly induced by the contamination of a spring or well with a neighbouring sewer. No matter whether the elements of putridity enter the system in a gaseous or a liquid form, they will in either case produce a like result.

It has been remarked that the summer of 1849 was not one of great humidity, but, on the contrary, an unusually dry season, less rain falling in latitude south of 53, than in the average of seasons, but more rain than the average in the north of England. A warm and dry season, however, is the one most favourable to the process of exhalation; and in marshy districts, and on the

banks of rivers there is always a sufficiency of aqueous vapours
to arrest the upward course of deleterious gases, and to hold
them in combination. Although the season was warm and dry,
Mr. Glaisher, of the Royal Observatory, Greenwich, tells us that
the period from August 20th to September 15th, when the
cholera was at its height in London, " was distinguished by a
thick and stagnant atmosphere, and the air was for the most part
close and oppressive." He adds, that the movement of the air
at the time was about one-half its usual amount.

"On many days, when a strong breeze was blowing on the top of
the observatory, and over Blackheath, there was not the slightest
motion in the air near the banks of the Thames ; and this remarkable
calm continued for some days together, particularly from August 19 to
24, on the 29th, from September 1 to 10, and after September 15.
On September 11 and 12 the whole mass of air at all places was in
motion, and the first time for nearly three weeks the hills at Hampstead
and Highgate were seen clearly from Greenwich. After the 15th of
September to the end of the quarter the air was in very little motion.
" From the published observations of the strength of the wind daily
at all parts of the country, it would seem that the air has been for days
together in a stagnant state at all places whose elevation above the sea
is small."

The fall of rain in August was less than has fallen in any
August since the year 1819 ; but heavy rains set in at the close
of September, and whether or not from their influence in preci-
pitating noxious vapours, and so purifying the air, the epidemic
immediately decreased in violence, and shortly after disappeared.

Another peculiarity of the late season has been an unusually
small development of insect life. A snow storm and severe frost,
the last week in April, would seem to have destroyed the *ova* and
the *larvæ* of many of the insect tribes. The turnip-fly was missing
in many districts, to the great relief of farmers, and butterflies
were scarcely seen. This militates against the theory which
attributes epidemics to swarms of *animalculæ*; a notion which has
no other foundation than the fact that immense flights of locusts,
and sometimes a rain like drops of blood (the red colour given
by animalculæ), have been occasionally observed at periods preceding pestilence.

An analogous theory produced some impression, in the alleged
discovery by Mr. Brittain and Mr. Swayne, of cholera fungi in
the intestinal canal: but many of the fungi described have since
been found to exist in every stale loaf ; and an able report, presented to the Royal College of Physicians, has shown that the
evidence is totally insufficient to establish fungi as a cause of
epidemics, although every form of disease may lead to the

production of fungi of a peculiar character, as a subordinate symptom.*

Another theory has attributed cholera to a deficiency in the atmosphere of *ozone*, a volatile product of hydrogen and oxygen, but with a larger proportion of oxygen than in water. Ozone has a deodorizing property, and is generated by electric action, and by combustion; on which account the exemption of Birmingham from cholera has been said to be occasioned by its great fires; but although the beneficent influence of fires to those who are within their influence, is not to be doubted, several towns in which the furnaces are as numerous as in Birmingham suffered severely; especially in the epidemic of 1832. Birmingham probably owes its comparative healthfulness to the dry and porous red sandstone on which the town is situated. The ozone theory, however, deserves some countenance from the fact that the season has been characterized by a low amount of electricity. This was observed by M. Quetelet at Paris, and by Mr. Glaisher, at Greenwich; and Dr. Adair Crawford states, that during the prevalence of cholera at St. Petersburg in June 1848, that "the electric machines could not be charged, and to a great extent lost their power," and that "the disturbed condition of the electricity of the air was also indicated by the peculiarly depressed and uneasy state of feeling which almost every body complained of, more or less: some entirely losing their sleep, whilst others slept more heavily than usual." †

The Telluric theory is founded upon the observations of earthquakes and volcanic eruptions, as frequently accompanying

* The following are the conclusions of the report, which is dated October 27, 1849.

"1. Bodies presenting the characteristic forms of the so-called cholera fungi are not to be detected in the air, and, as far as our experiments have gone, not in the drinking water of infected places.

"2. It is established that, under the term 'annular bodies' and 'cholera cells, or fungi,' there have been confounded many objects of various and totally distinct natures.

"3. A large number of these have been traced to substances taken as food or medicine.

"4. The origin of others is still doubtful, but these are clearly not fungi.

"5. All the more remarkable forms are to be detected in the intestinal evacuations of persons labouring under diseases totally different in their nature from cholera.

"Lastly. We draw from these premises the general conclusion that the bodies found and described by Messrs. Brittain and Swayne are not the cause of cholera, and have no exclusive connexion with that disease; or, in other words, that the whole theory of the disease which has recently been propounded is erroneous, as far as it is based on the existence of the bodies in question.

"WILLIAM BALY, M.D.   }   Cholera
"WILLIAM W. GULL, M.D.   } Sub-Committee."

† Official Circular, October 10, 1848.

epidemics, and from the death of fishes in great numbers, as if from the escape of gases, which have sometimes been seen after subterranean disturbances, bubbling up through the water. This subject is handled with great ability by Mr. John Parkin, in his treatise on the ' Remote Cause of Epidemics;' and we incline to the opinion, that the true cause of the changes in the condition of the atmosphere which produce epidemics, may be found in these internal commotions; but not so much in the escape of any subterranean gas, as from the variations they produce in the currents of electricity, of which at present we know little or nothing. Some new agent, which is only occasionally present, there must of course be to produce a sudden vitiation of the air, in the same place where human beings, a month or two earlier or later, might breathe with comparative, if not perfect safety. Subterranean disturbance producing an altered direction of the electric currents, is perhaps the simplest hypothesis by which the phenomenon is to be explained, and it is that which best agrees with the important fact, that the intensity of the morbific influence, alike in cholera and in marsh fever, is greater by night than by day. The following remarks upon this head are by Dr. Kelsall:—

"Any one who has witnessed the fearfully rapid course of blue cholera, can scarcely fail to be struck with the similarity of the disease to the symptoms of poisoning by some energetic agent; in fact, the patient appears to suffer from the effects of some specific volatile poison. Experiments have not supported the opinion that any peculiar electrical condition of the atmosphere has existed sufficient to generate a poison during the prevalence of the epidemic, but none have been instituted to ascertain the electrical condition of the earth's surface at the same period. It is true that, according to present theories, any electrical condition of the earth is supposed to influence that of the atmosphere, but such may not be strictly the case; and now, with this *petitio principii*, if it be permitted to suppose an electric current traversing the earth with some yet unknown relation to the magnetic meridians, the generation of a specific poison might be thus imagined.

"Cyanogen, prussic acid, strychnine, morphine, picrotoxine, and other vegetable poisons, are compounds of the four elementary gases, oxygen, hydrogen, carbon, and nitrogen, chemically united in various different proportions, each possessing widely different properties—the vegetable electricity of the laurel, the upas tiente, the poppy, the cocculus indicus, and the cinchona officinalis—each acting on these elements during the growth of the plants, to elaborate their several active principles.

"*A little variety in the proportions* of the union of these four elements, produces *vastly differing properties in the products*—for example, the elements of quinine are 20 atoms of carbon, 12 of hydrogen, 2 of oxygen, and 1 of nitrogen ; and strychnine, a substance very different in its properties, is composed of 30 atoms of carbon, 16 of hydrogen. 3 of oxygen, and 1 of nitrogen. The following table of five of these vegetable principles will render the matter more clear :—

Quinine is composed of			C^{20}	H^{12}	O^2	N
Strychnine	„		C^{39}	H^{16}	O^3	N
Morphine	„		C^{31}	H^6	O^{18}	N
Picrotoxine	„		C^{12}	H^7	O^5	
Hydrocyanic acid	„		C^2	H	N	

" The substitution of phosphorus, sulphur, &c. for one or more of these elements, would also be productive of other poisonous agents.

" The requisite for deleterious products being constantly at hand on the surface, or immediately below the surface, of the ground, if there always existed a power which should cause their chemical combination, the inhabitants of the land would never be free from the effects of some resulting poison. The vicinity of drains and fetid stagnant water is found by experience to be more favourable to the development of the cholera poison than dry open situations ; but the drains, cesspools, and putrid grave-yards of London have from time immemorial emitted the gases before alluded to, with sulphur and phosphorus, which in ordinary years have not resulted in the formation of this peculiar miasm, and there must be some reason why it should be so during the summer of 1849. A telluric electrical cause would account for the anomaly. In ordinary years the requisite elements are being constantly evolved, but remain inert because they are dissipated and blown away in the state of simple mixture : this year, if chemically united in certain unknown definite proportions, by the power of electricity, they may result in the formation of a volatile poison.

" But, although low and dirty localities evolve the requisite gases in greater abundance than cleanly situations, and so produce a greater amount of the miasm ; still as these gases must be present more or less everywhere, cholera would be liable to appear in every situation where the electrical stream should pass through, and this is borne out by the fact that no locality seems absolutely and entirely exempt from the visitation of cholera. If Birmingham or other places have enjoyed immunity from the disease, it is because the electrical current has not approached them.

" If it be allowed that the symptoms of cholera are caused by the absorption into the blood of a specific volatile poison through the medium of the lungs, then, in proportion to the quantity of poison inhaled, will be the malignancy of the consequent effects, which are abortive efforts of the nervous system to eject it from the circulation along with the serum of the blood, which is poured in immense quantities into the intestines, so that the patient may (in a manner) be said to bleed to death ; and those slight cases of cholera, called choleraic diarrhœa, are occasioned by the absorption of small doses of this unknown poison, of which the system can rid itself with comparative facility. It may be that the flocculent deposit in the watery fluid

ejected from the bowels *is the poison itself* in combination with particles of serum, which it has coagulated.

There may probably be this analogy between the poison of cholera
and that of common marsh fever. In swampy districts the electricity
accompanying the sun's rays, or the ordinary electricity of the atmosphere, may act on the gaseous elements evolved by the swamp, and
cause the chemical union of two or more of them in certain definite
proportions, and thus produce a peculiar volatile poison, difficult or
impossible to obtain by analysis, because it is composed of the same
elements as the atmospheric air which holds it in solution—*i. e.*,
oxygen and nitrogen, with, perhaps, carbon or hydrogen in such
infinitesimal quantity (as an atom or two of either) as to escape appreciation ; such a poison may occasion the phenomena of intermittent
fever. But if a stream of electricity traverse the surface of the earth,
either more powerful or of greater or less tension than that which
elaborates the poison of marsh fever, then a different poison—(*i. e.*, it
may be composed of the very same elements, but combined in different
atomic proportions) may be generated. In both cases the phenomena
of the diseases consisting in abortive efforts of nature to rid herself of
the noxious material.*

Upon the above, which generally accords with our views, we
have only to observe by way of further elucidation, that although
cholera does not appear in all places where deleterious gases are
present, the difference occasioned by altered currents of electricity
would seem merely to be one of greater or less intensity. We
are not to suppose that sulphuretted hydrogen can be breathed
with impunity, either in diluted or concentrated doses. It has
been rendered abundantly evident by the sanitary reports, that
the elements of putrefaction, wherever they are breathed, will
produce diseases of varying types and degrees of malignity. It
has been asked why cholera should have been absent, both in
1832 and 1849, from Lyons, one of the most ill-cleansed towns
in France, the lower parts of which are subject to annual inunda-
tions; the town being situated at the confluence of two rivers.
But Lyons is rarely free from typhoidal fever, and at the present
moment (December 1849), it is raging there in so severe a form,
that its identity with cholera is beginning to be asserted. To
account for apparent exceptions, we have only to remember that
the greatest danger is not necessarily in the place where the gases
are evolved, if rapidly disengaged by heat and dispersed by winds,
but where the mist which they impregnate *lodges at night,* and

---

* In one case where a patient recovered from cholera, she was shortly afterwards seized, *every third evening,* with the nausea, faintness, and sinking at
the epigastrium which characterized the original attack, and always at the
same hour; these symptoms quickly yielding to two or three doses of camphor.

this, although generally in the plains, may sometimes be on hill sides, or in the hollows and ravines of a mountainous country; or again it may be at sea, as in the case we have quoted of the attack of the crew of a steam-boat on the Goodwin sands. It appears by no means improbable, that the coast of Africa, at the embouchure of its great rivers, would not be found sickly to Europeans, if those who visited it adopted the precaution of sleeping at night in an elevated region. They are safe above what is there called the " fever level," whether by night or day; and the high table lands of South Abyssinia, although within ten degrees of the line, are stated by Dr. Beke to be as salubrious as any parts of England.

Following out these conclusions, we think it will be found that the mortality of hospitals has always been greatest, other circumstances the same, where they have been situated in a low and marshy neighbourhood, or near the banks of a river, as the Hotel Dieu at Paris.

In the cure of epidemics, the first step obviously is to escape from the cause that produces them. Where we are breathing a poisonous vapour no remedies can avail: to continue to breathe it must be death. The first care, therefore, of the patient should be, to change his lodging; and he will not require any table of levels for this purpose. A view about sunrise, from the top of any church steeple, will show him at a glance the level of the night mist. He should avoid that especially during the summer heats, as he would the white pall of the grave.

When a patient cannot change his lodging, or be suddenly removed, the next care should be, to raise at night, by a fire in an open chimney, the temperature of the room in which he sleeps, sufficiently to dry up the vapour and rarify any deleterious gases that may be present. Upon the more medical part of the treatment that should be adopted for cholera patients, we again avail ourselves of the pen of Dr. Kelsall.

"In the cases which I have observed where the patients did not sink irrecoverably at once, from inhaling an inordinate dose of the poison, the prognosis seemed to depend on one symptom, viz., the violence or long continuance of the serous purging and vomiting; other bad symptoms appearing to depend on these. If much serum was poured into the intestines, then the cramps, &c., were proportionately severe; the sufferer became blue, and sunk to a certain point, when a crisis took place, and he gradually and slowly rose again— the stage of recovery progressing according to his ability to bear the great depletion he had undergone; providing always that this stage was not officiously meddled with by the exhibition of food or physic. But if, with sufficient constitutional strength to bear safely the depletion, the alimentary canal was burthened with the weakest aliment, or what is more, with indigestible drugs, then the patient's only chance was often destroyed. In other words, a patient unencumbered with visceral disease and enjoying strong bodily vigour, being seized with cholera, the serous depletion, with its consequent symptoms, would continue until the whole of the poison was evacuated from the blood, and then a crisis would take place, and a restorative action commence. Such, I think, would be the course of the disease if the patient were left entirely to himself, and no impediments in the shape of aliments or drugs placed in the way.

" Throughout every phasis of this disease, from the premonitory diarrhœa to collapse, and throughout the typhoid stage which too often succeeds the state of collapse, the digestive function is totally suspended. The nausea, rigors, disgust at the sight of food, the rapid passage of indigested aliments, &c. through the intestines, are sufficient indications of the condition of the alimentary apparatus at the *commencement* of an attack of cholera. The dreadful sensation of sinking at the pit of the stomach, so invariably mistaken by the patient for the pangs of hunger, during the state of collapse, and subsequent typhoid stage, is known to be a morbid symptom and not hunger, by the immediate rejection of the ingesta in most cases, either by vomiting or purging—if the cold white tongue, or bilious vomiting, were not already a sufficient guide to the state of the digestive organs. To attempt to *force* nutrition while this state of things continues, is absurd as it is pernicious ; for as nothing which is introduced into the alimentary canal can be assimilated, it must act only as a cause of irritation, and aggravate the mischief already going on.

" If the stomach is not in working order we may as well expect sawdust to be digested as beef-tea, arrow-root, &c. and to the irritation of these aliments (?) during collapse, and subsequent typhus, I am persuaded that many persons owe their deaths, who would have survived had their stomachs been kept perfectly empty and at rest : indeed, it would be easy for me to quote some decided instances of the fact.

" The presence of a little milk and water in the stomach of a person suffering under this stage of the disease being productive of such aggravation, it would not appear to require much arithmetic to calculate the effects of the chalk, calomel, turpentine, laudanum, aromatics, astringents, brandy, &c., which have been so extensively " exhibited" for the cure of this morbid state of the alimentary canal. All that need be said on the matter is, that it would have been far better to have left the unfortunate patients alone than to have complicated their cases with the sufferings of indigestion, by stuffing them with these abominations. Those who survived this treatment have little to thank it for ; they got well in spite of the drugs, and should rather rejoice that the attack was originally a mild one- (perhaps aggravated by the physic), and that their constitutions could withstand the combined effects of cholera, and the empirical means used to cure it.

"Chalk mixture, &c., may do very well as palliatives, and even cure diarrhœa when this is occasioned by the presence of an acid in the intestines; but in malignant cholera the mucous membrane of the bowels is too busily engaged in pouring out serum to have time to think about manufacturing acids; and as to the stoppage of this flow of serum by means of astringents, the thing is impossible, their very presence adding to the irritation and increasing the flood of serum, whereby the chalk and astringents are quickly swept away. Opiates are indicated, perhaps, because the patient suffers, or is expected to suffer severe spasms, but as these spasms are merely one of the symptoms of the disease, to give laudanum is only to oppose a symptom, while the blood-vessels of the bowels may continue to pour forth their serum.

The exhibition of calomel is equally empirical and injurious, for besides that its presence in the stomach is a mechanical cause of irritation, it has no power whatever to alleviate any symptom: I have seen six or seven unfortunates during the stage of reaction, in a state of severe ptyalism, in whom the symptoms were just exactly the same as in others who had taken no mercury. That is to say, they still suffered from retching and vomiting of green bilious liquid, then bilious purging, extreme prostration, and superadded, the miseries of salivation, which might well have been spared, for they would have recovered without the use of mercury at all. One patient who had been under similar treatment ten days, and was then (when I first saw him) in a state of ptyalism, still continued to suffer, not only from retching and bilious purging every half-hour, but *the cramps had not ceased,* and though taking a daily abundant allowance of rice, sago, &c., he was rapidly losing strength. On stopping this man's allowance of food, the cramps disappeared in a few hours, and he absolutely gained strength on no diet at all. Observing a rigid fast for four days, the stomach and bowels became tranquil, and then an occasional teaspoonful of beef-tea was allowed, on which he thrived, and soon convalesced. Here, then, is an example, both of the inutility of mercury, and the impropriety of harassing the disordered stomach of a cholera patient with food.

"The premonitory symptoms of cholera generally commence by loss of appetite, sometimes attended by chills and flushes of heat. Thirst—a peculiar sensation of sinking at the pit of the stomach—rumbling in the bowels, like *"the fermentation of yeast"*—slight nausea—sometimes faintness—the tongue moist, flabby, generally whitish, and the point of the tongue cold to the touch; these are the premonitory symptoms of cholera, and if at this time camphor is had recourse to, it rarely fails to remove them speedily. If these first symptoms be disregarded, the patient soon becomes affected also with diarrhœa (often painless), occasional eructations, and disposition to vomit; but even when the disease has advanced thus far, camphor will yet be often the best remedy. It will, at all events, arrest the diarrhœa with more certainty than other aromatics and astringents, without the disadvantage of imposing any labour on the disordered stomach, because of its volatile property. But, from the first moment a patient observes the peculiar sensation of *fermentation in the bowels*, he should be cautioned to cease immediately from taking any kind of food whatever, and content himself with an occasional sip of cold water until all disorder of the bowels has disappeared."

The use of camphor in epidemics is of very ancient standing. It was recommended at the time of the Black Death by Gentilis of Foligno, an Italian physician of great celebrity. His theory of the epidemic of that period appears to have been the sound one—that it depended upon a pestilential state of the atmosphere, the effects of which might be best counteracted by disinfectants. He ordered, therefore, the cleansing of houses, sprinkling the floors with vinegar, and the healthy to wash with vinegar, to smell frequently of camphor and other volatile substances, and to maintain fires of odoriferous woods. Like other followers of Galen, however, he relied too much upon bleeding and purging at the commencement of an attack, and fell himself a victim to the disease, or to this mistake.

Upon the necessity of a total abstinence from food in cases of cholera, Dr. Kensall further remarks that—

"While cholera prevailed in London, the sufferers were almost universally recommended to take food, to *strengthen* them, of which we have seen the result; for to this cause, conjoined to the liberal 'exhibition' of indigestible drugs, much of the late mortality is due; and many a case of cholera, which ran to extreme length, would speedily have been cut short, had the digestive organs been left in a state of perfect rest. Among the premonitory symptoms of cholera, loss of appetite is a common one, which of itself is a strong hint from nature to abstain from food; but the English are a people who regard with instinctive horror the slightest allusion to this remedial measure, so that the very man who would complacently bare his arm to the lancet, and submit to the loss of some two or three pounds of his vital fluid, contemplates with surprising dread the imposition of a few days' fast, even though he may have no appetite to eat.

"If the disease continues to gain ground the patient will suffer from intense thirst, heartburn, and the feeling of loss of appetite will degenerate to an intense feeling of sinking at the epigastrium, which increases till it amounts to perfect anguish, a sensation which the patient mistakes for the pangs of hunger, and is probably owing to some morbid condition of the nerves composing the solar plexus. Sometimes even an intelligent patient is aware that this feeling is not hunger, yet he imploringly demands oranges, apples, ginger-beer, milk, broth, water, &c., in large draughts, and if these be given to him they aggravate his sufferings by causing increased purging and vomiting, and anguish at the epigastrium. They must be denied and withheld with firmness, a teaspoonful of plain water only being allowed him every few minutes, besides his teaspoonful of medicine. In a few hours, if his constitution be sufficiently strong to hold out under the trial, a crisis will take place, when the whole of the poison having been ejected from the system, the purging will cease, and with it the cramps; the pulse will begin to regain a little power; warmth will return to the extremities, and to the tongue; the extreme thirst and craving for food will diminish, and the first step towards recovery will have taken place, which must not be marred by giving him food. The tongue will at this stage be found more or less furred (generally loaded and flabby), a sufficient indication that the stomach is still not in working condition, and that it must be left for a while in a state of perfect rest that it may recover itself; and be it remembered that this cannot be effected by any medical legerdemain, for there is no drug in the pharmacopœia capable of conjuring away this atony of the alimentary canal. The poison of cholera is ejected through the mucous coat of the stomach and bowels, and by the liver; in its passage through these surfaces, it acts on them as it acts on the ejected serum which it coagulates, and nothing but perfect rest will enable the surfaces to resume their healthy condition. Abstinence from every kind of aliment must therefore still be persisted in until there is decided constipation of the bowels, and the tendency to retching has entirely ceased, small quantities of weak beef-tea may then be given in teaspoonsful at a time; but even then we must feel our way with great caution, and not commit the folly of attempting to *force* nutrition. If the tongue begin to clean, the more nutritious aliment may be given, disregarding entirely the constipation of the bowels; for these two things, viz., constipation and cleaning of the tongue, will be found to proceed together, notwithstanding any preconceived prejudices to the contrary, and the bowels will in due time open a passage for themselves without the use of purgatives.

" The worst and most fatal cases are those where the patient is overtaken with cholera on a full stomach (perhaps after eating a hearty supper), and is suddenly attacked with faintness, coldness of the tongue and surface, cramps, retching and purging of rice-water dejections, and other dangerous symptoms. In dealing with such a case the treatment had better be commenced by exciting full vomiting of the undigested aliment, by means of draughts of tepid water in which a few drops of camphorated spirit have been mixed. But with the single exception of clearing the stomach of undigested aliment by means of draughts of tepid water, the patient should not be allowed to drink, however urgently he may entreat. *The stomach must be kept empty;* the prime object being to check the vomiting and purging, but this will not cease if the stomach be distended with water, or, what is worse, by gruel, arrowroot, drugs, &c.

" When the cramps, purging, vomiting, coldness, &c., have ceased, the patient must not be considered out of danger. Rice water dejections may be succeeded by a thin, scanty, fœtid, peasoup-like diarrhœa; and if this continue, and be accompanied by cerebral symptoms, his condition is still very precarious. The skin is generally cool, pulse slow and marked ; but restlessness, slight delirium, or disposition to coma, and the furred or glazed tongue, show that he is far from being convalescent. This state strongly resembles typhus, and is probably occasioned by the great loss of serum which has taken place during the rice-water purging : few who unhappily degenerate into this condition survive—from seven to twelve days, however, will decide the patient's fate.

"Post-mortem examinations of these cases show that the mucous coat of the bowels is diseased, and the mesenteric glands sympathetically enlarged ; and, therefore, it is obvious that in such a state, the digestion and assimilation of food is impossible ; to feed the patient is consequently only to present a mechanical cause of aggravation to the organic mischief which has already commenced, and hasten his end, or destroy his only chance of recovery, while total abstinence will afford that rest to the diseased tissues which alone can enable the vital power to rectify the nascent lesion of the mucous membrane.

"I have witnessed the recovery of several patients who were rapidly falling into this dangerous state, by keeping them entirely without food (in one instance for thirteen days) ; they all continued to suffer the painful sinking at the epigastrium, which is almost characteristic of the disease, and craved more or less for "victuals ;" but when, after this long fast, the tongue began to assume a more natural appearance, indicative of a return of some tonicity to the stomach, this morbid craving for food ceased, the patients very contentedly desiring only the small quantities of beef-tea which were then allowed to restore them gradually, according to the well-known rule of giving small quantities of such diet to persons whose bodily powers are brought to a low ebb by shipwreck and starvation. Under these circumstances, a boy aged eight years, was sentenced to total abstinence, at the same time that a medical gentleman prescribed "a generous diet." He fasted six days, tossing about, and incessantly raving for victuals and drink, which his dry furred tongue, thin bilious dejections, and retching, warned his intelligent mother to withhold. Then, uneasy at her son's long fast, she gave him one single teaspoonful of arrow-root made with milk, which was followed in less than ten minutes by alarming vomiting and purging, increased anguish in the epigastrium and abdomen, and delirium, which convinced her that though starvation be an extreme remedy, in it consisted the only hope of saving the life of her child. After this she gave him nothing but a few drops of cold water at a time, for seven long days ; when the tongue began to appear natural, bowels and stomach tranquil, craving for food gone, and then, feeling her way cautiously with a few tea-spoonfuls of weak beef-tea, the boy slowly convalesced, and was ultimately restored to perfect health. Had she persisted in trying experiments to force a diseased stomach to do what it is incapable of, she would have experimented away the life of her son."

We have given insertion to the above as the opinions of an old member of the Royal College of Surgeons, whose treatment of cholera we know to have been eminently successful. It may be a drawback to the estimation in which they should be held, in some quarters, that Dr. Kelsall has become a convert to the principles of homœopathy; a debateable ground where we do not follow him. The doctrine of *similia similibus curantur*, and the new theory of the superior efficacy of medicines infinitesimally diluted, in their action upon the infinitesimal tissues of the mucous membrane, doubtless contain some element of truth, and are fit subjects for discussion; but recognizing as characteristic of human nature the general tendency of strong minds to extremes, we accept the advice of intelligent men, whether homœopathists or allipathists, when it approves itself to our judgment; confining our private faith in all remedial measures to those which we think we understand.

The assertion sometimes made, that the power of the globules of the homœopathists often depends upon the imagination of the patient, whether true or not, is suggestive of an undoubted fact, with which it would be well, in seasons of epidemic, if the public, and especially the clergy, should be made fully acquainted—that the mind acts upon the organs of digestion, in impairing or strengthening their functions, *through the nervous system.*

It was formerly taught by physiologists, that the process of digestion depended chiefly upon the action as a solvent of an acidulated saliva, called the gastric juice, secreted by the glands of the stomach; but it is now generally believed that the solvent properties of the gastric juice are chiefly derived from the food itself, and that the first part of the process is a chemical action induced by the nervous system, through which some portions of the food pass through the stages of starch, sugar, alcohol, or perhaps lactic acid, and the whole is converted into the pulpy state which is termed *chyme.* It has been proved by experiment, that by a separation in the neck of an animal of the *par vagum,* or eighth pair of nerves, the functions of digestion are interrupted, and almost entirely destroyed; and it is remarkable, as showing the connexion of the nervous system with the electric fluid, and perhaps of a low state of atmospheric electricity with diarrhœa, that digestion may be renewed for a considerable time, by exposing the mutilated nerves to the galvanic action of a voltaic battery.*

---

* This subject has been ably discussed by Dr. Robert Dundas Thomson, lecturer on practical chemistry at the University of Glasgow, in his '*Experimental researches on the food of animals.*' He remarks upon the influence of

348 *Epidemics.*

We may thus account, and with tolerable clearness, for the enfeebling and other fatal effects of fear, grief, and great mental anxiety. A shock is given to the nervous system, which interrupts the process of assimilation. The food taken ceases to nourish, and perhaps becomes converted into poisonous compounds. And, on the other hand, we may see why hope, joy, and great faith in a physician, act as restoratives to health. The wonted action of the nervous system is renewed, the functions of digestion are strengthened, and the waste of the solids and fluids of the system repaired.

We would have these facts brought before the attention of the clergy, because if incontrovertible, as we regard them, it follows that the efforts which were made by many of their body to procure the sanction of government for a national fast (which it is to the credit of the present ministry that it had the firmness to resist), and their successful efforts for local fasts in different parts of the

---

the nervous system, that the pulse beats quicker the moment food has been swallowed, and that when faint with hunger we feel immediately refreshed after eating, and long before the food can have been assimilated with the blood. He adds that—

"So remarkable is the influence of even simple food on the nerves, when abstinence has been practised for some time, that it may be interesting to quote the following case, in which intoxication was produced by the stimulus of oysters alone.

"In the well known mutiny of the *Bounty*, Captain Bligh was set adrift in boats, with twenty-five men, about the end of April, in the neighbourhood of the Friendly Islands, and was left to make his way to the coast of New Holland in such a precarious conveyance. At the end of May they reached that coast after undergoing the greatest privations, the daily allowance for each man having been one twenty-fifth of a pound of bread, a quarter of a pint of water, and occasionally a teaspoonful or two of rum. Parties went on shore, and returned highly rejoiced at having found plenty of oysters and fresh water. Soon, however, the symptoms of having eaten too much began to frighten some of us ; but on questioning others who had taken a little more moderate allowance their minds were a little quieted. The others, however, became equally alarmed in their turn, dreading that such symptoms (which resembled intoxication) would come on, and that they were all poisoned, so that they regarded each other with the strongest marks of apprehension, uncertain what would be the issue of their imprudence. Similar observations have been made under other circumstances. Dr. Beddoe states that persons who have been shut up in a coal work from the falling in of the sides of a pit, and have had nothing to eat for four or five days, will be as much intoxicated by a basin of broth, as an ordinary person by three or four quarts of strong beer. In descending the Gharra, a tributary of the Indus, Mr. Atkinson states ('Account of Expedition into Affghanistan, in 1o39-40,' p. 66), that on two occasions, during the passage, he witnessed the intoxicating effects of food. To induce the Punjaubees to exert themselves a little more, he promised them a ram, which they consider a great delicacy, for a feast, their general fare consisting of rice and vegetables, made palatable with spices. The ram was killed, and they dined most luxuriously, stuffing themselves as if they were never to eat again. After an hour or two, to his great surprise and amusement, the expression of their countenances, their jabbering and gesticulation, showed clearly that the feast had produced the same effect as any intoxicating spirit or drug."

country, were, like the processions of the flagellants at the time of the Black Death, the means of spreading alarm and fear, and therefore of aggravating the evils of the calamity sought to be averted. Very numerous have been the cases recorded of persons the most *nervously* anxious to secure themselves against the infection of cholera, falling among its first victims ; and the reason is now apparent.*

Dr. Johnson observes, that the influence of fear, anxiety, or surprise, will frequently induce attacks of asthma, which is another affection of the nervous system, producing a spasmodic contraction of the bronchial tubes ;—and it is again to be remarked that the attacks of this disease, as in cholera, are the most frequent in the middle of the night, or at an early hour in the morning ; showing an analogy in the cause of both. The cure, where there is no organic mischief, is found in removal to a purer air, and in cold water ablutions of the whole body, but especially of the spine, with active exercise afterwards. To this extent the hydropathic treatment is the best that can be adopted by all who would fortify the system, whether against asthma, or any of the epidemics which have been the subject of this paper ; and its invigorating effects in bracing the nerves and improving the tone of the stomach, will not be doubted for an instant, by any one who has tried the experiment and habitually repeated it.†

It would be a work of supererogation to enter into an exposition of the remedial measures recommended in the sanitary reports and by the Health of Towns' Commissioners, for increasing the salubrity of human habitations. The necessity of drainage,—of a continuous, instead of an intermittent, water supply,—of the abolition of the practice of intramural burials,— of the removal of city slaughter-houses,—and of the prevention of overcrowding, has now been universally discussed by the press, and is beginning to be generally understood. It is reasonable to believe that some legislative and administrative fruits may now be expected from the agitation of these subjects ; and we will therefore point out only two or three practical applications of the principles they involve, which should not be overlooked.

* Public fasts are entirely of Rabbinical origin. Moses instituted public *festivals*, but not a single fast. Christ emphatically condemned even the appearing to fast in public. National thanksgiving days, are of course, open on sanitary grounds, to no other objection than that, when not held on Sundays, they are often to the poor man, fasts in disguise, which, certainly, there is no authority in the New Testament to enforce.

† ' *The Domestic Practice of Hydropathy*,' by Edward Johnson, M.D. A work to be consulted by all who would investigate for themselves the laws of health, and dispense as much as possible with the very questionable aid of the apothecary.

First, with respect to drainage. We have seen that the greatest mortality is invariably found in the *lowest lying districts.* It is with them, therefore, independently of all considerations of outfall, that the work should begin. The work may be difficult, as in London on the Surrey side of the river, where the roadway is frequently below the level of high water, but it is the first difficulty with which we should grapple.

Second, with respect to the overcrowding of habitations. It is again in low-lying districts where this overcrowding is the most fatal. The lower the level of the habitations, the greater is the necessity for their thorough ventilation. We would, therefore, have the municipal authorities of towns form a fund, to be assisted where needful with government grants, to pull down at once the houses of all back courts and alleys situate on the banks of rivers, or about the same level. In a report by Dr. Laycock, on the sanitary state of York, he has shown, that a dark and filthy court thus situated, where the cholera broke out in 1832, was the very spot where the plague first appeared in that city in 1551 and 1604.* And it is satisfactory to find, that the destruction of similar nests of pestilence at Hamburgh by the fire of 1842, and the subsequent construction, under the superintendance of Mr. Lindley, of broad and well-drained thoroughfares, has led to the nearly total exemption from cholera in 1849, of the same localities which suffered so severely in 1832.† In connexion with this object, we trust it may be permitted us to hope, that the evaporating surface of the mud banks of the Thames may at last give place to a terraced embankment, worthy the metropolis of a great empire.

And lastly, with respect to *light.* From tenderness for the position of the Chancellor of the Exchequer, the Health of Towns' Commissioners refrained from reporting upon the baneful tendencies of a system of taxation which offers a direct encouragement, in the shape of a pecuniary saving, to the blocking out of light and air, and at the same time induces habits of personal uncleanliness. The evidence collected, however, upon this subject was printed, and the responsibility of neglecting it, after the late painful visitation, will, we imagine, be too serious to be longer incurred by any government; and we anticipate, if not the abolition of the window duty, at least its commutation into a house tax in the ensuing session. Let it be remembered, that without permission to open an unlimited number of windows, no system of ventilation can be rendered perfect. It is in the

---

* First Report of the Health of Towns' Commissioners, vol. i. p. 261.
† Official Circular for January 27, 1849 ; Mr. Grainger's Report.

cellars, closets, and roofs now rendered dark by the tax-gatherer that mephitic vapours are most collected, and to disperse them we require not merely the fresh air from without, stealthily introduced by ventilating apertures, but *the warmth of the sun* to rarify the gases there confined, and facilitate their escape.

Light is also a chemical agent, and the character of the gases evolved from various substances is dependent upon its action. In the respiration of plants less oxygen, and a greater quantity of carbonic acid gas, is given out at night than by day. In the germination of *seed*, carbonic acid gas is freely liberated; a process by which the starch of the seed is converted into sugar for the nourishment of the young roots; but the seed must for this object be supplied with moisture, and *deprived of light*. It is, therefore, quite certain that in all *dark* and damp situations there is a constant vitiation of the air from the germination of the seed of mosses, or fungi. Deprived of light, however, plants, after they have appeared above the ground, will not thrive: they grow devoid of colour, and without fibre, like the *celery*, which is made white and crisp for the table by earthing up the stem. *With light*, plants gain both colour and fibre, and it is most interesting to learn that the process by which this is effected is one which at the same time purifies the air, and renders it fit for animal respiration. The carbonic acid gas, says Dr. Carpenter, " is decomposed by the green parts of the surface of plants, and the solid carbon fixed in their tissues; while the *oxygen* is set free."*

Upon the action of light upon the nervous system, and its consequent influence upon human health, a treatise might be written. Every physician can testify to the restorative effects of a gleam of sunshine, and the corresponding depression of mind and body produced by living in a gloomy apartment. But enough has been said to induce reflection, and too much earnestness has now been awakened upon sanitary questions, to permit us to doubt the result.

---

* ' Vegetable Physiology,' page 176.

ART. V.—1. *Essays on the Philosophy and Art of Land Drainage.*—By Josiah Parkes, C.E.

2.—*A Microscopic Examination of the Water supplied to the Inhabitants of London.* By Arthur Hill Hassall, M.B., F.L.S.

3.—*Review of the Report by the General Board of Health on the Supply of Water to the Metropolis.* By Samuel Collett Homersham, C.E.

4.—*Reports of the Board of Health.*

ONE of the most remarkable advances of modern improvement, is grounded on the fact originally foreshadowed by Elkington, and since worked out in a practical form by the late Mr. Smith of Deanstone, and by the author of the Essays quoted at the head of this paper, namely, that perfect cultivation requires the most expeditious and certain removal of all moisture from the roots of the crop. Mr. Parkes' papers are directed especially to the advantages of deep drains—on which point, Mr. Smith was supposed to differ from him. We do not propose, at present, to enter into the discussion and respective arguments in favour of deep or shallow drains, or we should be running a tilt with the knights in the fable; the fact is, that both kinds have their advantages in the different localities of their application. We should be inclined to advise, where there is a doubt, always to lean to the advocates of deep draining; depth will cure evils which the shallow drainer will fail to remedy, and the prime cost of materials being the same in either case, a deep drain has a very small per-centage of additional cost against it, in an economic point of view. One important fact must also be remembered, which bears strongly upon the views which we shortly propose to discuss, viz.: that springs are very rarely seated at less than four feet from the surface, and unless these are thoroughly reached we cannot expect an efficient thorough drainage. These points are philosophically, and, what is better, practically, discussed in Mr. Parkes' Essays, leaving out, however, the considerations of the secondary effects which will be produced over the distribution of streams and rivers—almost over the geographical features of our island—from the simple but certain process which is taking place, shown by the wide streaks which we see during the winter months over the arable and pasture of all the better class of estates, and by the small red pipes which lie scattered ready for threading in their narrow cells—ready messengers to receive heaven's blessed showers, whose hours of *weeping* are the joy of the husbandman.

There are few now who are wedded to the quaint notion that water is no evil to the farmer; we trust that these good folks will ere long be consigned to the oblivion of Protection and Corn Laws—we leave them to travel by the night mail to Brighton, to insist upon riding in a hackney-coach in preference to a Hansom, —such men have not yet passed through the solemn ordeal of a Highgate tavern.

It would require more room than is now at our disposal, to discuss the cost of thorough draining, or its remunerative effect upon the farm; a question which must, after all, depend upon the locality and the nature of the soil, access to good tileries, and the extent of land to be drained in one operation. We have frequently also the expense of outfall to take into consideration, which may at once add two pounds or more per acre of land drained. Practical information upon these points, when required by the landowner, is best obtained from the professional engineer, whose experience, and habit of dealing with different localities, give him great advantage over the bailiff, or the steward, who has generally quite enough wherewith to occupy his time. If the landowner wishes to be clear of responsibility and details, and cannot charge his estate with a portion of the cost, there are private land-draining companies now established, who will generally be ready, for the sum of five pounds per acre at the utmost, to send down surveyors, who will design and map out every drain on an estate, arrange the necessary loans, and finally deliver the whole of the land with a perfect thorough drainage, and with a legal self-liquidating annual charge distributed over a period of years, so that the present expense is lessened, while there is the best outlay of capital, in making at once a complete and perfect work.

One of these Land-Draining and Improvement Companies has been formed for some years in the West of England, and is sufficiently established to test the advantage of this mode of working, both to the shareholder and landed proprietor. The strength and success of these companies must consist in the efficiency of the staff of surveyors and consulting engineers whom they keep in their employ; while the extensive experience which a company must give to its employées, would render them doubly efficient and useful to the landowner who may secure their services.

A considerable portion of Mr. Parkes' Essays is devoted to the discussion of the Dalton rain-gauge, kept by Mr. Dickinson, in the valley of the Colne; and his deductions bearing upon the amount of water absorbed by the soil and the influence on its temperature, are clever and practical. The Dalton gauge shows the quantity of rain which will percolate through three feet depth of soil, being arranged with a receiver and index, to show the daily effect of the percolating surface water. The following analysis of Mr. Dickinson's register is made by Mr. Parkes, to show the effect of rain-fall in winter and summer respectively:—

ANALYSIS OF THE DALTON GAUGE KEPT AT KING'S LANGLEY, FROM 1836 TO 1843, INCLUSIVE.

Total of each Year.			
Years.	Rain.	Filtration.	Evaporation.	Rain, per Acre.
	In.	Per Cent.	Per Cent.	Tons.
1836	31.0	56.9	43.1	3139
1837	21.10	32 9	67.1	2137
1838	23.13	37.0	63.0	2342
1839	31.28	47.6	52.4	3168
1840	21.44	38.2	61.8	2171
1841	32.10	44.2	55.8	3251
1842	26.43	44.4	55.6	2676
1843	26.47	36.0	64.0	2680
Mean	26.61	42.4	57.6	2695

April to September, inclusive.							
Years.	Rain.	Filtra-tion.	Evapora-tion.	Filtra-tion.	Evapora-tion.	Rain, per acre, filtrated.	Rain, per acre, evapo-rated.
	In.	In.	In.	Per Cent.	Per Cent.	Tons.	Tons.
1836	12.20	2.10	10.10	17.3	82.7	212	1023
1837	9.80	0.10	9.70	1.0	99.0	10	982
1838	10.81	0.12	10.69	1.2	98.8	12	1082
1839	17.41	2.60	14.81	15.0	85.0	263	1500
1840	9.68	0.00	9.68	0.0	100.0	...	980
1841	15.26	0.00	15.26	0.0	100.0	...	1545
1842	12.15	1.30	10.85	10.7	89.3	131	1099
1843	14.04	0.99	13.05	7.1	92.9	100	1322
Mean	12.67	0.90	11.77	7.1	92.9	91	1192

October to March, inclusive.							
1836	18.80	15.55	3.25	82.7	17.3	1574	330
1837	11.30	6.85	4.45	60.6	39.4	693	452
1838	12.32	8.45	3.85	68.8	31.2	855	393
1839	13.87	12.31	1.56	88.2	11.8	1246	159
1840	11.76	8.19	3.57	69.6	30.4	829	362
1841	16.84	14.19	2.65	84.2	15.8	1437	269
1842	14.28	10.46	3.82	73.2	26.8	1059	387
1843	12.43	7.11	5.32	57.2	42.8	720	538
Mean	13.95	10.39	3.56	74.5	25 5	1052	360

NOTE.—The quantities of rain in the columns headed Filtration, represent the required performance of drains in retentive soils. One-tenth of an inch of rain in depth amounts to 10.128 tons per acre.

Mr. Parkes shows from these tables that of the whole annual rain about 42½ per cent., or 11.8 inches out of 26.6 inches, filter through the soil, and that the annual evaporative force is only equal to 57½ per cent. of the total rain, which falls on any given extent of earth three feet in depth. In acknowledging the value of these deductions we are not disposed to allow so great a generalization of the experiments, because the amount of absorption must vary according to the nature of the soil; a sand, for instance, would pass water through it much quicker than clay; and rocky districts again are known to cast the falling rain far more expeditiously than either; again, if the water is once absorbed to any depth below ground, the effect of evaporation is in a great measure lost. It is highly desirable that these experiments should be repeated in various districts and at different depths, and if any contrivance could be made of a rain-gauge which should also indicate the surplus water which flows from the surface in flood time (neither penetrating nor evaporating), much more light would be thrown upon the disposal of the rain, dew, and moisture of our climate. Nothing would be easier than to thorough drain, say a rood or an acre of open field, and isolate it from the adjacent ground, leading the entire products into a cistern, where they could be measured at stated intervals; we should put drains in duplicate, say at six inches and four feet in depth, so that the surface discharge would be represented, as well the percolation below; we should thus have a magnificent rain-gauge, developing much more correct results, and showing the niceties of these meteorological operations in a manner to which the ordinary gauge of nine inches or a foot in diameter, is utterly inadequate.

Returning to Mr. Parkes' conclusions, we find that only about $25\frac{1}{2}$ per cent. of the rain which falls from October to March inclusive, passes back to the atmosphere by evaporation—the tables giving a mean of 10.39 inches filtrated during this period; whereas from April to September inclusive, about 93 per cent. is evaporated, or a mean of .90 inch filtrated during this period. If we follow out this generalization we shall easily appreciate the results which thorough drainage must have, both on the produce of springs, and on the variable quality of the discharge of rivers, as we shall take occasion to explain further on. In the meantime we will ask the reader to recollect that .90 inch of rain for six months will give a mean sum of eight cubic feet per minute for each square mile; while the winter filtration of 10.39 inches will give 91.7 cubic feet per minute for each square mile, for the six months, or half that quantity, if distributed during the whole year.

Several millions sterling must have been expended in England for drainage during the last ten years; probably not less than four millions, which would represent nearly a million of acres drained, or about one-thirtieth part of the entire area of England. Now, in discussing the effects produced upon the discharge of springs and rivers by the modern system, we have rather at present to endeavour to give an idea, not of what is actually sent down to the sea from the hills and the valleys, but the new form and manner in which the water is discharged from the surface. Assuming that 2 feet of water fall upon the entire surface of our island during each year—and this is probably a minimum average of our rain-fall—we shall have a mean theoretic discharge for each minute in the year of 10¼ cubic feet* of water for each square

---

* We give our measures in cubic feet, as more within reach of figures; a cubic foot contains 6¼ gallons; a square mile giving a minimum of eight cubic feet per minute, will afford about 70,000 gallons per diem, or a supply of 30 gallons per head for 2,333 people.

mile; but it is pretty certain that absorption of some kind will take up, waste, or evaporate about 1 foot of this amount;* the method is not clearly known. We shall then have an average quantity of 53 cubic feet per minute left as due to every square mile of ground in Great Britain. These calculations, however, are assumed on a basis of averages; we have other causes, which influence our streams, in the faults and fissures that may pervade the rocks; in the nature of the soil receiving moisture; and in the amount of local rain-fall, which varies from 5 and 6 feet per annum down to 16 inches in the small length and breadth of Great Britain. We happen to have experimented and gauged considerably, ourselves, over all portions of this country, and we find that the ordinary mean summer run of English rivers may be safely assumed as varying from 8 to 15 cubic feet per minute for each square mile; there are exceptions which give a much higher ratio, caused either by extensive mountain morasses at their heads, forming natural store reservoirs; and sometimes rivers are increased considerably in volume, relatively to the area they drain, by internal collections of water which pervade flat, or slightly-inclining stratifications, as the red sandstones, whose waters gush out in the form of springs at the line of weakest outward pressure, generally at some great fault or outcrop of the collecting stratifications. We will assume, then, that the mean summer run L. taken of any given stream—the Thames, for instance, at Staines, discharges in summer about a mean of 13 cubic feet per minute for each square mile of drainage area, representing 3 inches in depth of rain-fall per annum; but if 12 inches of rain pass off from the drainage area, there will remain an amount of 9 inches, or 40 cubic feet per minute, on a mean of the whole year, which is discharged at times when the river is above its ordinary run. But let us assume that by an extension of thorough drainage, one half the entire area draining into the valley of the Thames became subject to the increased velocity of discharge during wet weather, that will prevail when such an object is effected—if the summer storing power, so to term it, of the

---

* We would call the attention of meteorologists to a great discrepancy between the results of evaporation, according to ordinary experiments, when added to the quantity of water which is known to pass off any given district. Mr. Luke Howard's experiments show, on an average of three years, that while 23 inches of rain fall, 21 inches of rain evaporate; now it is certain that the above difference of two inches of rain would not supply springs, and loss from water passing off in form of heavy rain. Our experiments on a large scale would lead us to believe that much, or all, of the diurnal evaporation would not be supplied by dew, and that this action and reaction extends enormously beyond any recorded experiments; the ordinary rain-gauge does not indicate dew. We do not know any field of science less trodden than this.

valley of the Thames be worth 3 inches of rain per annum, it is certain that efficient thorough drainage would reduce this storing power by one half.

But to carry out the analogy still farther, we must bear in mind the fact, that the mean discharge of the Thames in the spring is probably equal to about the rate of 6 inches per annum during the four months of weather commencing with March (neither very moist nor very dry), when the effect of winter rains is still developing itself in the increased discharge of all the tributaries to the great arterial line of river. Now, if by increased facility of drainage, one half of this 6 inches be entirely delivered from the soil within a few hours on the occasion of rain-fall—which is a well-known fact on efficiently thorough drained estates, for the heavy spring-supplying rains generally fall in comparatively a few hours—we shall have a true idea of the revolution which may be effected by this small and slight process, when extended over a breadth of country.*   The above reasoning will easily show the conclusion, that an assumed increase of thorough drainage above-named, will have the effect of reducing the ordinary run of the Thames at Staines, during the four summer months, say of July, August, September, and October, by about 25 per cent.; and during the spring months by not less than 50 per cent., or a mean of about 33 per cent. loss of water-power during that portion of the year when it is most valuable. If we apply this to the minor streams, whose volume is not only used for power, but for the supply of water to our rapidly growing towns and cities, we shall readily see the difficulties and the remedies which will present themselves to the most superficial observer, and the danger of interfering with rivers without artificial assistance.

It is not altogether certain but that we shall experience, in regard to the laws which affect the discharge of moisture falling upon the earth, a revolution fully as great as that we have endeavoured to outline—the law of absorption by the earth under natural circumstances is entirely subversed when thorough drainage is applied, and a shower of rain is delivered from an acre of well-drained ground in as many hours as it had probably taken weeks to pass off, when in its pristine state—and thus the natural stores of water, formerly supplying the springs, are cut off, and they necessarily run dry.

---

* Not far from London, a few years since, some millers combined to cut for their stream a new channel through a small piece of boggy ground in the upper part of the valley; to their chagrin they found, shortly after, a visible difference in the supply of water-power, which has not since recovered itself.

These are not mere theories—they are strikingly exemplified in the hill-pasture districts and moors in North Britain, drained by the Tweed, Esk, Tay, Teviot, and other beautiful mountain streams of that many-showered country; there are few of these rivers that have not lost many of their bridges by floods, or *speats* as they are called; their districts are naturally subject to floods, especially in the Lammas period of the year (whence the term "Lammas floods"),—and with this, entire counties have been scored with "sheep drains" for improving the pastures—small open cuts, about 15 inches wide, and 12 inches deep, with the soil turned over on the down side. These drains follow across the steepest line of slope diagonally, at suitable intervals, and are again carried into intersecting drains, sloping at an easier angle to the nearest burn, or over the braes into the river itself; on every shower these drains pour out a flood with surprising rapidity, and away goes the river, as the author of the 'Handbook of Spain' describes of the floods of that country, like a *flight of stairs;* thus the Lammas floods of 1847 removed two considerable viaducts on the North British Railway, and did other damage; and on all the rivers of Scotland we are universally informed, that floods rise to a height and with a suddenness quite unknown in former years. It requires no great process of reasoning to perceive, that if water is delivered with this rapidity, there must be less of it at other seasons; or in other words, the equality of the stream must be very seriously affected by artificial drainage: and such is universally the complaint in the cultivated parts of Great Britain. If then there is an economic demand for water, either as mill power, or as supply to a town, new considerations have arisen out of the modern practice of drainage of a wide-spreading character, that only require generalizing to gather a true force,—a revolution arising out of a simple, and, in detail, small operation; we have only to add to this element of our problem the enormous increase in the use of steam power, the consequent growth of manufactories into and around populous districts,—they again begetting a populative action and reaction—engine succeeds engine—power accumulates power—factory and loom demand their tiny attendants—push forward together in the relentless march of competition; but all must be fed, both steam and human engine, and to each the staff of life is water—we have attempted to depict a cycle of necessities, a great revolution in our means of life—the corn land must be drained to enable the farmer to feed us, but the river must not be permitted to run dry, or the mill which grinds will stop; and the population which has risen like magic upon its banks, will be deprived of their supply.

Concurrently with this revolution, it becomes requisite for the sake of purity to collect higher sources of the stream, and to call in artificial aid to remedy the sudden discharge of floods; if it be necessary to continue the mill power the same steam engine which has tended to the change, can be applied as a far more efficient substitute for the water power, which is either lost or abstracted. Thus to remedy, in an artificial manner, the sudden discharge of water and consequent falling off during droughts, we should as necessarily require enormous reservoirs to store perhaps three months' of our demand, as our village neighbour requires an ample barrel to catch the rain from the eaves, which, without such precaution, would run to waste all the valuable soft water thrown from her roof. Hence any system of rendering available, on a great scale, the purer upland waters, will be total failures, unless accompanied by the above named useful but costly water-butt. Away then at once with the fiction—that for supplying water to the greatest metropolis in the world, we are to drain and delve after the imaginary springs of 100,000 acres of sands, which would fluctuate in supply like an April shower—at rainy periods when a metropolis requires but little water, having an over due supply, and in droughts when, from the peculiar habits of a London season, sometimes 40 per cent. more water is required than the mean demand, having empty services —not to mention the deficiency which would occur in years of extraordinary demand, such as may take place during the exhibition of 1851, if accompanied by a hot summer.

To add to these elements of the problems of sanitary adaptation to the wants of an overwhelming population, we have only to look at our own noble river, and mark the progress of its defilement —now where a thousand sewers are pouring their fœtid contents, where gas works uncontrolled are sending their noisome refuse on the banks, the slightest agitation serving to develope the imprisoned gases of decomposition—we had in our youth a fine stream of water, which was potable as far as London bridge, if not at any portion of its course. We give this as a flagrant instance of the general fact, that the once brawling streams, laughing and glittering over pebbly beds—where the village Rebecca might be seen at the fountains—are rapidly disappearing wherever population and manufactories are on the ascendant; and we must go to the Eskdales of North Britain, or to the bright streams of Cambria, to witness any longer the natural application of our rivers to the economic purposes of a scattered population. In seeking, then, for a supply of water for our populous places, we are driven by the force of circumstances to search for our sources, and to design their adaptation under new conditions, and there is nothing novel in the profound and sagacious proposition, that the *nearer* the source the *purer* the supply; the novelty perhaps would lie in the possibility of such a *non-sequitur* as the following,—that the *nearer* the source the more *plentiful* the supply. These problems are not always synonymous, and they pourtray the exact point where the theorist, the chemist, or the microscopist, and the civil engineer are apt to differ.

If we take nature for our guide, we shall find that excessive purity of water is never continued far beyond the first ebullition of the spring from its bed. The tendency to growth of all kinds of microscopic animal and vegetable species in very pure waters, is only checked by large volume, or by hardness caused by salts of lime or other minerals in solution; we shall therefore invariably find, that when the slopes of rivers are sudden and quick, and water is plentiful, it is generally soft; but on the other hand, when we get into the plains where the streams are sluggish, and not great in volume, they become hard, —a beautiful natural check upon the tendency to vegetate, which would otherwise rapidly choke up and spoil the supply. We are far from advocating the use or selection of a hard water for town supplies, but we feel that an unscrupulous advocacy of soft water, will be likely to lead us into evils of a worse tendency.

Mr. Hassall's book contains some clever and ingenious pictures of the denizens of the waters, pure or impure, which metropolitan hydropathists are condemned to drink. He pourtrays visible reasons for condemning some of the sources of water; but, from not being acquainted with the engineering features of the various water-works, our author's conclusions are frequently drawn from supposed arrangements, which were discontinued and remodelled twenty years since. He would have done great benefit to science by his facts, if he had given us chemical analyses of the several waters experimented upon, so that the constituent elements of the Fungi, Algæ, Diatomaceæ, &c., should be determined; and we should then have known the chemical nature of the inhabitants of our waters. In each imperial gallon of the general chalk-district waters supplying London, we have about a grain of silica, forming the delicate reedy fragments which flit across the microscopic field, relics of the bamboos and palm-trees of this invisible world, and forming miniature coal-fields and shales, at the bottom of our tanks. The entire of the remaining objects under Mr. Hassall's microscope appear to be represented in the chemical analysis, by from half-a-grain to two grains of " organic matter," which is not detrimental to health according to the general opinion of toxologists. The remaining chemical constituents of the better class of

London waters are, common salt about two grains, and carbonate of lime twelve to fourteen grains; making, with minor constituents, about eighteen grains *in toto* of solid matter, per imperial gallon—this predominant *bi-carbonate* of lime, of all others, is the one most readily precipitated by boiling, and one whose substitution by other constituents is most to be avoided.

We find, on a careful perusal of the analysis of the various waters flowing from the Bagshot sands, made by Professor Brande and Mr. Warrington, that they contain from ten to twelve grains of solid matter per imperial gallon, of which one to four grains are common salt, one to two grains are carbonate of lime, one to two and a half grains form organic matter, with one to two grains of sulphates, which chemists generally regard with suspicion; the remaining constituents being silica, carbonate of soda, magnesia, &c. But a more flagrant contrast between the chalk streams which supply London, such as the Lea, the Coln, and the Darenth, is shown in what any observer can practically believe, that these streams are bright, pure, and limpid, fit for use by the most capricious; while in following the Bagshot streams to their source, we find them perfectly unfit for use; so much so, that the inhabitants of their localities are unable to use them for domestic purposes, when flowing at their very doors.*

The eminent chemists whose report is before us have the following remarks generally attached to their numerous specimens of Bagshot-heath waters which they have analyzed,—" *Turbid, opalescent, of an ochreous tinge ;—depositing ochreous matter—inodorous, vapid :*" again, " *Opalescent, dark ochreous tinge, and a large flocculent ochreous deposit —inodorous, soft, slightly chalybeate.*" It would throw great additional light on the microscopic nature of these extremely soft waters, if Mr. Hassall would examine and give in his next edition a picture of the cause of the *opalescence* here referred to ;—it is a common property of the Bagshot class of waters. We ourselves visited the scene of the speculations of the Board of Health, during last summer, and found the waters black, turbid, and filthy, on the day after a slight rain, and fully bearing out the above description.

The sole point of doubt, then, between the waters, *as they might be* conveyed to London, under *improved plans or modern adaptations*, consists in the comparative softness of their different sources ; *even if other things were equal* as to mode of collection and delivery, we have merely a loss of soap to the disadvantage

---

* Mine hostess at Bagshot complains most loudly of the iron-moulded state of her snowy aprons " since she left Windsor." We fear that no good housewife would wish to save soap on such terms.

of the chalk waters. The Board of Health and their engineers appear to have forgotten—it is perhaps, after all, more a matter for the laundress—that water loses about two-thirds of its chalk in boiling, without which process this useful personage is not in the habit of attempting to remove the smoke of London, at all events.

Mr. Napier, in his improved edition of the Board's scheme, lowers the softness of their proposed water supply from about four degrees of hardness to one degree—a quality which would render the supply absolutely poisonous and dangerous unless we were to spend at once two or three millions sterling in removing every leaden pipe and tank in the metropolis, substituting, we suppose, some pipes of glass or earthenware—a scheme similar to one for stone pipes which ruined some companies when attempted about thirty years since.

It is easy to get up evidence upon any view of a case if there are no opponents ; but facts are stubborn, and the actual poisoning of families—the ready proof which any one may obtain for himself, by putting a piece of lead for a few hours into a glass of rain water—are worth a hundred sublimated theories drawn from returns of the soap duties, and the statistics of the China trade and the tea-pot.*

A public Board, with a staff of paid servants at their command, has a great advantage in promulgating any peculiar doctrine or impracticable theory ; the chief has only to assert that small pipes will carry as much water as large ones, and away starts forth a band of apostles who preach little pipes to the wondering officers of the local Boards, not to mention the extraordinary magic of an internal glaze which lasts through perhaps a week of practical operation. Say gathering grounds are to give you water, and you

---

* Remarkable evidence has been adduced of impurity of water, by producing eels and other strange *tenants* from the mains of waterworks—these are occasionally obtained in London where nothing can have got into the pipes more than one twelfth of an inch in diameter. Strange to say, in the limpid streams which flow from the wells near Trafalgar-square, fish are sometimes found ;—a fact which has sometimes caused suspicion on the part of water companies whose works they approach—the fountains are clearly enough supplied from wells—the origin of fish is somewhat mysterious. Well-water from the chalk is very remarkable in its extraordinary power of generating Algæ, which formed a serious nuisance in the Orange-street cisterns, and also in the Naval School Baths at Greenwich, both supplied from very deep wells. The only solution of this remarkable phenomenon is, that myriads of the imprisoned seeds are washed out from the crevices of the chalk and sand beds, and germinate on their exposure to light. This beats mummy wheat hollow—and carries one back to the actual shedding of seeds in the heated climate of a former age : still remaining fruitful although gathered from the vast morasses where saurians were accustomed to wallow, and when yet our coal beds were uncarbonised.

must universally adopt the idea like the tailor in the Flying Island. "Trial works" are to be adopted regardless of expense, and in defiance of all practical experience; while their successors are to spend as much in their demolition and reconstruction, as may be witnessed at this moment in various parts of the metropolis. If we were not a *practical* people it would be impossible to account for any success in great national works, considering the extraordinary nature of appointments which are occasionally made; but for this it would be impossible to carry on the engineering executive control of the Board of Health (whose powers are supposed to extend to the smallest sewer in every town in England and Wales), without placing it under the management of some skilful and experienced man who should have the penetration to divide theory from practice, and to sift out charlatanism from common sense; such services are to be bought, and would save their annual cost every week, when the real expenditure in drainage works had commenced. At present, swarms of sappers are located in the rural towns, extending their expensive operations around them, where, unless each becomes a Manchester, there will be not a building within a hundred years. The present style of management of these sanitary outriders may do very well for the provinces; but the metropolis will require something more practical for the improvement of its water supply, than is contained in the document issued from Whitehall.

To test the capacity of government water schemes, we need not travel further than the establishment at Trafalgar Square, where well water was once supposed to be of unlimited quantity and undoubted quality; as to the latter, it is found to contain 70 grains of salts per imperial gallon; as to quantity, there have been great and expensive works recently added with a view of increasing the supply. According to the statements of the advocates of the well system, more than about 100 cubic feet per minute is scarcely expected, or the amount due to twelve inches of rainfall upon two square miles of area; while the excessive pumping of these wells has been alleged to cause serious damage in abstracting or lowering the water in the neighbouring ones. The history of the Trafalgar-square water-works would be an instructive one for the political economists of the Cobden school, to whom we commend this field for their industry and reform. The Chelsea Company supplied various government establishments at a moderate rental, and offered to include the fountains for an addition of £400 a year : however, it was thought that an expenditure of £18,000, with an annual charge of £350 per annum, would supply the fountains and all the Government establishments with an ample supply of water. The works were executed ; mains were laid in all directions, many of which were destined never to receive water from the new source ; the Chelsea Company must now have got back much of their rental ; the government have spent perhaps £40,000 on their pet project, and the annual expenses must be nearer £800 a year than the original estimate—making, with repairs and liquidation of capital, an annual charge of about £3,000 per annum, to effect a saving of, perhaps, £1,000. It would be impossible to find dearer, or, chemically speaking, more impure water than is afforded by this specimen of central management.

The importance of supplying London with a large and pure supply of water, demands a searching inquiry, by a legal and impartial tribunal, who can take proper evidence upon the subject from those who are competent to offer opinions and measure the difficulties of the subject. Indeed it is almost an insult to common sense, to offer to the public opinions and designs— such as have been issued from Whitehall—entirely without that foundation in practical experience but for which our great public works would be nonexistent, and we might be still travelling express to Manchester at nine miles per hour.

We have, first, the ' Report of the General Board of Health on the Supply of Water to the Metropolis,' heralded by the trumpet of expectation ; a new district is discovered, and soft water is to reward the patience and pertinacity of rate-payers ; thousands of pounds are to be saved on soap ; not to say the reform in our laundresses' bills by diminished scrubbing of our linen ; all which is faithfully calculated and deposed to, in this singular document, by witnesses who are all on one side*!! The whole style of this report is well exposed in Mr. Homersham's pamphlet, which also contains some valuable remarks from Mr. Toulmin Smith the barrister, on the illegal and unconstitutional manner of getting up one-sided evidence after the fashion of these reports. This document is now so thoroughly dead that it is useless and ungracious to waste words upon it ; sufficient condemnation of it is to be found in Mr. Napier's report, whose *new light* completely extinguished the Bagshot scheme for supplying London with water, by broadly admitting that there is not a possibility of forming reservoirs to collect the rain-fall, which was to have been artificially gathered together by a system of pipe drainage. The new plan is to draw together the springs,

---

* The only practical and independent suggestions in the report, which bear upon the sources and modes of supply, are those by Capt. Vetch, R. E., shown upon general map attached, but which are not neglected or carefully slurred over in this report.

pure from the fountain head, over a tract of country probably 30 miles long, and 15 to 20 wide;* the surveyors *appear* to make out a case of *quantity*, but possibly have forgotten, after tapping the barrel, to await its running out; springs rising out of sands are not *free*, and we suspect that they have been opened out for gauging, but that this operation has not been extended so as to ascertain what their real *minimum* supply may be.

This indeed has always proved the weak point of previous attempts, to supply towns from springs—they fail when most required; and it has been universally found in any system of collecting springs, that unless we have reservoirs of ample size, the whole will turn out a failure. We happen to have a striking instance of the failure of the exact method of collecting springs, now proposed for London, in the mode originally adopted for the supply of the City of Edinburgh. The Pentland-hills are only from 7 to 9 miles distant from the city, and those portions of them more immediately available, are about 20 square miles in extent; their geological form is highly suited to the full development of springs, and the feeling of the executive of the water company (established about 30 years since), was strongly in favour of collecting springs in precisely the manner proposed by Mr. Napier. This was done to a great extent, with the additional aid of a very large reservoir for catching floods, constructed in a gorge of the hills, which in point of fact, gave on the average about three times the discharge of the springs of the district; in spite of this aid, and an average rain-fall double that of Middlesex, the supply in dry years totally failed. The company, however, would not be taught by experience, and again extended the system over an adjoining district with a different drainage area; never-failing springs were reached, and glazed pipes duly conveyed to the city, water of a very high character and quality; again with the present autumn have the works entirely failed in their powers of supply. Fortunately the error was arrested in time, and an Act of Parliament was obtained for extended reservoirs (not yet completed), which will enable the city to be securely and amply supplied; but the evidence upon which the new act was granted, after a most

---

* The new gaugings include springs twenty-five miles apart (as the crow flies), which would require independent conduits, thirty miles and twenty-five miles in length respectively; the estimates for conducting all the springs could be disproved by the merest tyro in engineering; a brick tunnel is to convey the water to Wimbledon, at a high level, for £168,000; this would be twenty-five miles in length, and about seven miles would be eighty feet above ground. To give London springs which supply Dorking is a shrewd notion—to offer compensation would be like passing an Act to make it lawful to be robbed and murdered on Bagshot Heath.

searching ordeal and opposition by rivals, was that the really magnificent springs belonging to the company were occasionally liable to failure. The entire produce of the springs extending over 15 square miles of mountain, has fallen as low as 300 cubic feet per minute, without *estimating compensation* to mills and other sources of water privileges which must be especially provided for in extreme droughts.

This amount of 300 cubic feet per minute, is equal to a supply for 90,000 people; we can therefore easily reckon what population could be supplied from a district of ten times the area, but having about one-third the rain-fall over the higher water-bearing strata. To give a stronger turn to Mr. Napier's proposition, he gravely proposes to allow the metropolis a reservoir holding 4 days' supply; with the minimum above stated in the Edinburgh case, there were reservoirs capable of holding about 200 days' supply. The fact is, that any dependence upon springs for water required in a wholesale way, has universally failed; springs are cut, a volume of sparkling water is poured out, and the imagination supposes the supply inexhaustible—to be disproved by the reality of the absence of rain, and drought, which generally comes in a cycle of years in these temperate climates.

To endeavour to bolster up a project, which to themselves was evidently incapable of supplying sufficient water, the Board start a novel proposition, containing, of all others, a doctrine the most dangerous to a beneficial supply of water, viz., that the quantity necessary for London can be enormously reduced below even the present limited supply, with advantage to all parties; grounding their opinion on some reports made to them of the quantity of water passing through sewers, which are wholly irrelevant to the purpose. Mr. Homersham exposes this fallacy, so as to show the extremity to which we should be reduced, according to the new projectors; "if, as according to the Board, 45 million gallons of water per day be delivered into the metropolis, and 30 million gallons are daily wasted, it would follow that 15 million gallons is the actual daily consumption. Deducting from this 15 millions the 5 millions conjointly used for the supply of the wholesale consumer, for the watering of roads, for the flushing of sewers, and for the extinguishing of fires, there will remain 10 millions for the domestic supply of the 270,581 houses shown to be supplied by the metropolitan companies, or 37 gallons per house per day, which at $7\frac{1}{2}$ persons per house, comes to 5 gallons per head; from these 37 gallons per day let there be deducted 15 gallons as the ordinary supply of a water-closet to such a household, and only 22 gallons per house per day remain for private baths, horses, stables, washing carriages of all kinds, and frequently the

watering of gardens, independent of washing, drinking, and culinary uses; for, under the title of house or domestic consumption,
the water supplied by the companies for all these purposes is
included. 22 gallons per house corresponds to 3 gallons per
individual per day, which is manifestly insufficient for all the
purposes above enumerated."

We forbear to enter into the expense of collecting springs, and
the frightful claims on compensation and damage where water is
thus taken in detail, claims which, in the neighbourhood of the
metropolis, would be necessarily very serious. The loss of capital
in this plan of proceeding, may be found in papers presented to
Parliament in the case we have quoted; all which we beg to
offer to Mr. Napier's consideration when he amends his estimate,
containing £100,000 for land and compensation.

Having thus freely expressed ourselves on the plans proposed
by the Board of Health for supplying London with water, we
would most carefully guard ourselves from being misunderstood,
as *advocating* the cause of the present companies, and their
modes and sources of supply. There is, undoubtedly, much to con-
demn; but we are far from thinking that the mutual check of these
great bodies, who are extremely jealous of each other, may not be
valuable to the consumers. The consumption of water is not ex-
pansible, nor is it a manufactured article, like gas; any attempt
at coalition and centralization will have its attendant evils, and
certainly the most recent and successful attempts at amalgamation, that of the Southwark and Vauxhall Companies, was not
by any means advantageous to the public, although so highly
paraded by the Clay school of economists. Imagine that within
several years two companies should have united, to do no better
than erect works for pumping from the Thames below Battersea-
bridge, with a suction pipe, opposite the Ranelagh and King's
Scholar's pond sewer, and only half a mile above the great gas
and bone-grinding establishments at Vauxhall—*ecce signum*—
in the tall clean standpipes and chimneys near the Nine Elms
station. We should earnestly advise the present water companies to beware of paying high dividends, and rather to reserve
their surplus profits to meet the spirit of the times and the unavoidable march of events and of improvement. The steward-
ship is an important one, and we believe that there is every
reasonable chance of such an extension of the metropolis, as to
make either new efforts by the present companies, or new companies for the outlying districts, a certain and safe investment
of capital, with the additional advantage of doing common justice
to the water-rate payers, who are entitled to be heard in their
cry for reform, although one may be not disposed to accede to

them a vote in the management of concerns which require careful attention, and that kind of energy and control which is only to be found successfully applied by those with whom it is a pocket question.

Let us for a moment sketch the geological features of the districts encircling London, as the question of water supply must at all times be contingent on the economic position of the town to be supplied, in relation to the surrounding country. Proceeding a short distance from the Tring station of the North Western Railway, we shall find ourselves on the line dividing the waters flowing north and south, from the chalk range called the Chiltern-hills — their summits are, like all the hills which surround London, from 300 to 500 feet above the sea, and having few water-courses, but *apparently* absorbing a great deal of the rain which falls upon the surface. Travelling westward, we shall find that the back or north of the Chiltern-hills drains into the river Thame, which flows westwards for many miles, and gradually sweeping round, joins with the Isis near Oxford, and forms the Thames-Isis, or Thames : this river passing on by the town of Reading (where it receives the Kennet, which is to a great degree shed from a chalk and lime-bearing country), cuts through the edge of the chalk basin in the beautiful valley extending from Henley to Maidenhead, and consequently obtains all the chemical characteristics of a chalk stream.

Recommencing at Tring, and travelling eastwards, we have the heads of the various streams issuing from the chalk hills, and the vast natural filter-beds of sands and gravels which cover the whole of East Hertfordshire, from 5 to 20 feet in depth. These streams, gathering strength as they go, converge to a point within a short distance of Hertford, where they all collect and form the river Lee, on the banks of which Izaak Walton loved to ramble, and whose pure waters are proverbial. This river falls into the Thames *below London*, and thus renders any abstraction for the use of the metropolis, an aid to the general scouring power of the Thames; an object which is rather lost sight of, by those who advocate the abstraction of this more important river at a distant point, by carrying it at a high level into London, and thus would despoil the main river of a valuable share of its volume, for a distance of forty miles.

Passing across the Thames at Blackwall, we reach the district formed by the chalk ranges of North Kent, having a character somewhat similar to those of Hertfordshire, but more destitute of the capping sands and gravels; they do not form great leading valleys like those of the Lee, but rather shed their waters direct into the Thames, and thus are more difficult of application for affording water for London. On the Darenth and the Cray there are, nevertheless, opportunities of obtaining water, rendered somewhat difficult by the establishments which their volume and purity have created on the line of stream. The foregoing characteristics lead us up the Thames as far as the mouth of the Wey, near Hampton Court, which drains a large chalk district, and partakes of the usual hard character of these waters. This river bears some of the waters draining from the Bagshot sands, which fill the area of country remaining between the chalk valley of the Thames at Henley, before described, and the high ground forming the last appearance of the chalk range between Guildford and Farnham. It is this gap, covered with the Bagshot sands, and having an area of about 100 square miles, which contains the enormous supply of water reported to the Board of Health— a quantity which is entirely contradicted by the gaugings of Mr. Rennie and Messrs. Mylne and Fulton, and not borne out by any streams, rivers, or feeders to justify such an assumption; and, as we have before pointed out, having no natural capabilities for forming reservoirs where the falling rain might be caught and stored by any artificial system.

We have here endeavoured to describe generally a circuit of some 120 to 150 miles round London, as if swept by a pair of compasses, with a radius of twenty-five miles on the north and north-western side of London, extending the length to thirty miles in the Bagshot direction, and contracting our available reach of water-shed to fifteen or twenty miles on the southern side, where the ranges which turn the streams into other valleys are somewhat nearer home. The reader will perceive that any *economic considerations* of conveying water from its source, or from above the influence of the sewerage of the various towns and villages round London, must be much influenced by the distance to be traversed, and the height at which water can be drawn from the hills and delivered in London ; in fact, that the *cost of the article* is a matter which requires judgment, as well as *the quality*, otherwise we could recommend no better plan than a grand chemical establishment for distillation, or other doctoring process. The London water-rate payer will require an *ample and constant supply of good wholesome water*, at a price not higher than the lowest scale now charged by any existing company, and we believe that the demand of manufacturers, and the increased charge which the wealthy class of houses are always, on principle, made to pay for their more luxurious modes of supply, should enable companies to offer the poor a far better supply than is now given. For if the rich man, who has servants at his command, requires water laid on, and, in effect, all the advantages of constant service, how much more the poor man, whose time is essentially his daily bread,—who has poverty to contend with, and the consequent absence of those adventitious aids and assistance which wealth can purchase! We believe that much amendment might be at once made in the supply of poorer tenements by improved and extended powers of the Building Act, over the third and fourth-rate class of houses; a little practical philanthropy exercised in this direction would be quite as useful as speculations on the possible saving in soap, or the reasons why a hard-working man prefers beer to water—and the probability of his resorting to teetotalism, if we could give him very soft water to drink.

Among the numerous schemes which have been prepared for the next session of Parliament, for better supplying water to the whole or part of the metropolis, it is singular that the Board of Health project, although open to the public, has not found any one to pay the expense of the necessary plans, so as to give it a position before the Legislature. We are to have pure spring water from Watford on the north; on the south the Wandle is to be relieved of sewerage, and pumped up for supplying the district which it traverses; in the west, the Thames is to be delivered from Henley; and in the east, immense reservoirs are to be formed in the valleys of the Lee, while the *Old* New River is to be straightened, enlarged, and shortened in its windings, by twelve miles out of forty, so as to carry the great additional volume of water, which would be available for London, at the elevation of Islington. This plan is designed to give, by means of the reservoirs, that amount of soft water stored at flood time, which, mixed with the pure chalk-borne streams of the district, would offer a moderately soft water to the consumer, in lieu of the present undoubtedly hard supply. The principle of this project was in fact to a great extent sanctioned by the legislature during last session. We will leave for the present the discussion of these several plans, feeling assured, that Parliament will not allow another session to pass, without deciding fairly on the merits of each, and all of the rival schemes.

THE CONTAGIOUS CHARACTER OF CHOLERA.*

THE author's object in this little volume is to establish that doctrine which denies any contagious character in the present epidemic, and refers its propagating causes to those which are annually in operation. He also denies the existence of any new features in the disease, excepting what belong to an increased severity of their form ; several epidemics are referred to as having created much more havoc than the cholera, and it is assumed that this and the last year have been singularly unpropitious for physicians, notwithstanding the cry of " cholera ;" old medical writers are cited, who are said to have known the disease in this country ; and its Asiatic origin, in 1817 or 1818, is, of course, denied.

This is all very well, and does credit to the author's reading ; but it has entirely failed in attempting to convert us from our belief, and dispelling our fears, of the epidemic being of a *communicable* nature. All infectious diseases differ in the degree and mode of communication ; and while cholera is perfectly capable, we believe, of becoming infectious or contagious, it does not appear to be so in as high a degree as other diseases ; and yet even the most virulent do not affect all constitutions at all times : Nature, while she permits mankind to be afflicted with diseases of an epidemic and infectious quality, provides us with the property of counteraction.

The more we see and hear of this remarkable disease — so sudden in its invasion, and so rapid in its course — the more we feel convinced of its Asiatic origin and new character, and the more we are disposed to place confidence in the sanitary regulations recommended. At the same time, we doubt the efficacy of the quarantine laws, and are disposed to think lightly of the parade of fumigating baggage, cloths, stuffs, &c. &c. We are but little if at all informed as to the nature of this disease, and its laws of propagation ; and frequently we see instances of its breaking out independently of any direct source of infection, at least such as can be demonstrated. Apparently we are no nearer ascertaining the exact laws of its propagation than we were before the disease appeared ;

but when we attentively study its progress, we cannot refuse our admission that it is identified with the spasmodic cholera which first made its appearance in central India about the latter end of 1817 or the beginning of 1818. Has it appeared at distant places in various quarters of the globe simultaneously ? Certainly not ; and if we regard its progress, it has generally come when expected, according to past observation. We trace it gradually from Russia to Hamburgh ; and then, the country being filled with alarm and in full expectation of its appearance, it breaks out upon *the opposite shore of Great Britain*, having no interposed land to rest upon, just as it has now broken out in America, having reached the western ports of England and the coast of Ireland.

We question not the fact on which Dr. Webster insists, that fruit and other indiscretions in diet, as to quantity and quality, predispose to or excite cholera. These causes have so operated constantly, and produce violent but less fatal symptoms, which, from their resemblance to the premonitory symptoms of the epidemic, have caused the latter to be distinguished by the same appellation. Dr. Webster, &c. may, however, write and say what they please upon the question of the newness of the disease to us, but they never will persuade us that it is merely an exaggerated form of the ordinary bilious cholera. Its main symptoms and peculiarities are quite distinct and perfectly novel, and most strongly force upon us the conviction that patients labouring under the Asiatic form of the spasmodic cholera have imbibed some morbid poison ; but whether from the air alone, or the air tainted by the presence of the cholera, and from what peculiar state of the atmosphere, we are unable to determine. Several suggestions have been made upon this point, but none that have been conclusive.

In the north of England, flights of insects, of excessive minuteness, are said to have been observed in places where cholera raged, to have preceded it in infected places, and to have had, at their departure, a coincident decrease and subsidence of cholera cases. Dr.

* An Essay on the Epidemic Cholera, being an Inquiry into its new or contagious Character ; including Remarks on the Treatment, &c. &c. By John Webster, M.D.

Prout examined the weight of the atmosphere about London, and found it to be specifically heavier than usual.

While, however, we must believe the present cholera (evidently on the spread) to be a different one from that which usually becomes frequent in the fruit season, it is quite evident that the same causes may excite both, and that a neglected state of the digestive organs under irritation is a very common foundation of the complaint, leading to its premonitory symptoms; while, if these last be not stopped, the patient may fall into a complete state of the Asiatic or blue cholera.

" On the 18th of May, clean bills of health were issued to the ships, the cholera having subsided," says Dr. Webster; and we ask him where is it *now*, or, rather, where is it not? It has been and is in the north, and in the east, and is now getting south and west; — it has been and is now in Paris, sweeps Belgium and the Prussian frontier, and has entered Holland; — it has pervaded the river-sides of London and other districts, and is now pervading the higher and more remote quarters of the city and west end, without regard to persons, the rich and the poor alike having experienced its attacks, among whom are some melancholy examples; and to the friends and families of these Dr. Webster's book will afford no confidence or consolation, nor will it be likely to persuade them that we have no great or destructive epidemic among us, and that we may congratulate each other on the great healthiness of the season, and the little havoc cholera is making.

Upon the great question of *quarantine*, we so far agree with Dr. Webster, that it is, in our opinion, attended with more inconvenience than advantage. We really do not believe that the cholera is to be kept out of a town, district, or country, by any practicable quarantine; but we do see the propriety of very strict measures of prevention being every where practised, and of great attention to the separation of the sick.

As to the treatment, we have little to say upon this part of the book before us, because the learned author himself has had no experience to guide him, and goes, therefore, only upon analogy; in which, so far, he displays judgment. Unfortunately, this disease is not one which admits of very clear reasoning in

relation to symptoms; and practice built upon the prevalent indications is but little successful; and when recovery takes place, it seems to do so more in obedience to a natural propensity than to the interference of medicine. Hence, perhaps, have arisen the most opposite ideas: *cold*, *heat*, *sedatives*, *stimulants*, have each successively been popular; and now the great tide of prejudice sets in with the *saline* treatment, as it is triumphantly styled; and for the application of which, at the Coldbath-fields prison, the magistrates awarded Dr. Stevens 100*l.*, with which the conscientious physician walked off, no doubt laughing in his sleeves at the gullibility of the glorious bench of the county unpaids. And well he might; for when government directed members of the Board of Health at Whitehall to look into the affair, the greater part of the *cures* had never been cholera cases at all, and some mere diarrhœa. It was farther reported, also, that the use of the saline system had not been attended with that degree of success which afforded any flattering hopes of its being more effective than the ordinary course of proceeding, adopted by the central board as having best succeeded in Russia. Those who are interested in the inquiry as to the Coldbath-fields prison, may see the whole correspondence, and the statements of the cases, published in the medical weekly gazettes, &c., in which statements it appears that the governor was either a willing or unsuspicious tool in returning cases as cholera which were not so. Among this falsified list, one girl's name absolutely appeared who had only complained of the tooth-ache! Moreover, it appears that several of the inmates had *feigned* cholera, for sinister motives. So much for this the newest humbug that has arisen out of the cholera mania. It appears, however, that in North Britain the practice of injecting large quantities of salt and water has been attended with very frequent restoration of the pulse in the collapse stage; and if this be true to any flattering extent, it bids fair, *conjoined with other remedies, perhaps*, to prove a very effective improvement in practice. But, in reference to the Coldbath-fields affair, we consider Dr. Stevens's bubble to have burst. We believe, after all, that the best treatment is that which is most consistent with sound sense, skill, and experience, and that kind of judgment which a well-educated and sensible medical man possesses ; for it is evident that *no specific* has yet been discovered for curing *Cholera Indiana.*

People in general are very anxious to know what to take when seized with cholera ; but the difficulty is, in knowing when you are so. The first symptoms are merely premonitory, and resemble ordinary complaints of the stomach, rendered irritable by heat, or some error of diet, perhaps. We, however, feel disposed, especially when there is a disposition to nausea or vomiting, to advise the immediate taking of an emetic, followed by calomel and opium pills, and weak brandy and water, warm, with ginger. The rest had better be left to medical advice.

We regret to see fears so rife as they are at present. Fear, if only used for the sake of caution, is good ; because it keeps people from taking liberties with their constitutions, and makes them guarded in their diet, and forces attention to their health. But, if fear acts as a dread of the disease, we know of no causes much more powerful in disposing the constitution to the prevailing epidemic, be that what it may.

It may perhaps be interesting to read what our transatlantic neighbours think of the epidemic, and the chances they have of sharing it with the inhabitants of the old world. The writer of a letter in the *Montreal Gazette,* of June 9, is extremely facetious upon the subject, and very confident in his opinions. But scarcely was his writing printed off, we believe, before some thousands were laid down in the malady, to which he affixes no infectious quality. Yet, how got it over the Atlantic, and why did it not arrive sooner ?

From a Correspondent of the Quebec Mercury.

Sir,—" 'The height of nonsense,' says an Irish proverb, ' is to try to keep out the tide with a pitchfork ;' and, though less in degree, the attempts made here and in Europe to arrest the progress of cholera, are very nearly allied to the edifying exercise above mentioned.

" I have only been two days in your city ; but, from the awful note of preparation which has been sounded far and wide —the tons of chloride of lime—the appointment of boards of health—and the instalment of a chapter of knights, of the order of Cloacina, I suppose, whom I see parading the streets in their spick and span new red ribands—the establishment of Grose Island as a grand lazaretto— and, above all, the profuse grant to pay

for all this nonsense, convinced me that you were going to run ram-headed against some absurdity. And, lo ! I have not been disappointed ; for as some of the ships that arrive in the course of the season will, no doubt, bring out typhus fever, measles, scarlet fever, small-pox, and other diseases, which are indubitably infectious—and as each vessel so doing will club its quota of mercies for the behoof of the denizens of Grose Island, prepared, as their bodies must be, for the reception of disease by the privations of a long voyage—you will throw a body of distempers into these colonies worse than the cholera at Calcutta in 1817-18. But as I have no hope that my feeble voice will be heard against the uplifted shout of the collective wisdom of the province, I shall confine myself to a few facts concerning the disease, which fell under my own observation, or which were related to me by people on whose truth and judgment I could depend, during a residence in Bengal, in the very worst times of cholera, namely, the years 1817, 18, 19, and 20.

Asiatic cholera is a disease of congestion ; whether it proceeds from the brain and nerves, or from the arterial system, I do not know, and I do not care ; for it is quite enough for us that we know how it operates, and, from that, how its operation can be counteracted. The spasms, which are common to the Asiatic and European cholera, and which are given to totally dissimilar diseases the same name, to the great confusion of terms and botheration of the faculty, are only symptoms of the disease, which is merely a contraction of the extreme vessels, causing the blood to rush inward upon the brain and abdominal viscera ; so that nine times out of ten the patient dies of apoplexy. My friend Mr. Marshall, in his work on the Medical Topography of Ceylon, (which work, like its author, though diminutive, contains a deal of good sense,) states, that on *post mortem* examinations, the pia mater was so turgid, that, when removed and thrown into a basin, it looked like one homogeneous clot of blood. The question then is, how to remove the pressure on the brain, and restore the circulation to the extremities ; for when you have done that, you have cured the cholera.

" With Europeans we found an early use of the lancet of great benefit ; but it must be a very early one, for if the attack has been of fifteen minutes' standing, you can get no more blood out of the patient's arm than out of a turnip. Our next reliance was on brandy and opium, in very large doses, and very often repeated.

" I once saved an over-scrupulous Mussulman, who refused to take any medicine, by means of a sinapism, covering about as much of his body as the cuirass of a life-guardsman ; and he told me afterwards that, if he took it again, he would rather die than undergo a second time the pain of such a cure. And I have heard of an amateur practitioner, somewhere up about Agra, who was a great advocate for decided practice, and who relieved many patients by pouring a tea-kettle of scalding water over their abdomen. But I would not recommend either of these being inflicted on his Majesty's lieges. Yet I should think rubifacients to the skin, and perhaps the hot bath, would be valuable auxiliaries in restoring the equilibrium of the circulation. The great secret, however, in treating the disease, is to get at it in time ; if you do so, little difficulty will be found in treating it. I was for nine months in charge of 1500 men (natives) in the year 1819, when the cholera was raging. My mode of management was this : each Serang (head of a gang) was provided with a bottle of brandy and laudanum, mixed in the proper proportions, and a measure holding exactly a dose for an adult ; his instructions were, on the first symptoms˙ of the disease, to give the patient a dose, and run with all speed for me. If he came in time, of which I could judge pretty accurately from the appearance of the patient, as well as from his testimony and that of his fellows, I gave him a rupee ; if he had neglected his duty, he was treated to a sound whacking with a bamboo. So that, with the two strongest motives to human action, hope of reward and fear of punishment, I was speedily apprised of danger ; and during that season, though many were attacked, I did not lose a single patient.

" One singular circumstance attendant on this disease is, that when it has been some time in one place, its force and virulence seem to be expended. Nothing will cure it on its first arrival, while any thing or nothing is held as ' the sovereignest thing in life' for it, after it has continued for three months ; so that we may expect that infallible remedies will be discovered in Sunderland, which will be found totally inefficacious in London.

" Is cholera contagious ? The *Quarterly Review* says it is—I say it is not ; and as the *Quarterly* never had the cholera in its life, and I had it twice, I think I should be the better judge of the two. Besides, is there any surgeon who has seen it in both countries says it is contagious ? Does Jock M'Whirter—does Marshall—does Daun—or Robin Badenach ? Not one of them : and why ? Because they know the disease, have seen it for years, and have treated it in thousands of cases : while the alarm-ists and contagionists are theorists, who never saw it in their lives. But what can be expected from a set of people who can foist on the public such nauseous hog-wash, as that a man should be smitten with the pestilence in consequence of scraping the pitch off the bottom of a ship that had been in Sunderland harbour ? But suppose all these good people, and half a hundred more besides, should assert that it was contagious, I think I can prove, from unquestionable facts, that it is not. So to the proof.

" When the Marquess of Hastings was narrowing the circle which he had been eighteen months extending, to hem in the gigantic Mahratta and Pindarree conspiracy, Sir Lionel Smith's division was occupying a pass in the Ghauts, in advance of Poonah ; his army was attacked by the cholera, and the hospital tents were pitched on a small hill, close to the camp. Whenever a man was taken ill he was conveyed over to the hospital hill, accompanied by a comrade, a wife (or some one *conomine*), and in no one single solitary instance was any of those who accompanied the sick taken with the disease ; now if they could have been infected, surely they had a better chance of catching the disease than by staying in the camp. But if a proportion of the hospital attendants had taken the disease, it would only prove that the people were liable to it in both situations ; but when people attending the sick (not being regular hospital attendants, mind ye), to a man or woman, as the case might be, escaped, it is, to me, a full proof that there is no contagion in the question.

" When Lord Hastings moved on from Mhow, he was encamped by the side of a brook (or nullah, as it is called in that country), and his body-guard (consisting of two squadrons of the finest heavy cavalry I ever saw, except the Life-Guards) were encamped two troops on one side of the brook and two on the other. Those on the one side were attacked severely with cholera, while the squadrons on the other entirely escaped. The same phenomenon was observed in many villages through which it passed, where it seemed to divide the village by a direct line, the one side being infected and the other safe. I was witness to a similar circumstance in Calcutta, where one part of the town alone was infected, and so virulently, that I was called up to see a gentleman's bearers, of eight of whom six had taken the disease, and five were dead before I arrived. Yet, though many in that quarter took it, and most of them died, it did not spread to another quarter of the town, until it nearly left the city altogether, and on its return broke out in another quarter.

" The sloop Curlew, Captain Dunlop, was three years on the Indian station, and during that time lay frequently at every port on both coasts, while the cholera was raging ashore, and an unrestricted communication was allowed between the ship and the shore, but not a single case occurred on board. At the end of this period the sloop was sold out of the service, and Captain D. and half his crew ordered round to the Malabar coast, to get the Termagant frigate, which had been built there, ready for sea, and to bring her home. On the 4th day after leaving Colombo, the cholera appeared on board, and nearly one-sixth of the crew were taken simultaneously, and in the end it went fore and aft the ship,—so much so, that at one period, to man a 28-gun frigate there were only eight men in one watch and nine in the other, including the captain and officers. Now, had cholera been contagious, would it not have attacked some one or other of them while exposed to its influence, and not nearly the whole of them after they were out of its range?

" But if you will not believe me, will you believe the disease itself? Had a contagious disease been introduced into Sunderland, would it not have gone all round like the circles formed by a stone thrown into a lake? But did cholera do so? No; it reached the banks of the Forth before it crossed the Tees; and things must be strangely altered since I left Scotland, if the stream of travel does not set more from north to south than in the opposite direction. Going north in a straight line (as it usually travels) we would trace its steps from village to village, and from town to town: this looked a little like contagion; but what are we to say when we hear of it taking a hop step and jump from the bishopric of Durham to the county of Kent, and thence to the city of London, leaving the midland and some of the northern counties untouched; and to the last hour we have not heard one syllable of its travel-

ling towards Whitehaven. Would an infectious disease act thus?

" Will cholera come here? I think it will, but not for some years. From the year 1818 I was clearly of opinion that it would traverse the whole world; and in 1822, I, together with a medical friend of mine from Tabriz, who had traced its progress through Persia, where he was surgeon to the embassy, made out a calculation of its progress, and were kind enough to chalk out for it the most convenient route, namely,—through Egypt, and along the northern shore of the Mediterranean, across from Ceuta to Gibraltar, so through Spain and France; thence, per packet, from Calais to Dover, by which route we supposed it would arrive in the metropolis about the beginning of 1830; but we never thought cholera would be so bad a general, with the example of Napoleon before his eyes, as to penetrate into the north of Europe, where, as we believed, like his great prototype, his force would be destroyed by frost and snow.

" What the d——l could have caused all this contagious alarm?—more especially here in his majesty's strong fortress of Quebec, the metropolis of the wide-spreading province of Lower Canada, and the wisest and fairest of all the cities of the earth; for surely there has been nothing to lead to the adoption of such measures, unless indeed the embargo placed on the Sunderland colliers by Gaffer Grey's administration, while they let the mail and stage coaches go without question, be looked upon as a pattern of wisdom instead of an example of folly. So keep up your heart, my dear Mr. Editor: take your glass, and don't alarm yourself, and give the same advice to your friends. If cholera is not coming here, so; if it is, the Grose Island cordon will hardly prevent it. So, that you may be preserved from the pestilence of cholera, the mania of anti-cholera measures, and the plague of blundering devils and compositors, is the sincere prayer of your affectionate friend,   Q. HY."

The writer of the foregoing letter is no other than the facetious TYGER, whom we introduced to our readers last month as the Backwoodsman. Whatever may be the professional knowledge or experience exhibited in this epistle, the talent and singular humour of the author cannot but render it most acceptable. We deem ourselves fortunate in obtaining a copy so early, and in giving a place in our columns to a production of no common literary *gusto* and merit. But although, in one respect, the fact of the cholera appearing at Quebec, almost contemporaneous with the publication, seems contrary to the doctor's opinion, the truth will, perhaps, be found to lie half way between the contagionists and anticontagionists; for it by no means follows, that a contagious disease is not also epidemical. We have heard a curious illustration of the progress of the cholera, in which it was supposed that the infection went floating along through the air, like oil in veins that remain unmixed with water. The inference from which is, that only those take the pestilence on whom a film of it had lighted; or can transmit the taint, unless they have previously received it, either from another, or from the atmosphere.— O. Y.

FRASER'S MAGAZINE

FOR

TOWN AND COUNTRY.

No. CCXV. NOVEMBER, 1847. Vol. XXXVI.

THE SANITARY COMMISSION, AND THE HEALTH OF THE METROPOLIS.

WE look forward with much interest, and some impatience, to the appearance of the blue book which is to embody the labours of the new Sanitary Commission. As a general rule, we have little confidence in commissions, unless they contain one man qualified and determined to take the lead. However respectable and intelligent the individual members may be, the inquiry entrusted to them is too apt to degenerate into a series of conversations without aim or point, and the Report to possess too much of that quality which is familiarly known as "milk-and-water." But the name of Chadwick re-assures us. We call to mind the sanitary reports of 1842 and 1843, and are satisfied. The same vigorous hand which held the pen in Somerset House will guide it in Whitehall. The mysteries of London will be revealed; the secrets of "local self-government" laid open; and that gigantic accident of brick and mortar, the metropolis of England, will be placed before us in all its fantastic proportions. Under the guidance of this modern Asmodeus, we shall be able to take a bird's-eye view of the great city, to track the footsteps of the pestilence which walketh in filth and darkness, and to

watch the stealthy inroads of scrofula and consumption in the wretched hovel of the labourer and the crowded workshop of the artisan. We shall learn the secrets of the obstacles that block our thoroughfares, and of the worse impediments which obstruct the flow of the dark streams that own the control of the Commissioners of Sewers. Marylebone shall be stretched upon the rack, and the City groan under the torture; and all the world shall see what sort of a home for two millions of human beings this boasted centre of civilisation is.

We congratulate the public on having once more secured the services of Mr. Chadwick. We thank the government for giving us this earnest of their good intentions; and we felicitate Mr. Chadwick himself on having escaped from the thankless service of a miserable system of palliation to the more genial work of prevention, in which he has already attained to such proficiency.

Of his associates in this useful inquiry we can also speak with approval. Dr. Southwood Smith's services in the sanitary cause are too well known and too generally appreciated to need any praise of ours; Lord Robert Grosvenor is a benevolent and patriotic nobleman; Mr.

Owen, a comparative anatomist of the first order; and Mr. Jones, a fitting representative of the interests and prejudices of the City. We are glad, too, to see the name of Mr. Austin, who has so long and so ably discharged the duties attaching to the office of honorary secretary to the Health of Towns' Association, figuring as the right hand of this sanitary quintette.

If we were disposed to be hypercritical, we might take exception to one, at least, of these appointments ; but, provided that Mr. Chadwick be allowed full play, the constitution of the Commission will be a matter of secondary moment. We hail the appointment of Professor Owen, however, as evidence that the Smithfield Market will not escape unscathed. The health of cattle, as affected by a sojourn in town, with all its agreeable accompaniments, is an inquiry for which he is admirably fitted ; and a city, which has not a solitary stream of water to cool the tongue of a dog, much less to slake the thirst of the droves of cattle that crowd its leading thoroughfares, will afford a theme more spirit-stirring than all the monsters of the antediluvian world. If we are not misinformed, Professor Owen is, or has lately been, at Paris, collecting materials for instituting a comparison between the abattoirs of that capital and the slaughter-houses of London. A more striking contrast it is scarcely possible to conceive : the one all order and cleanliness ; the other, a slovenly scene of filthy confusion. There is here an opportunity, which ought not to be lost, of placing side by side the economic beauties of consolidation and the costly defects and deformities of that repellent system of self-will and accident which has made this giant metropolis the chaos that it is.

To shew how this chaos may be reduced to order, to point out how its scattered and mis-shapen parts may be made to coalesce into a form of health and beauty, is the work which the Commission is called upon to perform. The undertaking will prove laborious and difficult, and many obstacles will have to be encountered ; but the main difficulty will arise when the inquiry is finished, and the Report laid before the public. The inevitable remedies for the ma-

lady under which the patient labours will be any thing but palatable. A radical change of system will have to be prescribed. The quackery of local self-government must be abandoned, the best advice of the state-physician must be resorted to, and steady and constant surveillance must be substituted for the self-willed irregularity which has set all system and method at defiance.

We foresee that our refractory patient will not be easily induced to take this reasonable course ; and we, therefore, offer our humble services in the way of persuasion. We flatter ourselves that we know something of his malady, and we are not without hope of being able to address to him some convincing arguments. But this metaphorical style will not do. This giant of brick and mortar must be dealt with in plain prose.

Let us sit down, then, with map in hand, and the best authorities, historical, statistical, and sanitary, open before us, and endeavour to form some idea of the metropolis of England, not as a great centre of commerce, not as the gay resort of fashion, the abode of royalty, or the seat of government, but as the home of two millions of human beings. Is it a decent, cleanly, wholesome home ? There is but one answer to this question, and that, unhappily, in the negative. London can boast of no superiority — of none, at least, which is not purely accidental—over other large cities. Like them, she has done all she could, by carelessness and negligence, to justify the uncomplimentary epithets with which large towns in general have been assailed. She has been made, or has been suffered to become, one of the " graves of mankind ;" a " foul and pestilent congregation of vapours ;" a " huge accident of brick and mortar ;" and, indeed, any thing and every thing that she ought not to be. It is in vain that she parades her public buildings, and multiplies her statues, and builds up long lines of imposing streets, with gorgeous mansions and glittering shops. We know that this is all treachery and deception,—the mere outside-splendour of the whited sepulchre, concealing revolting scenes of corruption and decay. What are her leading thoroughfares but so many showy screens, run up to hide from sight the manifold nuisances which abound in their immediate vicinity ? Her squares, and public places, and fashionable quarters, what are they but oases in a worse than desert ? The noisy tide of fickle fashion and bustling trade flows through them, all unconscious of the sad contrasts shut out from view by a narrow barrier of brick and mortar. These highways constitute the town and the world of nine-tenths of the rich and fashionable. " Where are the people ?" is a question which not even the example of an emperor can prevail upon them to ask. The people! There is in that idea a bewildering vastness, an oppressive grandeur, an awful sublimity, which brings the frivolous and thoughtless to a sudden pause. Its presence mars enjoyment. It casts too broad and deep a shadow across the path of pleasure. But it will sometimes force an unwilling entrance through the sullen barrier of indifference, startle the sleepy conscience, and arouse the apprehensions of the bravest. The people! What a grand, concrete idea! The passions, the sorrows, the trials, the struggles, the labours, of one man multiplied by millions! The rivulet swollen to the stream, the stream to the river, the river to the mighty ocean!

This idea is, so to speak, embodied in the great town. It assumes a visible and tangible shape. The units of the living sum are brought close together. The population of a county or a kingdom is compressed into the space of a few square miles. This it is which lends to the large city a character of sublimity. It is this which renders a residence amid all its noise and bustle so grateful to men of large and comprehensive views. It was this feeling which possessed Samuel Johnson, when he expressed his indifference to the country and all its quiet attractions, lauded the superior charms of Fleet Street, and gloried in the full tide of human existence flowing through its narrow channel. All honour to the great lexicographer for the human sympathies which made the great metropolis so dear to him! and honour to all those who labour to make it a fit object of interest and attachment!

Let us, then, consider the metropolis in this light, as the dwelling-place of the People,—the scene of their toils, and sufferings, and pleasures,—their work-place, and their home. And again we ask, Is London what it ought to be ? Has it been constructed with a view to its proper uses as a place of habitation ? Have its streets been so laid out, its workshops, shops, and dwellings, so constructed, and its municipal laws so framed, as to economise to the utmost all those things which are most valuable to its inhabitants — time, temper, money, health, and life ? Have suitable provisions been made for the recreation and instruction of the people, for their elevation and refinement ? If these questions could any where be answered in the affirmative, it ought to be in this metropolis,— the royal, legal, legislative, commercial, and fashionable centre of the United Kingdom,—the largest and richest city in the world,—the home of two millions of human beings! To every one of these important questions, the answer is an emphatic negative. Be it our easy task to prove the truth of this statement in all that concerns its sanitary condition.

The leading principles which have been established relative to the health of towns are grown so familiar, that it is not necessary to prove them in this place. We shall, therefore, take them for granted. As a general rule, towns become more unhealthy as they increase in size. But that this rule is subject to exceptions, the metropolis itself is a striking proof. Though the largest city in the world, it is by no means the most unhealthy. Compared to the capital cities of the leading European states, it may even be pronounced healthy. It occupies the same place among them that England does among those nations themselves. England is the healthiest among leading states, as London is among populous capitals.

Nay, more, if we measure the sanitary condition of the metropolis by the rough test of the proportion of deaths to the living, it will be found to be more favourable than that of the whole of Prussia, Austria, or Russia; for while the metropolis sustains an annual loss of 25 in the thousand, Prussia loses 26, Austria 30, and Russia 36.

So, also, if we compare the metropolis with other large English cities, it will be found to have a similar advantage in a sanitary point of view; for while, with its 2,000,000 inhabitants, it loses 25 in the thousand every year, Birmingham, with its 150,000 inhabitants, loses 27 ; Manchester, with its 200,000, 32 ; and Liverpool, with its quarter of a million, 35 in the thousand. It also enjoys a similar superiority if compared with the large cities of Scotland and Ireland.

The metropolis will also be found to hold the same favourable position with regard to the large towns just mentioned, if we employ a standard of comparison of most unexceptionable accuracy, namely, the average age of death, which would obtain, if precisely the population of London, with its own peculiar proportion of inhabitants of different ages, were supposed to be transferred to the towns in question, but to retain the rate of mortality at each age proper to those towns. From these accurate comparisons, the following averages result :—

```
Metropolis............29·06
Manchester...........27·37
Birmingham ..........26·82
Liverpool ...........25·07
```

So that, one with another, the inhabitants of London live nearly one year and three quarters longer than the same population would live in Manchester; two and a quarter years longer than if it were transferred to Birmingham ; and as nearly as possible, four years longer than if it were removed to Liverpool. Multiply these several differences by the deaths taking place annually in the respective towns, and we have a very fearful sacrifice of life on the one hand, and a very marked advantage of the metropolis in a sanitary point of view on the other.

London, therefore, though the largest city in the world, is by no means the most unhealthy ; and if Englishmen could only be content to compare themselves and their cities with other people and other towns, they might sit down and fold their arms in silent and idle self-complacency. But this is not, and we trust never will be, the habit of Englishmen deserving of the name. Our standard of comparison must not be even the best governed, most prosperous, or most healthy among foreign states, or the most flourishing among modern cities. The standards of comparison of a great people ought to be, if not ideals, at least the best and noblest realities of ancient or modern times. The history of the past and present ought to be diligently studied, and each wholesome usage, whenever and wherever it obtained, be copied as nearly as is consistent with convenience ; and, if improvement be practicable, improved upon.

If we may believe Herodotus and other ancient writers, Babylon of old had within its walls one hundred square miles of open space for exercise and recreation. The city, which was a square of fifteen miles on each side, had fifty streets, each 150 feet broad, and fifteen miles long. They all ran in straight lines, and crossed at right angles, so as to cut the houses into 676 squares of half a mile in the side. No two houses touched each other, or were without spaces between them ; and the middle of each square was laid out in gardens and pleasure grounds. Here, then, is an ancient city, built nearly 3000 years ago, which may be fairly held up to imitation, as affording an instance of large and liberal provision for the exercise and recreation of its inhabitants, and for ensuring, by free external ventilation, the utmost possible purity of atmosphere. What a contrast does this mighty city of old form with modern London! If we estimate the builded area of London at fifteen square miles, and add five square miles for parks and recent additions, we have a total of twenty square miles, which forms but a fifth part of the mere exercising ground of the inhabitants of ancient Babylon. Not to pursue this comparison further, we insist that this is such a standard as we should always keep in view, and to which we should approximate as closely as possible.

It is true that this metropolis could not, without an impossible sacrifice of property, have main streets opened out of 150 feet in breadth, and inferior streets of proportionate width. Nor could our present system be so far altered, that no two houses should touch each other, or our tortuous streets be straightened out, and made to cut each other at right angles. Nevertheless, we may so far approximate to our standard, as that open spaces for exercise and recreation may be secured wherever the spread of buildings threatens a long unbroken encroachment on the country; the present narrow and winding thoroughfares may be gradually widened and straightened; blind courts may be converted into streets; and provision be made for constructing all future increments to the giant city on a well-considered plan.

As to the proper mode of laying out those large and growing additions, which may be justly regarded in the light of new towns, rather than in that of increments of an ancient city, we may find our standard and exemplar in more recent but still ancient times. The Romans might be our teachers in this matter. We are informed on good authority, that they were in the habit of regarding the construction of a city as a great religious rite, justly deeming, that a proceeding in which health and life were so intimately concerned, had something sacred about it, and required to be set about in a solemn and thoughtful spirit. Accordingly they used the greatest circumspection in the choice of a site; and, under the imposing sanction of religious ceremonies, carefully examined the livers of the animals sacrificed upon the spot, and did not enter upon their work till they had satisfied themselves by this test that the water and soil were salubrious. When the external walls were planned, the enclosed area was carefully laid out; the streets were arranged so as to exclude winds injurious to comfort; and all the sewers and drains were well considered. Convenient and commanding situations were selected for the public buildings; and care was taken that the foundations should be adequate to their support. Laws were also enacted to prevent individuals from doing anything which could interfere with the public health or enjoyment.

We must turn to a contemporary standard for our guidance in the adaptation of the existing structural arrangements of London, to the more enlightened views and wants of the present period. Paris has solved the problem of the reconstruction of an ancient city, in such a manner as to create the least possible inconvenience and interference with property; and Paris, therefore, in this, as in one or two other points, ought to be our standard and guide. The scheme to which we refer is as follows:—A comprehensive plan of the city accessible to the public, and approved and sanctioned by the municipal authorities, indicates the improved and widened lines of streets to which houses when rebuilt must conform. Compensation for the ground ceded for this widening of the streets is fixed by juries of " experts ;" and we are told, that their mode of assessment gives rise to few complaints.

This gradual process does not produce such grand and striking results, at first, as our own more vigorous method of procedure; but it has the great advantage of spreading the blessing of wide streets and relieved thoroughfares equally throughout the city, instead of creating a heap of ruins by dispossessing the poorer classes of their homes, and throwing them in crowds upon the already dense populations of the immediate neighbourhoods.

Paris, again, may be cited as a fit model of imitation in another matter to which we have already referred : we mean the establishment of abattoirs in the environs, as substitutes for the existing slaughter-houses which lie so thick about the great parent nuisance of Smithfield.

In the vital matter of a supply of water, we must go back again to ancient Rome, and imitate in the spirit, if not in the exact form, of her arrangements—the city of aqueducts ; or, crossing the Atlantic, take instruction from New York, with her unequalled mechanical arrangements for pouring a river of the pure element in refreshing streams through every part of the city, for every purpose to which it can be applied.

Thus would we make the whole world, and all times, ancient and modern, tributary to the great metropolis; combining in her and for her every arrangement which experience has shewn to be conducive to the health, comfort, and well-being of the inhabitants of cities. In this way only can she be made a worthy

centre of attraction to her own people, and a reflex of the humanity
and civilisation of England.

From the details into which we
have just entered it will be inferred,
that though London is undoubtedly
the most healthy of capitals, and an
exception to the general rule, that
towns become more unhealthy as
they grow larger, it owes its superiority, not to the perfection of its
structural arrangements and sanitary
regulations, but to the circumstance
that all large towns, in every part of
the world, are built on unsound principles, and in ignorance or forgetful-
ness of the models of a remote antiquity. In municipal laws and regulations there is no doubt that modern
nations have very greatly degenerated,
and that they have yet much to learn
of that noblest of human arts and
sciences—the art of preventing disease and preserving health.

The causes of the favourable sanitary state of London, when compared
to that of other large cities, are for
the most part to be found either in
its position or in circumstances which
are purely accidental. Neither its
inhabitants nor the government can
justly claim any credit for having
brought about its existing superiority. Its situation on the two
banks of a large river conduces
to health, by promoting ventilation
and by facilitating drainage. The
river, in fact, is a wide open space
which cannot be built upon, and
upon which the air is generally in
motion; and it constitutes a large
open sewer, in which the refuse of
the town is diluted by so large a
body of water as to lose all its injurious properties, except where, from
any cause, that refuse stagnates on
the banks. From this great natural
drain the land upon the north rises
at first abruptly, and then by more
gradual ascent, to Hampstead, Highgate, Primrose Hill, and Pentonville;
on the south-east to Greenwich,
Blackheath, and Shooters' Hill; on
the south-west there is also a sufficient slope, leaving only the southern
and western parts of the metropolis
on a level at all unfavourable to
drainage. Westminster and Southwark are situated at so low a level,
as to offer serious impediments to
drainage; but the greater part of the
metropolis is probably more favour-

ably circumstanced, in this respect,
than most of the large cities of England or of the Continent. The convenience of commerce has placed
most considerable cities on the sea-
shore, or on the banks of rivers, but
few have been more fortunate in the
general disposition of their surface
than London. Without entering into
a description of the geological formation of the soil on which London
stands, it may be stated, in general
terms, to be also favourable to the
health of its inhabitants. With considerable facilities for drainage, that
most important operation has been
carried out on a larger scale than in
any other city; and though it has
been done without much order or
method, under the management of
seven distinct commissions, which
have not often acted in concert, and
under the authority of an ancient
act of parliament, which was adapted
solely to the drainage of a marsh,
the results, on the whole, have been
beneficial, and have tended decidedly
to the preservation of the health of
the inhabitants.

Another cause of the superior
healthiness of the metropolis is the
large space of ground which has been
appropriated to the inhabitants, taken
one with another, when compared to
that which has been assigned to the
populations of some of our own large
cities, and to most of the continental
towns. This fortunate result, again,
is not to be attributed to any deli-
berate intention of preserving the
health of the people. It is one of the
happy accidents of a city no longer
enclosed within walls, and in which
ample space has, in some way or other,
come to be considered as a luxury by
the rich, and wide thoroughfares as
necessary to intercourse. The parts
of the town inhabited by the poorer
classes, and especially those most remote from the great lines of traffic,
will gain little by a comparison with
Birmingham, Manchester, or Liverpool. Thus, if we take the total
area of the large towns just mentioned, the metropolis has 27,423 to
the square mile, and Birmingham
33,669; while Manchester crowds
83,224 into the same space, and Liverpool 100,899. If we take the builded
area, however, London has about
50,000, Manchester 100,000, and
Liverpool 138,224 to the square mile,

while Birmingham has only about 40,000 in the same space.

London, again, as being neither exclusively manufacturing nor exclusively commercial, but having a due mixture of all classes of men among its inhabitants, does not suffer in an extreme degree from the evils of either system, but presents that average state of health due to the admixture of the several classes and ranks of men.

Add to these causes of a good sanitary condition, a high rate of wages, and a consequent command of an abundance of wholesome food, good clothing, and sufficient shelter, and facilities of amusement and recreation, which tend to a more moderate use of alcoholic liquors than obtains in other large towns, and we have the principal causes which have tended to render London more healthy than other capital cities and populous places.

But, as we have already intimated, we ought not to be satisfied with comparing London with other large cities, and especially with such notoriously unhealthy ones as those which we have just selected. In order to judge correctly of its true sanitary condition, we must adopt one of two standards of comparison,— the mortality which obtains in other towns of considerable size, not more favourably circumstanced than itself, except in points obviously admitting of improvement; or that which exists in some neighbouring district operated upon by the same general influences, and differing only in the same manner. Now, in the year 1841, there were no less than thirty-seven English towns, some of them of considerable size, and differing widely from each other in soil and situation, and in the occupations of their inhabitants, in which the annual mortality did not exceed two in the hundred. The only particular likely to influence the health of their inhabitants, in which they differed from the metropolis, was the space that they had at their command, and the more perfect external ventilation which naturally results from it.

It is, therefore, fair to conclude that, by making more liberal provision of space for the pent-up inhabitants of London, and by putting in force every obvious means of improvement, the annual mortality might be reduced to the same favourable point ; a point, be it recollected, many degrees below that of the more healthy English counties, and still more inferior to that of healthy rural districts. Assuming, then, that the mortality of London does admit of being reduced to two per cent, it will be very easy to calculate the annual loss which we sustain by the neglect of those sanitary measures by which the capital admits of being placed on an equality with the towns to which we have referred.

The annual number of deaths in London fluctuates according to the season, between about 46,000 and 53,500. The first number of deaths occurred in the years 1839, 1841, and 1842, and the last in 1838. The deaths in 1845 amounted to upwards of 48,000, and in 1846 to more than 49,000. Allowance being made for increase of population, the deaths for the later periods will have to be somewhat reduced, for purposes of strict comparison ; but if we take the average of the seven years, 1838–44, of which 1841, the year of the census, was the middle term, and assume that the population in the first three years as much exceeded that of 1841 as the population of the last three years fell short of it, we shall have an average annual mortality of 48,553 ; and, on the above assumption that the rate of mortality admits of being reduced to two per cent, an annual waste of upwards of 10,000 lives. The exact number is 10,232.

The mortality of the current year is high beyond example. The deaths in London for the first quarter amounted to no less than 15,289 ; the greatest recorded mortality for the same quarter in any previous year being 14,528 for 1845. The deaths in the second quarter were 12,361 ; the greatest number previously recorded for the same quarter being 11,621, in the year 1843. It would appear, therefore, that London is now suffering under an unexampled mortality, which there is too much reason to fear may be still further increased by the visitation of the pestilence, which is advancing with rapid strides, by its old familiar route, to add to the arguments in favour of a prompt and stringent measure of sanitary reform.

We believe that those who have given most attention to the subject of the public health, will not charge us with exaggeration if we estimate the average annual excess of deaths in the metropolis above a fair standard of health at upwards of 10,000, being nearly 200 a-week, more than twenty-eight every day, and more than one an hour. So that every hour that strikes, tolls the knell of at least one victim of the fatal system of neglect to which we have so long struggled in vain to put an end. The standard of comparison which we have hitherto employed in our calculations is the moderate average mortality of two per cent, which, as we have stated, actually obtains in English towns of considerable size. The Registrar-general, in his return for the first quarter of the present year, employs, as his standard of comparison, the mortality in the Lewisham registration district, which comprises Black-heath, Sydenham, Eltham, and Lewisham itself; and he shews that, measured by this healthy standard, the excess of deaths in London in the seven years, 1838–44, was not less than 97,872, or 13,981 a-year; of which number 58,961, or 8,423 a-year, were under five years of age, and, therefore, unaffected by those un-wholesome occupations to which a part of the high mortality of adults is justly attributed.

Reverting to our first moderate estimate of 10,000 deaths a-year over and above a favourable, but not extremely low rate of mortality, we invite our readers to pause for a moment, and contemplate with us this fearful sacrifice of human life, with its melancholy accompaniment of equally unnecessary sickness (commonly estimated at twenty-eight times the amount), and the sorrows and sufferings which sickness and death entail.

If we suffered ourselves to think seriously on these matters,—if, as we are bound to do, we looked upon these totals not as dry figures of arithmetic, but as sums of which every unit is the life of an immortal being prematurely brought to a close,—we could not persevere in our present indifference, nor our municipal and local authorities in their course of vexatious opposition. It is because we are still steeped in indifference, it is because

they have not yet abandoned their cruel opposition, that it behoves us to endeavour to place this annual sacrifice, of which every hour claims at least one victim, in the strongest possible light.

Let us first suppose these 10,000 men, women, and children, thus wantonly destroyed, instead of being scattered, as they are, over the wide area of a vast metropolis, to be brought into one spot, to be the inhabitants of a single town, and then to be offered up, hour by hour, amid the burning tortures and fierce delirium of fever, or the slow, wasting, sufferings of consumption, to the system of *laissez faire*, the god of our idolatry, till not one of them remained; or let us suppose a town of the size of Liverpool, every inhabitant of which is delivered up once in each year to one unnecessary attack of sickness, with its burden of sorrow, suffering, and expense; let us view the matter in this light, and we must throw off our fatal indifference, and give up our most unworthy and selfish opposition.

If this mode of representing the annual sacrifice of health and life fail of making an impression upon us, then let us look upon the work of destruction as upon a warfare, in which 10,000 unconscious and unwilling soldiers fall in a hopeless conflict with disease on a field without glory, and amid sufferings keener far than sword or cannon can inflict.

It may help us to form a more vivid conception of the amount of the annual sacrifice of life in London, if we compare it with that which has taken place upon some of our most famous fields of battle.

The number of killed in the battle of Waterloo was 3,587; the wounded amounted to 7,769; the missing to 1656;—making a grand total of 13,012 casualties. So that the number of killed was little more than one-third of the annual slaughter in the metropolis; and all the casualties put together, fell short of the annual excess of deaths during the last seven years, according to the estimate of the Registrar-general.

The impression which this sort of comparison is calculated to make may, perhaps, be strengthened if we take a more recent example. In the four great Indian battles of Moodkee,

Ferozeshah, Aliwal, and Sobraon, the total loss in killed was 2,133, or little more than a fifth of the annual slaughter in London; the wounded were 5,330, or about half that annual sacrifice; and the total of killed and wounded 7,463, being considerably less than the yearly excess—above two per cent—in the most healthy of the seven years to which we have referred. According to the more liberal estimate of the Registrar-general, the deaths in these great battles would be somewhat less than one-seventh; the wounded, more than a third; and the killed and wounded, taken together, upwards of one-half the excess of deaths taking place every year in London.

It is not pretended that this comparison is in all points exact and fair. The slaughter on the field of battle is an affair of hours or days, that which has the wide metropolis for its theatre extends over an entire year. The comparison is intended to apply solely to the extent of the sacrifice, for the slaughter of the battle-field seemed better calculated to arrest attention than any other form of wholesale destruction. It might not, perhaps, be uninteresting or useless to point out other differences besides that of time. The soldier's battle is fought by men hired to do that work of blood, and entering upon the career of an honourable profession with their eyes open. With comparatively few exceptions, too, they are men without wives and families, and whose death entails the minimum of sorrow, suffering, and expense on the community; but in this fierce and fatal battle with disease, the motley group of warriors enter upon the inglorious and unpaid conflict with an unseen enemy —if not against their will, at least without their consent — and their death inflicts the greatest possible amount of sorrow and suffering on others, and on the community a very serious total of expense.

Would that by these, or any comparisons, we could succeed in arousing the people of this country from their present indifference! They have been told, over and over again, that typhus fever is more fatal than the sword of the enemy, but still they cannot be induced to take those steps which may banish this ever-present foe. They have become so accustomed to this civil warfare that they scarcely heed it; and the friends of sanitary improvement are beginning to hail the threatened approach of the cholera, in the hope that the invasion of a strange and mysterious enemy may strike them with that salutary terror which our own familiar pestilence fails to inspire.

But we must not satisfy ourselves with the general statement we have made, that the metropolis loses every year from 10,000 to nearly 14,000 lives over and above those which would perish in the common course of nature, were sound sanitary measures in universal operation. It will be both interesting and instructive to examine the several districts of the metropolis, with a view to determine the seats of that excessive mortality; for it may happen that there are parts of this great city which are in a peculiar manner fatal to the health and lives of the inhabitants, and on which it will be both just and expedient to fix the charge of the neglect that has occasioned that result.

The Registrar-general, in his Report for the first quarter of the present year, presents us with a valuable table, in which the number of deaths at the several periods of life out of 1000 living at those periods, is given for the several registration districts of the metropolis. Taking the period from birth to five years as on the whole the best test, we shall be able to throw the several districts of the metropolis into three classes — the healthiest, the medium, and the unhealthiest—and thus to form a very fair estimate of their relative sanitary condition.

The *healthy* class, comprising the districts in which the deaths among female children do not exceed 70 in the 1000, consists of the registration districts of Lewisham; Hampstead; Hackney and Camberwell; Wandsworth and Islington; Poplar and Greenwich.

The *medium* class, in which the deaths range from 70 to 90 per 1000, comprises (we place them as before, in the order of their healthiness, beginning with the most healthy) Newington; St. Pancras; Kensington, Chelsea, and Stepney; Lambeth; City of London; St. George's, Hanover Square, and Shoreditch; Bethnal

Green; Rotherhithe; Clerkenwell; and the Strand, Bermondsey, and Marylebone. The *unhealthy* class, in which the deaths are from 90 to 109 per 1000 (arranged as before, *i.e.* beginning with the most healthy), consists of Holborn and St. Martin-in-the-Fields; St. James, Westminster, and St. Luke's; St. Margaret, Westminster; St. George's-in-the-East; St. George's, Southwark; Whitechapel; St. Saviour and St. Olave; East and West London; and St. Giles.

A glance at these instructive groups will shew what are the districts least and most fatal to health and life, and least and most in need of sanitary improvement. The *healthy* districts are the thinly peopled and half-rural environs of London; the *medium* districts consist, as might be expected, of a mixed group of out-lying parishes, in which the density of population is not carried to a very extreme point, such as Newington, St. Pancras, Kensington, Chelsea, Stepney, Bermondsey, and Rotherhithe; and the fashionable parishes of St. George's, Hanover Square, and Marylebone. The *unhealthy* class contains almost all those districts which any man of observation would point out

as being most densely peopled and most neglected. It is not to be wondered at that St. Giles should close the list, or that the parts of the metropolis which have been pointed out as lying lowest, and being least susceptible of efficient drainage, namely, Southwark and Westminster, should be found to figure in this group of most unhealthy districts. The noisy and busy parish of Marylebone, as might naturally be anticipated, does not hold a very favourable position, for it stands with Bermondsey on the verge of the unhealthiest group; and the aristocratic region of St. George's, Hanover Square, is exactly on a level with the plebeian district of Shoreditch. East and West London stand where the loud boastings of the City would lead us to expect them—in a position only more favourable than that congenial abode of the Irish, St. Giles.

The general and broad inference to be drawn from a careful study of these facts is, that the mortality is greatest in those districts which are most crowded. Thus, if we take the first and last of each of the three groups, and compare their area with their population, we have the following striking result:—

Registration district.	Population to an acre.	Deaths per 1000 females under five years.
St. Giles	270	109
St. Martin	94	91
St. Marylebone	92	85
Newington	87	70
Greenwich	16	65
Lewisham ...... less than	1	47

Over-crowding, then, is *the* great concomitant and cause of the mortality of the most unhealthy parts of London,—over-crowding of streets—over-crowding of houses—over-crowding of rooms, shops, and work-shops; and that over-crowding, itself the parent of so much disease, destitution, and demoralisation, is the child of that cruel system of *laissez faire*, against which we must raise our voice, till every hovel in the land echoes back the cry. Men cannot live under the tyranny of perpetual negligence. There is no help for them but in the liberty of stringent laws. This nuisance of over-crowding must be abated, before we can hope to see any real improvement in the physical or moral condition of the

people. But—mockery of mockeries! cruelty of cruelties!--we not only do not take any steps to mitigate this fearful evil, but, under pretence of improving the thoroughfares of the metropolis, we destroy the dwellings of the poor by thousands, without making any sort of provision for their accommodation. We give facilities to carts and horses, but as to human beings, they may find house-room where they can. We don't build houses for the poor. We leave that to chance, and the tender mercies of supply and demand. We build prisons and workhouses. That is the only architecture worthy of a nation. As to the habitations of the poor, they are beneath our notice. But if our system had happened to be a different one,—if it had only occurred to us to enact, that for every third or fourth - class hovel destroyed by a metropolitan improvement a real house must previously be built on the nearest available space, and that, till this preliminary was arranged, carts and horses, cabs and carriages, might twist and crowd through the crooked thoroughfares as they would, we should have done more than all the charities or joint-stock companies, with all their zeal and energy, will effect for half-a-century to come. We should have called into existence real houses enough to have shamed all the pigsties in London into the occasional use of whitewash, and a moderate outlay on the means of decency and comfort.

The most cursory inspection, however, of the table to which we have just referred, must convince us that over-crowding is not the sole evil to be corrected, ere the metropolis can attain to a good sanitary condition ; and that a neglect on the part of the authorities, on whom the duty of widening our thoroughfares has devolved, to provide accommodation for the ejected tenantry of that hard landlord, the Public, is not the only act of omission of which the effects are traceable in the figures of the Registrar-general. The over-crowding has many unwholesome concomitants, which account for a great part of its fatal consequences. In those densely peopled districts, every act of negligence which authority can ommit is brought to bear on the unhappy inhabitants. The Commissioners of Sewers, the Commissioners of Paving, and the Scavengers forget and neglect them, and the Water-Companies are not required to supply them with water, except after the fashion of cab - stands, by stand - pipes in the courts and alleys pouring forth a slender stream for an hour or two three times a-week. With lanes, alleys, and courts, built without a plan, and houses without a purpose, —the victims of universal neglect,— a prey to every species of physical corruption, who can be surprised to hear that those to whom the means of decency, comfort, and health, have been denied, should sink to the lowest depths of misery and degradation, and that these scenes of filth should

become hot - beds of disease, and haunts of crime ? We will not offend the taste and delicacy of our readers by descriptions of these miserable abodes of miserable men. Some items of the description, indeed, are too gross for ears polite ; but if any of our readers doubt our statements, the pages of the Reports of the Sanitary Commission are open to them, and the publications which are daily issuing from the press will enlighten them. Nor let our fashionable readers suppose that these scenes are only to be found in the low neighbourhoods of St. Giles-in-the-Fields, or St. George's-in-the-East. They bask under the very shadows of the cathedral and the palace. They are profusely scattered, in all their festering foulness, through the aristocratic parishes of St. George, Hanover Square; St. James, Westminster ; and the best parts of St. Marylebone. A stone slung at hazard from any one of our most fashionable thoroughfares would scarcely fail to reach them. But for the sound of your own carriage-wheels, and the noisy hubbub of your fashionable frivolities, you might almost hear the mutterings of the fever patient, or the moanings of the consumptive ; and, but for a narrow screen of shops or houses, your own eyes might see the things we speak of. Nay, we are not sure that such scenes are not nearer to you still, as any man of moderate means, who has sought for a really decent habitation in your fashionable neighbourhoods, could easily testify ; and the records of the Fever Hospital would, if we mistake not, prove that the basements of houses of the best exterior are not altogether guiltless of breeding and nursing pestilence. We would accuse you, if we could, of indifference to what is going on about you ; but the condition of the streets in which you live, and of the houses which you yourselves inhabit, absolves you from every charge but that of ignorance. But as the palace of our queen has been built upon a swamp, and in the lowest level of the lowest district of London, you do but follow the fashion if your own abodes are not models of wholesomeness. We trust that the Sanitary Commission will not confine their inquiries or their teachings to the hovels of the poor.

The so-called houses of the rich—or, at least, of the professional and mercantile class—might be inspected with great advantage, and would figure pleasantly in a Sanitary Report.

Let us hope that these things have had their day, and that history will record to our honour that, after having for about ten years written much and talked more about the necessity of doing something for the health of the people, and having bandied the matter about in speeches from the throne, debates in the legislature, and abortive acts of parliament; and encountered and tired out the opposition of parish vestries, local boards, and irresponsible commissions; we were permitted at length, about the middle of the nineteenth century, to give an authoritative definition of a house; and that thereupon the era of housebuilding did commence in earnest, and the people at large were suffered to enjoy the same privilege which the more intelligent among our agriculturists have long awarded to their cattle.

Let us hope, too, that the same veracious chronicler will set forth how, about this time, John Bull, awaking like a giant from a dreamy sleep, became conscious, all at once, of the barbarisms by which he had surrounded himself, and of the barbarities which he had unconsciously perpetrated; how he began to look upon the smoking factory and steamer as a waste of fuel and an intolerable nuisance; on the manure of our towns thrown into the sea as a virtual destruction of his children's food; on the cattle-market, the graveyard, the slaughter-house, the laystall, and the offensive manufactory, planted in the midst of a crowded population, as worthy of the times of gross and unlettered ignorance; how he determined to display that vigour which he had hitherto exercised solely on the battle-field, or on his own peculiar element, against the domestic foes who had combined to poison and oppress his children; and how he had laughed to scorn and put to flight the aiders and abettors of " local self-government," consolidated the "heptarchy of foul waters," routed the paving-boards, controlled the water-companies, and brought about that much-desired union of centralisation and parochialism, under whose enlightened and vigilant sway so many blessings had been conferred upon the nation.

From this period of time we are convinced that history will date the commencement of England's real prosperity. Taking a large and comprehensive view of the acts and principles of a bygone age, she will pronounce the one to be the rude efforts of uninstructed and undisciplined vigour, or the happy accidents which strew the path even of thoughtless negligence, and the other as the warm impulses of a generous spirit awaiting the correction of a more mature experience. The charities which, in innocent self-satisfaction, had been paraded before the world as evidence of a rare humanity, will then appear in their true colours as the offspring of a listless indifference, which could only be moved by the contemplation of its own inevitable results; the almsgiving, which had grown into a huge system of temptation to the worthless and encouragement to the idle, will be recognised as the mere letter of the divine law, of which prevention is the spirit; and the gigantic system of compulsory charity, which diverts the wages of labour into the hands of idleness, and holds forth a perpetual temptation to the neglect of the duties of kindred and relationship, will be acknowledged on all hands to have been based upon a principle which Christianity never recognised, and which is directly opposed to the teaching of an inspired apostle. In place of the doctrine that no man shall be permitted to starve, and the cruel tyranny which pronounces that all men, without distinction of character or conduct, have a claim on the fruits of other men's industry, will be substituted those acts of prevention and foresight which will make the want of the necessaries of life an event so rare, that the spontaneous charity of a small fraction of the people will be amply sufficient to meet every real case of destitution; for though we are taught on authority we dare not question, that "the poor shall never cease out the land," we are nowhere taught that their number does not admit of being reduced from millions to thousands.

For our own part, we are confident that the only sure way to bring the present appalling mass of destitution and crime within reasonable and manageable limits, is by the universal practice of simple and well-considered measures of prevention, and by the gradual, and ultimately complete, disuse of all measures of palliation, which are not properly the province of the State, and not the highest privilege or function even of the Church.

Sanitary Reform, which is alone capable of achieving these great results, is, from first to last, a grand scheme of preventive charity; a practical application, on a large scale, of the soundest principles of humanity and economy. It is neither the dream of an enthusiast nor the panacea of a quack. Its plans are too sober for the one, too multifarious for the other. It opens the view of a new moral world through the agency of a physical reformation. It dispenses the pure elements of nature by the best contrivances of man's ingenuity, and proclaims a universal equality in the enjoyment of air, light, and water. It deals chiefly with the town, because the town stands most in need of improvement, and is most likely to influence the country by its example; and it looks with peculiar interest to this great and growing metropolis, as the best teacher and exemplar of physical improvement, as the centre from which England best fulfils her mission of teaching the nations how to live.

The object of the sanitary movement may be summed up in a few words, — a sewer in every street of every town and village; a drain for every house; a constant and unlimited supply of good water to every family; pure air at any cost; the application of the refuse of towns to the purposes of agriculture; and, lastly, to secure these blessings, the removal of every impediment, phy-

sical and moral, and the destruction or reconstruction of every form of local administration which does not work well towards these righteous ends.

That the inhabitants of the metropolis ought not to be excluded from a participation in these good things, no one will be bold enough to deny; that they can miss them, if they are only true to themselves, no one will believe; that the Sanitary Commission will ably plead their cause, we cannot suffer ourselves to doubt; and we are sure that the government is sincerely desirous of conferring upon them the benefit of a good sanitary measure. There will be some local resistance to overcome; but we think that we see signs of repentance in quarters where the outcry against Lord Morpeth's Bill was loudest, and some slight misgiving, which may ripen into a wholesome scepticism, as to the virtues of unmitigated local self-government. If this repentance and this misgiving really exist, the revelations of the new Sanitary Commission cannot fail of giving strength to these feelings. But if, unhappily, we are mistaken, and the old opposition to Sanitary Reform is to be revived, let no one forget at what cost of health, life, and money the luxury of resistance must be purchased. Ten thousand lives, a quarter of a million cases of unnecessary sickness, and waste or misapplication of some three millions of money, is the heavy tax which the inhabitants of London will be called upon to pay every year to parochial perverseness and municipal mismanagement. Let the rate-payers look to it. We are pleading their cause. Let the working-classes lay it to heart, for they may rest assured that they are more interested in Sanitary Reform than in any or all of the nostrums with which political quacks love to perplex and tantalize them.

THE PUBLIC HEALTH BILL: ITS LETTER AND ITS SPIRIT.

THE 'solitary sheaf' of the session of 1848—somewhat thin in the ear, and slightly damaged by the rough handling of those unskilful and talkative labourers, Sibthorp, Urquhart, and Drummond — has been safely garnered, and is destined, as we hope, to furnish seed which shall bear fruit a hundred and a thousandfold. We turn aside once more from the flowery and more seductive paths of literature to survey this new field of practical science, to examine its capabilities, and to feast our fancy with the destined fertility of the waste we laboured to reclaim. This language of metaphor is not altogether inappropriate to a measure which promises to ensure abundance, no less than to preserve health. The Bill which is to be the agent of all this good, after undergoing more transformations than we care to number up, has at length put on the more enduring form of an Act of Parliament. Thanks to the patriotism of that invaluable check to popular prejudice and local perverseness, the House of Lords, the Act is not a bad Act. It establishes a central authority, it appoints superintendent inspectors, organises a local executive body with ample powers, imposes upon it some wholesome checks, and appoints a corps of useful officials:—in a word, it is an Act which, in honest, firm, and willing hands, is capable of working a complete physical revolution in the disease-smitten towns of England. The clause to which we refer with most satisfaction is that which places it beyond the power of the local bodies to prevent the application of the Act where it is most called for. A mortality of twenty-three in the thousand is to be in itself a sufficient ground for bringing it into operation. For this boon the working people of England have to thank the hereditary branch of the legislature. The Act also gives some important and much-needed facilities to small towns. Deficiencies, of course, it would be easy to point out. The Smoke nuisance, we are sorry to say, is to continue without abatement, so that our large towns must still submit, for a time, to wear their costly mantle of unconsumed fuel; and we fear that scarcely power enough is given to the Central Board, or local bodies, to obtain in all cases a sufficient supply of water. But, deduction made for these and other deficiencies, we have much ground for thankfulness and satisfaction. We may now look forward with confidence to the time when England shall possess real towns, approximating in completeness of structural arrangements to the cities of old Rome, revelling in the wholesome beauty of running waters, open everywhere to the life-giving influences of sun and air, with perfect mechanical appliances for removing all things which can offend taste or endanger health, and conveying them, suspended in the waters of a mimic Nile, to the surrounding agricultural districts, where they will cover cultivated lands with unwonted verdure, and make desert sands and barren moors to blossom as the rose. In the Public Health Act there are the necessary powers for accomplishing this, and much more. Such things are, so to speak, latent in the letter of the Act. But the spirit of the Act — the idea that is striving for expression and developement — the broad generalisation which has this for its first substantial embodiment — what is it but the divine wisdom which has clothed itself in the homely English proverb, PREVENTION better than CURE? This is the spirit which animates those material forms, the Model Lodging-house, the Bath and Washhouse, the Ragged School, and all the mighty works of the New Philanthropy, mighty even now in accomplished good, mightier still in promise. The carnal eye sees in these model lodging-houses mere improvements in structural arrangements; but the spiritual vision discerns a series almost infinite of combinations and associations for bringing about in sober seriousness all that is good or desirable in the benevolent schemes of Owen and Fourrier: first of all, association for cheap and wholesome accommodation; next, association for economical consumption; and, lastly, perhaps (but this is much less desirable and much more difficult), for cheap production. To what extent this principle may be carried out, and of what developements it is susceptible, no man living can form a just idea; but every one must see the intimate bearing which a good sanitary bill must have upon it, in the large facilities which it affords for all structural improvements.

In one point of view, to which we have already briefly referred, this Bill is peculiarly important. In common with the Metropolitan Sewers' Commission Bill, it gives the necessary powers for dealing with those mines of liquid wealth, the guano streams of England. Their waters, rich in all the elements of fertility, can now be conveyed to the land for the production of food, and to the confusion of face of all who hold to the dispiriting theory of the pressure of population on the means of subsistence. Already the first steam-engine is erected, and the first pipes laid down, for the distribution of the fertilising fluid among the market-gardens of Fulham; indeed, but for unforeseen obstacles, this important experiment would long since have been made, and one of the greatest questions of the day would have been solved. But rumours are rife that obstacles have been raised and difficulties created by the Commission of Sewers, acting under the inspiration of one to whose industry and ability in collecting evidence and high administrative talent we have already borne willing testimony in these pages—we mean Mr. Chadwick. We fear that these rumours are not altogether without foundation, and we feel it to be a duty which we owe to the Sanitary cause to warn Mr. Chadwick of their existence. He must not conceal from himself the unwelcome fact that in entering upon the responsible duties of the Central Board, of which it is understood that he will be the paid member, he will have to encounter a greater amount of suspicion and mistrust than has hitherto fallen to the share of any public man. That suspicion and mistrust may be without foundation, but certainly no surer means can be devised to confirm these unfavour-

able sentiments than the placing of obstacles in the way of a public company established for important public purposes, its object having been sanctioned by the Report of a Parliamentary Committee, its powers conferred by Acts of Parliament, and guaranteed by a clause in the recent Metropolitan Sewers Commission Bill. The legislature plainly intended to give to this company the use of the sewage of a certain defined district; and it is anything but creditable to the Commission, or the Committee to which this business may have been referred, that they have left no device untried to defeat the intentions of the legislature, and to set its authority at nought. It would be most unfortunate for the cause which Mr. Chadwick is so capable of serving, if, acting under the stern compulsion of a theory, or the sinister influence of some favourite crotchet (for no one, we believe, has ever accused Mr. Chadwick of being swayed by mere personal considerations), he should be tempted to counsel or commit an act of tyrannical injustice. It is not likely that one who took so active a part in the establishment of the defunct Towns' Improvement Company, which, had it succeeded, would have grown into the most gigantic monopoly of the day, can be conscientiously opposed to companies as such. Indeed, it would argue the greatest ignorance of the history of civilisation in England if the services of companies were overlooked, their operations impeded, or their future formation discouraged. It is, we know, the fashion to inveigh against the unsound system and exorbitant profits of the water-companies. But though we are far from putting ourselves forward as their apologists, we can never forget the services they rendered to the population of our towns before Sanitary Reform was thought of, or Mr. Chadwick born. It was, doubtless, the recollection of these services which induced the legislature, in framing the Public Health Bill, to deal tenderly with the water companies, and to trust to the public spirit which is in them, and which is always ready to display itself when they are not made the subjects of unjust vituperation or attack. Now, if these companies are compelled to witness acts of tyranny and injustice put in force against a body which has so many points of similarity with themselves, they will be little disposed to expect at the hands of the active instigator of those acts that wise policy of forbearance and conciliation to which they are richly entitled.

Let the explanation of the obstacles thrown in the way of the Metropolitan Sewage Manure Company be what it may, the public will certainly draw from the perseverance of the Commissioners of Sewers in the course on which they have entered, inferences highly unfavourable to the smooth and successful working of the Public Health Bill. Men who busy themselves in driving coaches and six through Acts of Parliament, and in trampling the scattered fragments under foot, and who amuse themselves by imposing five-hundred-pound fines on companies constructing harmless works, after fair notice, on their own free-

holds, are not likely to be very agreeable colleagues ; and we shall not be surprised to hear that Lord Morpeth has to encounter greater annoyances in Gwydyr House, than fell to his lot in St. Stephen's. He would certainly find his comfort greatly promoted by the presence at the Board of a man of firm nerve and tried decision of purpose ; and we trust that Lord Ashley, who is understood to have been appointed the third Commissioner, will not shew himself deficient in those qualities. Mr. Chadwick, we repeat it, has high administrative talents ; but, that he may exercise them to our advantage, he must recollect that England will not suffer even an enlightened and benevolent despotism. She looks to find in all her public servants the tolerant and forbearing spirit of the nineteenth century. He and his noble colleagues have a great work in hand, and everything depends upon the spirit in which they enter upon it.

CHOLERA GOSSIP.

WHEN, some twelve years since, the nation, putting faith in facts, determined to know something definite about the movement of its population in the important matters of births, deaths, and marriages, and to this end established the office of the Registrar-general, it is probable that very few even of the clearest-sighted and farthest-seeing of the philosophers of that day had any definite idea of the useful purposes to which the new institution might and would be put. We need not go back to the discussions on the proposed measure in and out of parliament to know what men thought of it. Like a many-sided mirror, the subject was, of course, made to reflect the prejudices and prepossessions of those who approached it. The recalcitrant admirer of the middle ages started back aghast at the thought of so great an innovation; a few solitary fanatics shuddered at the remembrance of the sin and punishment of the Psalmist in numbering the people of whom the God of Israel had undertaken the defence; the economist turned pale as he summed up the tens of thousands of pounds which the new establishment must cost; and the spirit of chivalry glanced indignantly from the glistening eye of those who, to parody the language of Burke, saw the glory of Europe departing amid the dusty clouds of facts and figures to be raised by the labours of future 'sophisters, economists, and calculators.' The most sanguine statist was probably prepared to rest satisfied with an accurate and accessible record of births, deaths, and marriages, available for legal purposes, and a faithful tabulation of the ag-gregate results, as an aid to the researches of the political economist and the calculations of the actuary. If no greater result than this had been realized, we should still have had no reason to regret the creation of a very considerable corps of new officials, at an annual outlay of 60,000*l.* But the nation has had the singular good fortune to secure the services of men who took a larger view of their duties and opportunities, and who, to an excellent capacity for the routine duties of their office, have added a ready apprehension of the wants and requirements of our times, and a philanthropic zeal for the furtherance of that great cause of sanitary reform which is the highest and best application of the labours of the statist. Accordingly in the weekly, quarterly, and annual returns of the Registrar-general, we see abundant evidence of a desire to supply materials and means of instruction to every class of minds; to the statistical inquirer who revels in massive columns of figures, no less than to the light skirmishing man of single facts, who has the same objection to big tables that the great majority of mankind have to big books. From these single facts, fresh from the pens of the registrars and sub-registrars of town and country, we propose to select the chief materials of our Cholera Gossip.

By 'Cholera Gossip,' be it clearly understood, we do not mean a careless and trifling handling of a grave subject. On the contrary, we would speak with a seriousness worthy of so awful a theme; but yet so as not to weary, by an array of formidable tables and sustained discussions, such readers as may be in the habit of opening these pages, if not for mere amusement, at least for relaxation.

And yet if we were mere triflers, what countenance and support might we not fairly claim from multitudes of persons of very grave pretensions; from the old women of either sex who waged war against fish, fruit, and vegetables, up to the potent journalists who threw open their columns to all the absurdities of all the propounders of marvellous remedies and infallible methods of cure? Of certain microscopic triflers we would speak with tenderness. Though they came with haste to wrong conclusions, they are not to be classed with the credulous folk who fancied that every cholera patient who got well under their hands recovered *because* of their treatment. And what warrant, we would ask, had they for expecting that a remedy would be found for a disease which has as yet paid us only two short visits, when our old familiar maladies, small-pox, fever, scarlatina, and measles, to which we believe we may safely add consumption, still continue to baffle us in our search after remedies? The merest tyro, in the first year of his apprenticeship, knows that we possess no cure for any of these maladies. Why then expect to find a cure for cholera? It is much—very much—to be able to combat its premonitory symptoms with success. But here, though at the risk of being deemed over-sceptical, we cannot refrain from giving expression to a doubt whether the large proportion even of these cases would have gone on to cholera; in other words, whether they were not strictly analogous to the attacks of that slighter indisposition so prevalent every year in the warm season, and so unjustly attributed to the abuse of fruit. We must not, however, suffer ourselves to linger any longer amid scenes of doubt and conjecture, for we have before us matter which will better satisfy our curiosity and repay our trouble.

The history of the cholera in 1848-9 is in many respects the counterpart of that of 1831-2. The two epidemics have, in some parts of their long journey, followed nearly

the same course; the same places have often been attacked in the same order, at the same season of the year, and even in the same month; and the districts and parts of towns which severely suffered, or were lightly visited, or altogether spared in the first visitation, have been similarly affected or have enjoyed the same immunity during the present attack.

And yet there have been some noticeable differences between the two visitations. Like a traveller already acquainted with the road, the cholera has this time advanced more rapidly and lingered less by the way. Where, however, it has found suitable accommodation, and its unsavoury tastes have been duly studied, it has shewn itself in no haste to depart. London, which in 1832 had been forward to welcome the expected guest, took great pains in the long interval of seventeen years to add to its attractions; and was rewarded, as it deserved, by an earlier visit and a longer stay. So with Edinburgh. On the first occasion, nearly three months elapsed after the arrival of the cholera in Sunderland before it took up its abode in the capital of Scotland; but in 1848, it had fairly established itself there within a week of its appearance in the ports of London and Hull. Its visit to Dublin, however, was postponed for more than four months beyond the date of its arrival there in 1832. Portsmouth, Bristol, and Plymouth were visited, on both occasions, at about the same interval of time after its arrival in England, but this time Liverpool has been spared for upwards of three months. From the sea and river-ports of England, Scotland, and Ireland, inwards towards the more inland towns and districts, seems to have been, in 1849 as in 1832, the general direction of its incursions.

A quicker march, a longer sojourn, and a greater tendency to subside and reappear, seem to have almost everywhere characterized the recent epidemic as compared with that of seventeen years ago. A still more interesting and important peculiarity is its wider prevalence and increased fatality. In 1831-2 the cholera attacked upwards of 400 places in England and Scotland, and destroyed more than 31,000 persons; in 1848-9

3 B

it has already visited nearly 650 places, and carried off more than 47,000 victims. In London, in 1831–2, the deaths were 5275 ; but in 1848–9 close upon 15,000. Making every

allowance for increase of population, it is clear that the recent epidemic has been much more fatal than its predecessor. A rough calculation gives us the following result :—

	1831–2.	1848–9.
England and Scotland	1 death in 440	1 death in 380.
London	1 death in 280	1 death in 145.

The cholera is now nearly extinct in the metropolis, and fast subsiding in the provinces. The weekly report of the Registrar-general has dwindled down from a small volume into a folded paper of four pages; and the deaths by cholera from upwards of 2000 in a week scarcely more than two months ago, to less than the weekly average of the season.

The weekly report of the deaths from cholera in the provinces is also much less formidable than was the daily bulletin a few weeks back. For the present, then, the cholera seems to have nearly finished its allotted task. But the question is beginning to be anxiously mooted, Whether our present comparative exemption is to be looked upon as the lull of a tempest, or as settled fine weather? Will the cholera break out again? If we follow the single precedent of 1831–2, we must answer in the negative ; but if we look only to the history of the recent epidemic, and call to mind the somewhat startling fact that after the cholera had fairly set in in London at the beginning of October 1848, it underwent a very marked remission during the whole month of December, and that during no less than ten weeks (from the third week in March to the last week in June 1849), the deaths from this cause never exceeded ten in the week, and thrice fell to a single unit, we must confess that we feel by no means confident that we are fairly released from the presence of our unwelcome visitor. As wise and prudent men, we ought to choose the safer of the two alternatives thus set before us, and act as if the destroyer were merely sharpening his arrows and replenishing his quiver in readiness for a new campaign. Fortunately for us, we have been taught that if we cannot quench his fiery darts when once they have pierced us, we may throw up very efficient defences, built of materials ready to our hands.

There is an impression abroad that

the cholera attacked chiefly the poorer classes. Is this impression justified by fact, and if so, to what extent? We happen to have the means of answering this question as far as it relates to the metropolis, and its adult male inhabitants. On referring to an analysis to which we have access, we find 135 deaths set down as occurring among gentlemen and men of independent means, 34 among members of the learned profession, and 56 among the members of other professions and persons above the rank of the shopkeeper. The tradesmen of London have lost 558 of their number, and the working men about 3489. Now, at first sight, these figures seem conclusive as to the excessive mortality from cholera of working men, and the comparative immunity of those who have the advantage of being in more easy circumstances. But when we come to compare the number of deaths in each class with the number of its living members, the difference between one class and another proves to be much less considerable. One person of independent means, for instance, died out of about 200, and one member of the learned profession out of about 300. The remainder of the professional class lost about 1 in 200. The mortality among tradesmen was about 1 in 150, and among working men 1 in 120. It is true, then, that the cholera did attack the class of working men with the greatest severity; but the difference between them and their neighbours was by no means so great as has been generally supposed. The list of deaths comprises those of three clergymen of the Church of England and three ministers of other persuasions, of thirteen lawyers, and sixteen members of the medical profession. The clergy and the medical profession suffered in nearly the same degree; the lawyers were comparatively exempt. The first two classes were brought into contact with the sufferers ; the last was not. An argument this in favour of contagion ; but not conclusive, inasmuch as clergymen and doctors are not merely brought into contact with the sick, but also into the places in which the sickness originated. But there is another inference which we are disposed to draw from this comparatively slight disparity between rich and poor. The fact that the class of gentry and men of independent means lost more than half as many members as the working class, though in a very much less degree exposed to the acknowledged predisposing causes of the disease, establishes a sort of probability that, *cæteris paribus,* the richer members of society are more susceptible of the attack of cholera. They lost a smaller number in proportion, because they were placed in more favourable sanitary conditions ; not because they were of stronger frame, or less susceptible of morbid influences. This theory harmonizes with another favourite doctrine of ours, to which we attach some importance—that when the working classes shall enjoy a sufficiency of air, light, and water, they will be much healthier and longer-lived than their superiors. It is so even now in the rural districts ; why should it not be so hereafter in our cities ? In support of the opinion that the prevalence of cholera among the working class is attributable much more to the unwholesome influence to which they are commonly exposed, than to any constitutional liability arising out of the nature of their employment, we would instance this most consolatory fact, that out of the large population inhabiting the model lodging-houses now scattered over the metropolis, only one death took place from cholera, and this in the person of a very old man, at the model lodging-house in George Street, St. Giles, within a stone's throw of that source and centre of infection, Church Lane. We may mention incidentally that the mortality from cholera is greatest at the very age (between seventy and seventy-five) which this man had attained, and least from five to fifteen. Up to about twenty-five years of age it is also greater in males than in females, but after that age the proportion is reversed. But we forget that

such details somewhat belie the title we have chosen.

Line upon line, and precept upon precept.' Such is the merciful reiteration with which we are taught in temporal as well as in spiritual things. We are dull and inattentive scholars in the low form of human knowledge, as in that highest class of heavenly wisdom. In both how complete the means and appliances of instruction, how slow, sluggish, and perverse the scholars ! If we will ' work out our own salvation,' we are denied no necessary means to that end—on earth no lack of materials, in Heaven no stint of grace. But we must put forth our hands to grasp and mould the one, our faith to lay hold of the other. Industry, the rule of both worlds ; idleness, the thing abhorred both on earth and in Heaven, by the diligent Creator and upholder of all things. That we might work, and live by working ; and if we work aright, with right ends, and from right motives, be saved by working ; see what Providence has done for us. What a wonderful world for working and struggling in is this home of threescore years and ten ! All we possess has been, at some time or other, gained by a conflict with overwhelming physical forces, victorious not by brute strength put forth to meet the emergency or the danger, but by previous preparation of the means of conquest. The wild beast which preys upon our destined food must be slain by the arrow or the bullet, or captured in the snare ; the tempest must be baffled by the harbour ; the flood controlled by the dyke ; the lightning conveyed harmlessly away by the conducting-rod. And so it is with that invisible enemy—disease. The ague must be banished by the draining tile ; plague and typhus fever ignominiously driven out by soap and whitewash ; and smallpox disappointed of its prey by a weapon from its own armoury. No otherwise does it fare with us in moral matters. Crime is as the wild beast preying on the fruits of peaceful industry, a perpetual call to watchfulness ; the insurrection of the multitude, the threatening tempest ever suggestive of measures of wise precaution ; ignorance and sloth the pestilential marsh whose stagnant waters must be changed by education into flowing and irrigating streams; sin the plague to punish our neglect; dissent and difference of opinion in secular and religious matters the necessary stimulants to a sluggish and careless nature. And mark how things good and evil cluster about each other; how Idleness and Neglect overwhelm themselves with unexpected consequences; how Industry reaps rewards he never bargained for. Drain a marsh for health's sake, and you shall be rewarded with contingent plenty; do it for plenty's sake, and health shall be given you into the bargain. On the other hand, fold your hands and leave things to take their own course, and disease shall be added to famine, and demoralization to both. Such is nature's law; such, in an eminent degree, the lesson taught us by this new pestilence.

Its origin, birthplace, cause, and nature, shrouded in the mystery which hangs about all its kindred pestilences, raging furiously in bodies of armed men and crowds of pilgrims (as in 1781 and 1782 among the troops at Ganjam, and at Madras; in 1783, among the pilgrims at Hurdwar), then disappearing, or not being heard of, for the space of a generation, till it sprang into renewed life and activity from the steaming swamps of Bengal; its first victims the squalid and miserable Pariahs of Jessore, the first territory it claimed as its own the sunderbunds of Bengal, extended and enlarged by the inundation of the Ganges. During fifteen years of most strange journeyings, east, west, north, south, along river-valleys, across burning deserts, up lofty mountains, now with favouring winds, now against the monsoon itself, in every season, and in all weathers, by land and sea, hidden away in caravans, stowed in the holds of ships, does this mysterious and most puissant pestilence fulfil its mission of destruction.

Then comes a respite of another fifteen years or so, during which time the pestilence is still busy on a small scale in India; and again choosing a new point of departure in Persia or Cabool, sets out on its second errand of destruction. But

we must not lose sight of those sunderbunds and the poor squalid Pariahs of Jessore. There is a lesson to be learnt there which is worth all the theories of cause and cure which have been puzzling, exciting, and disappointing us for nearly twenty years. Let us not forget that the cholera of 1817, whatever may have been the history of its birth and parentage, had a swamp for its cradle, and poor Indian serfs, earning twopence halfpenny a-day, broiling under a vertical sun, and living, doubtless, as poor workmen live in more favoured lands, after a very miserable and squalid fashion, for its first victims. If we had conned this lesson well in 1832, we should not have had to record so many thousand deaths in 1849. We should have recognized in every part of England worse swamps than those of Bengal, and more likely victims than the Pariahs of Jessore. We present our readers with a few illustrations from the recent quarterly and weekly reports of that Prince of Gossips, the Registrar - general. Hear what the registrar of Portsea Island reports to head-quarters concerning Fountain Street and Nance's Row:—

Fountain Street has the main sewer of the parish passing under it, which having been ' blown,' during the wet season of last winter, the whole place was inundated with its contents, so that the poor inhabitants were obliged to wade through fourteen inches deep of foul refuse. Here the cholera first appeared, and here it raged most severely. Nance's Row contains about twenty mean crowded houses, and is situate in an open field. At the end of this row there is a junction of the four parish watercourses, about six feet deep, where a vast accumulation of foul stagnant water is formed, and here the cholera appeared in its most fatal form, twenty-two persons falling victims in the seven northern houses, and not a single case in any of the others.

Hear next the voice from Windsor:—

In Windsor, out of twenty-six deaths from Asiatic cholera and four from diarrhœa, fourteen were in Bier Lane and the courts adjacent. The medical attendant remarks of one of these courts that the houses abut on a black ditch, and are filled with disgusting odours from this source at all times; and that other nuisances are in the neighbourhood. There have been, within a radius of twenty-five yards of this part of Bier Lane, ten deaths from cholera in the last month, and cases of diarrhœa have occurred in every one of the houses.

The Report from Huddersfield shews that swamps haunted by cholera are to be found even in elevated situations:—

The first case of cholera was registered on the 3d of August; the second on the 9th, when the fearful pestilence made its appearance on an elevated part of the district, containing about fifteen or sixteen labourers' dwellings, situated on a hill-side, without drainage, the refuse thrown on the surface, with open cesspools, and malaria rising from a dirty fish-pond, which has not been cleaned out for thirty years, full of slime and aquatic vegetables, the water for the last four months having been drawn off, and the slimy deposit and decaying vegetable matter left exposed on the surface to the action of the sun and atmosphere. This pond presents about 1500 square feet of evaporating surface, and is situated within 150 or 200 yards of the dwellings on the hill-side, where the cholera has been most intense; every house in this district has been infected, and for two days before the cholera the wind blew directly from the pond into the dwellings. In this particular locality twelve deaths have occurred, some of them among nurses who have gone from other districts, and been attacked while on the ground. There have been other cases in other parts of my district, but all in badly-drained and filthy localities.

So much for cholera - fostering swamps in the provinces. Let us see what the Registrar-general has to tell us about metropolitan swamps. The south side of the river, as every body who knows London will readily believe, is one inhabited swamp from Greenwich in the east to Battersea in the west. In some parts the land lies two feet below the level of high-water, in others it is on the same level, but everywhere lies low as compared to most of the districts on the north side. In the absence of machinery the water must either flow back into the sewers at every tide if they are untrapped, or their contents must be retained for hours together if otherwise. Under these circumstances one may easily imagine the unfortunate condition to which the inhabitants must be reduced in

times of high tides or heavy rains. The result, as regards the prevalence of cholera, may be guessed at by what has just been said concerning the provinces. The mortality from cholera on the south side of the river has been three times as great as on the north side. This disproportion would probably be increased if the deaths which have taken place in the hospitals on the north side were distributed over the places from which the patients were sent; for though the eastern districts on the south side of the river have easy access to those two noble establishments, Guy's Hospital and St. Thomas's, the districts lying to the westward seek their hospital accommodation in St. Bartholomew's, King's College, Charing Cross, and Westminster. The proportion of three to one, therefore, is rather under than above the truth.

If the southern districts are entitled to be considered as the sunderbunds of London, we shall find its Jessore in the district of Rotherhithe or Bermondsey. An able writer in the *Morning Chronicle* * has very aptly christened a certain 'Jacob's Island,' in the last-named district, as the 'Capital of Cholera,' 'the Jessore of London.' We earnestly commend the description of that frightful spot, and still more fervently a visit to the place itself, to all our readers. We could not abbreviate the description without injustice: we dare not, for fear of consequences, transfer it to our pages. It is too loathsome to trust to the chance of its being read aloud. If such the mere description, what the reality? Once more we say to every man who has an atom of sanitary curiosity in his composition, 'Go and see.' Let all who cannot see with their own eyes task their imaginations to the very utmost to conceive all that is most disgusting to every sense, most revolting to every feeling of propriety and decency, all the hideous barbarisms of Church Lane, St. Giles,† exaggerated by the addition of a foul tidal ditch, and the unseemly necessity of drinking water drawn from the Thames as it flows past London, pushed to the last conceivable point of sicken-

* September 24, 1849.   † See No. 219 of this Magazine: March 1848.

ing loathsomeness. In the district cursed with this ' Venice of drains,' 163 in every 10,000 inhabitants were cut off by the cholera,—a mortality only exceeded in the adjoining district of Rotherhithe, where 225 in the 10,000 perished. On the other side of the water, Marylebone, Hackney, and Clerkenwell, lost 15 in the 10,000, and even notorious St. Giles only 48.

As an illustration on a smaller scale take the following report from the registrar of Greenwich East:— 'North side of the district, chiefly below high - water mark, and (Greenwich Hospital excepted) badly drained, 102 cholera, 12 diarrhœa. South side of the district, a rising ground and healthy, 28 cholera, and 21 diarrhœa.' Such is the penalty we pay for swamps and their concomitants ; so fearfully does cholera prove its identity of character on English and on Indian soil. The main difference is that we make our own swamps in England, and compensate for a hotter sun by fouler water, which water, let it not be forgotten, we drink.

Of this disgusting habit, or to speak more truly, necessity, the cholera has also in its own convincing way proved the danger. The water was found to be polluted with the foul contents of drains in one of two adjoining courts leading out of Thomas Street, Horsleydown ; in that one the cholera committed great ravages, the other experienced a comparative immunity. The same cause was ascertained to be in existence at Albion Terrace, Wandsworth Road, the scene of a frightful mortality. In Jacob's Island, as we have stated, the impurity of the water is carried to its extreme point, and there, too, the cholera was most rife. It is more than probable that the high mortality which occurred in Millbank Penitentiary was not unconnected with the use for drinking purposes of the waters of the Thames. In the entire southern district of London this cause may be presumed to co-operate with the low level and consequent want of drainage.

But swamps and polluted water are by no means the only circumstances favourable to the spread of cholera. A close and impure atmosphere, the result of faulty structural

arrangements of streets and houses, and overcrowding of rooms, has played a very conspicuous part in fostering the pestilence. Witness the appalling tragedy at Tooting, unparelleled since the days of the Black Hole at Calcutta ; and due mainly, though not exclusively, to overcrowding of pauper children. As such a lesson ought not to be thrown away, let us collect the statistics of that frightful mortality.

In the very first week in January, 1849, no less than 47 fatal cases of cholera were reported from Mr. Drouet's establishment. In the second week of January there occurred in Mr. Drouet's establishment 69 fatal cases of cholera and 8 of analogous diseases, and in workhouses to which the poor children had been removed, 9 deaths from cholera. In the third week of January, the deaths from cholera in the house at Tooting were 27 in number, and in workhouses to which the children had been taken, 6. Four fatal cases occurred at a later period. *A hundred and forty-seven* fatal cases of cholera in the establishment, 15 in workhouses to which the pauper children had been removed, and 8 deaths by analogous diseases—making a grand total of 170 deaths — such is the statistical summary of one of the most awful cases of wholesale homicide by omission hitherto placed on record.

The absolute immunity from cholera enjoyed by the inmates of Christ's Hospital contrasts most favourably with this frightful destruction of life, as does the similar freedom from the disease of the inmates of the several lodging-houses now happily scattered over London with the loss of life occurring among the very class of persons by whom they are inhabited, when less favourably circumstanced in the important matters of air, light, and water. Even the solitary case of cholera which, as we have stated, occurred in the person of an aged inmate of the model lodging-house in George Street, St. Giles, out of a population of about one hundred single men, may be fairly regarded as a proof of the preventive properties of fresh air, good drainage, and pure water, when it is borne in mind that the house in question is literally within a stone's throw of Church Lane, where the cholera raged so furiously as to put to flight numbers of its squalid occupants.

It would be a curious illustration of the destruction of life, which may be brought about by a law enacted for the express purpose of saving men from one form of death, starvation, if we could bring together into one sum total the deaths by cholera and other epidemic diseases which have happened in workhouses, in excess of the natural mortality of their inmates. The single establishment at Tooting (to say nothing of the recent outbreak in the Taunton workhouse, and the mortality in the poorhouse at Market Drayton, which caused the local authorities, in a fit of desperation, to raze it to the ground) occasioned a loss of life not to be compensated by the most ingenious device for quartering one class of the community on the industry of the remainder. What is true of cholera in 1849 is true of typhus fever and other contagious disorders always. In the Tooting establishment cholera has wrought the same destruction in 1849, which in Marlborough House, Peckham, the union workhouse of the City of London, typhus fever has been occasioning for years past. Do what we will, workhouses here and there will be exposed to the serious inconvenience of overcrowding; do what we will, poor-laws will often be harshly administered; do what we will, the local authorities will neglect their duties of supervision; do what we will, they will remain conscious of the significant fact that one class of persons is living in idleness on the industry of another. A practically humane poor-law is not in the nature of things; and we do not hesitate to express our firm conviction that poor-laws always have destroyed, and always will destroy, more lives than they save. We believe that this has been the case even in Ireland; we cannot doubt that it has been so in England.

In most instances more than one acknowledged unwholesome influence will be found to have co operated towards the production of cholera as towards the spread of fever. Bad drainage, foul air, and polluted water, are natural concomitants, working together to the same end. We sub-

join a few illustrations from the Reports of the Registrar-general, some referring to the metropolis, others to the provinces.

The registrar of Shoreditch tells us that the greater proportion of cases of cholera have occurred ' in the narrow streets, courts, and alleys, with which the district abounds, and which for the most part are very badly drained and ill-ventilated.' In the Trinity sub-district of Newington there were 308 deaths from cholera, and thirty from diarrhœa. The registrar says, ' The most important local causes I believe to be the very defective drainage, and the over-populated and ill-ventilated habitations of the poorer class.' From Lambeth we learn that Spring Place and the small streets adjoining, near the Wandsworth Road, which suffered very severely, are thickly populated and badly drained. Several fatal cases of cholera occurred in Little Gower Place, close to University College. The place is described as ' ill-ventilated,' the air being ' shut out at both ends,' and the house-surgeon of the hospital has been tempted to report the place to the Board of Health as being in ' a filthy condition,' and a source of supply of numerous fever cases.

From the rural districts the reports are to the same effect. From Mortlake, Surrey, we learn that twenty cases and upwards of Asiatic cholera ' have arisen principally from defective drainage, deficient ventilation, over-crowded habitations, and intemperance,' and that 'the drainage is very bad.' From Gravesend the report states that ' cholera has prevailed in the same and similar localities as those that were severely visited with fever in the September quarter of last year;' that there ' are no available common sewers,' and that ' the whole of the surface and underground drainage falls into rudely constructed cesspools.' At Edmonton the pestilence broke out in a row of eight filthy houses, to which there are no back yards: there were eleven fatal cases. Three cases of cholera at St. Alban's are reported to have occurred in houses with an open cesspool close to the back doors.

The cholera prevailed to a very alarming extent in the town of Great Marlow (Bucks), but 'the disease was confined to the poor and over-crowded, ill-drained, and ill-ventilated part of the town.'

One of the registrars of Norwich reports that of fourteen cases of Asiatic cholera, ten occurred in a small yard, underneath some of the houses of which runs a most abominable sewer.

One of the registrars of Sunderland, after reporting twenty-nine fatal cases of cholera in his district in the last quarter of 1848, says,— 'There is a great deficiency of light, air, and water. Many passages and staircases are quite dark, and windows are built up' (hear this, ye Chancellors of the Exchequer) 'to escape the tax.' The registrar of St. Paul's district, Bristol, says,—'The twenty-five cases of cholera occurred within ten days, and were confined to an area of a few hundred yards, consisting mostly of three densely crowded courts, the houses in which were found to be ill-ventilated, almost without drainage, and abounding in filthy accumulations.' In St. George's district, Clifton, eighteen fatal cases of cholera occurred in eleven houses in little more than a month. Most of the houses are described as being 'badly ventilated,' and some as having 'neither door nor window in the back.' In the district of Charles the Martyr, Plymouth, 'the majority of the sufferers' are stated to be 'living in close, ill-ventilated apartments, herded together in a manner almost incredible.'

The frightful mortality which the cholera occasioned when it broke out in towns and villages where such unwholesome influences exist in their greatest intensity, will be understood from the following examples :—

At Wreckington, in the parish of Gateshead, four miles from Newcastle, where the disease broke out on the 9th of September, 1849, 120 deaths from cholera took place in a population of 1000, of which number no less than nineteen occurred in a lunatic asylum containing forty inmates. This gives the high ratio of one death in about eight inhabitants. About the same rate of mortality occurred in the little fishing-town of Kingsand, in Cornwall, the deaths from cholera being ninety-three in a population of 719, or about two deaths in every seventeen inhabitants. At Noss Mayo, in the parish of Revelstoke, and district of Plymp-

ton St. Mary, Devon, the disease committed still more fearful ravages. The deaths from cholera were forty-eight in a population of 300, or one death in little more than six inhabitants. This greatly exceeds the highest mortality recorded in 1831-2. Dr. Buckland, in his sermon at Westminster Abbey, gave an example, on a small scale, of a still higher mortality.

Want of space alone prevents us from multiplying illustrations of the ravages of cholera in places destitute of common aids to health, decency, and comfort.

Is cholera contagious or infectious? If we were to poll the medical men of London, we believe that the majority would answer the question in the affirmative; if we were to take the votes of the country practitioners, we are inclined to think that an overwhelming majority would range themselves on the same side. The reason of this difference, if it exist, would be found in the great difficulty which there is in tracing the communication of one sick person with another in so large a city as London, and the comparative facilities for such inquiries in the country. We regret that want of space prevents us from citing from the last quarterly report of the Registrar-general a considerable number of instances in which the cholera is affirmed, with more or less confidence, to have been imported into country towns by sailors, travellers, Irish labourers, and vagrants. One fact recorded by the registrar of Market Drayton we must quote, for the edification of those good-natured folk who club together their pence in highways and doorways to support a travelling corps of purveyors of typhus, smallpox, scarlet fever, and cholera :—

The deaths (he says) would have been considerably below the average of previous corresponding quarters, had not the cholera (by which seven persons have died) unfortunately been introduced into the union workhouse by an itinerant mendicant, said to have come from Wolverhampton, who was picked up in the streets labouring under the disease.

Truly the inhabitants of Market Drayton ought to be much obliged to the charitable individuals whose judicious outlay of small coin set up this 'itinerant mendicant' in business as a hawker of pestilence. We could furnish several analogous cases, substituting typhus fever, smallpox, and scarlet fever, for cholera. But we abstain, partly from want of space, and partly because we have little hope of converting from the great error of their ways the imbeciles who are suffered to go about without keepers, spilling money in the streets at the sight of every idle vagabond who chooses to disguise his worthless carcass in rags and filth.

It is time that we brought our gossip to a close. Last month* we took occasion to revert to the days of humiliation, and the merciful removal of the cholera which followed so fast upon them; and in doing so, insisted on the value of a sincere practical repentance, as opposed to that general and indefinite regret for sins past, with which nations no less than individuals are so apt to rest contented. We have now had a day of national thanksgiving, characterized, we rejoice to say, not less by an orderly and pious observance on the part of the people, than by the inculcation of sound practical doctrines on the part of the Church. The Bishop of London, to whom the sanitary movement was already under the greatest obligations, addressed to the clergy of his diocese a pastoral letter, which may be regarded as a complete and authoritative recognition of the great truth, that cholera in common with other plagues sent by Providence to punish sinful nations, derives much of its fatal power from the unwholesome conditions to which man exposes his fellow man. A very fair proportion of the metropolitan clergy, we are glad to find, followed the wise example thus set them by their diocesan, and acted upon his advice in appropriating the whole, or part, of the collections made in their churches, to the improvement of the dwellings of the industrious classes. This is a new and most welcome acknowledgment of the value of that policy of prevention so often advocated in these pages.

There are one or two peculiarities of the recent epidemic which appear to us to call for remark, as special grounds of national gratitude and thanksgiving. It is quite conceivable that the disease which was sent to us as a chastisement, might have been purely a chastisement without a single element of instruction in it. It might have been not merely a very fatal disease, but a highly contagious one, communicated rapidly from person to person, and inspiring an extremity of fear. closely akin to the most heartless selfishness. Under the compulsion of such fear, the churches might have been crowded with worshippers during the visitation, to be abandoned without improvement as soon as the danger was over. The cholera, on the other hand, though calculated to inspire apprehension into the stoutest heart, gave no encouragement to selfishness, but rather, by revealing physical conditions which contributed to promote it, roused us to the unselfish exertions necessary to remove them. Again, the cholera might have been allowed to take up its abode among us as a naturalized plague; in which case its more sudden attacks would have come to be regarded in the same familiar light as so many apoplectic strokes, and the more chronic cases as the typhus fever, which we have so long viewed with such supreme indifference, though divinely commissioned to teach us the very same lessons as the cholera itself. That cholera has been made to obey a different law, is also a ground of thankfulness. Before we had grown familiar with its horrors, it has been suspended or removed, that on the occasion of another visit, it may still inspire the same salutary terror. Such are a few of the considerations which have occurred to our minds as calculated to heighten our gratitude, as a nation, for the removal of the cholera. If we continue to shew our thankfulness in acts of wise and merciful prevention, we shall reap a rich reward either in the permanent removal of the cholera from our shores, or in the comparative harmlessness of its next visitation. But if we persist in our health and life-destroying negligence, then it will be unreasonable to expect that the next epidemic of cholera will as much exceed in virulence that which seems to be now passing away, as this pestilence of 1849 has surpassed in violence that of 1832.

---

* 'Work and Wages.'

QUARANTINE.*

THE recurrence of the visitation of cholera to the north-eastern regions of Europe, and its consequently dreaded reapproach to Great Britain and the adjoining countries, have revived attention to the Report of the General Board of Health on quarantine ; and the agitation of the great question of contagion or non-contagion which it involves, seemed some months ago about to be renewed under the threat of an impending practical solution. The appearance, also, within the last month, of yellow fever on board of two of the West India mail packets; and a reported fatal case of it at Southampton, necessarily excite considerable public anxiety as to the measures to be adopted by Government in the present conflicting state of opinion between the executive Quarantine authorities and the Board of Health, as evinced in the Report of the latter on yellow fever. The first Report, with which alone we are to deal in the present article, received on its appearance in 1849 the usual cursory commendations of the newspapers, and its originality, philanthropic spirit, and beneficial tendency certainly entitle its authors to some public admiration and gratitude. An authoritative essay, which in an agreeable style, and displaying extensive knowledge, appears to advocate the principles of humanity and common sense against an alleged revolting system, established in ignorance and maintained by prejudice and perversity, cannot fail to gratify and console its readers; and except to the very few who minutely inquire into its postulates and deductions, and examine and *cross-examine* the evidence on which they rest, must carry complete conviction of their soundness and incontrovertibility. The general reading public, whose knowledge is derived and whose opinion is formed exclusively from the laudatory articles to which we have alluded, naturally concur in their correctness, and thus quarantine, by a union of apathy, amiability, and imperfect information, is doomed by decree of the General Board of Health, to irrevocable extinction, as a barbarous, inhuman, inefficacious, and pernicious system, the tendency of which has ever been, and still is, to foster rather than prevent pestilential diseases !

The subject, however, is too important to be left to these indications of public feeling, and although it will be obvious to those readers who are acquainted with it, that its magnitude precludes the possibility of its being treated with adequate comprehensiveness in our limited space, we shall endeavour to compress in it as much useful information as such space will admit ;

* *General Board of Health—Report on Quarantine*—Presented to both Houses of Parliament by command of Her Majesty, 1849.
General Board of Health—Second Report on Quarantine. Yellow Fever. 1852.

happily, no technical or professional knowledge is required for discussion of it,* and we can try the question at issue by the tests upon which alone it is repeatedly stated to rest, namely, evidence, observation, and experience. It is due to ourselves, however, to say, that in analyzing, with the view of commenting on this Report, we have encountered great difficulty from its very defective arrangement, and the want of any continuous line of, argument, or specification of points upon which objection can be fixed; and above all, from an indiscriminate use of the most important words, such as fever, contagion, and infection, without regard to their separate meanings, while the necessity of guarding against such indiscriminate use is in other parts distinctly pointed out.

The Report, which is understood, we believe correctly, to be the exclusive work of Dr. Southwood Smith, originated in an investigation by the Board into the Quarantine Regulations enforced in English ports upon the appearance of cholera in 1848, and unquestionably, such glaring instances of absurdity and abuse as are there exhibited have seldom been submitted to public reprobation. Here truly the proposition for which the Board contends, of the inutility of quarantine, as enforced in England, is clearly made out (Appendix to Report, No. 1), but the Report immediately generalizes the conclusion, and maintains the like inutility of quarantine for prevention of the spread of any disease whatever. By assuming that there is such a resemblance in all diseases—typhus, scarlatina, influenza, plague, yellow fever, and cholera—as to render them all alike dependent on certain atmospheric and other stated conditions, the proof of the inapplicability of quarantine to any one of them is held to be conclusive with regard to all. It is on this generalization and assimilation of disease, this entire extinction of contagiousness, that we think the doctrine of the Board untenable, and the evidence and arguments adduced in support of it inconclusive; and it

is obvious to us that by reasoning throughout on this assumption, the Board has afforded to the supporters of quarantine the means of refuting the entire principle of the Report, by the mere proof, which we think glaring, not only of the dissimilarity of the specified diseases, but of the impossibility of their possessing in common the characters which the Board has attributed to them. These characters or common properties of all diseases are stated to be as follows:—

They are all fevers; they are all dependent on certain atmospheric conditions; they all obey similar laws of diffusion; they all infest the same sort of localities; they all attack chiefly the same classes, and, for the most part, persons of the like ages; and their intensity is increased or diminished by the same sanitary and social conditions.

Now, with the exception of the first of these attributes, which is little more than saying that all diseases are illnesses, we question if any medical man in Europe will admit this dogma without qualification, and to our unprofessional perceptions the concurrent existence of the above characteristics in all diseases seems contradictory, and is, to say the least, subversive of established notions on such subjects. We have always understood typhus to originate in famine, cold, and vitiated human effluvia, and to be entirely independent of atmospheric influence; influenza to be produced and diffused by atmospheric influence only; yellow fever incapable of diffusion outside the tropics or within a certain temperature never durably experienced in England; scarlatina highly contagious and indiscriminate in its attacks both of locality and person; cholera not contagious, but conveyable in atmosphere; and plague simply contagious, without dependence for its diffusion on atmosphere, locality, class, or circumstance. These notions are no doubt all controvertible, and many of them are most strongly controverted, particularly on the points of contagion or non-contagion, but where the object of quarantine is stated to be to prevent the introduction from one

---

* 'It is not a technical question, but one of evidence, on which a person capable of observation is as competent to judge as any physician.'—*Report*, p. 20.

country into another 'of such diseases as are propagated by contact,' is it logical or fair to class under one category, and to reason upon it as a ground for the *entire abolition* of quarantine, diseases in which not only contact but all other means of personal conveyance are on all sides held to be nugatory—(such as influenza, against which quarantine was never even by implication levelled)—with diseases such as plague, against which quarantine is chiefly aimed, or cholera, against which experience seems to have shown it inefficient ?

Having established this in our opinion very unsound basis, the Board propounds its general, its all pervading principle, that 'sanitary measures,' by which we are to understand cleanliness, ventilation, pure and abundant air and water, thorough drainage, and destruction or removal of all noxious substances, are the sole means of prevention of the introduction or the spread of disease, such measures 'tending to prevent or remove certain conditions without which pestilential diseases appear to be incapable of existing.' The existence of disease at all is stated to depend upon the presence of a peculiar state of atmosphere, which there was evidence in the cholera season spread over thousands of square miles, and yet affected only particular localities, and in these localities the conditions (which we infer are filthy, low, close, undrained, and unventilated sites and dwellings), were found visibly and offensively to prevail.

It follows that our true course is to make diligent search for all localizing circumstances, and to remove them, so as to render the locality untenantable for the epidemic. But quarantine makes no such search, and leaves all localizing conditions untouched and unthought of. —*Report*, page 6.

Admitting the truth of this and every other similar allegation against the power of quarantine over atmosphere or locality (pages 6, 8, 10, 12, and 16), to which power we never heard, nor is it insinuated, that it pretends, and admitting as we cordially do, the wisdom and, where practicable, the efficiency of the recommended 'sanitary measures,' what argument do they afford

against the true and the sole object of quarantine, which, as already stated, is, in the words of the Report, 'to prevent the introduction of epidemic diseases from one country into another, and its regulations are based on the assumption of the contagiousness of the diseases with which it deals, it being supposed that such diseases are *propagated by contact*, direct or indirect, of the unaffected with the affected!'

'Contagiousness,' to which alone the power of quarantine is here justly held to be limited (although the assumption of its blind neglect of collateral preventives is unwarranted), is defined in the following most important passage, and we entreat our readers to adhere to the definition, which in spite of its obvious necessity, and the Board's own recommendation, the Board itself most assuredly has not done :

There has been much confusion of terms in respect to the use of the words contagion and non-contagion. We have had instances of professional men who avowed their belief of the contagiousness of typhus, and stated that they had experienced it in their own persons. When asked for the evidence on which the belief was founded, they have usually related some circumstances such as those described, showing, not the contagiousness, but the infectiousness of the disease. Contagion is a term applicable to a different set of circumstances. According to the hypothesis of contagion, no matter how pure the air, no matter what the condition of the fever ward, if the physician only feels the pulse of the patient, or touches him with the sleeve of his coat, though he may not catch the disease himself, he may communicate it by a shake of the hand to the next friend he meets; or that friend, without catching it himself, may give it to another; or if the physician wash and fumigate his hand, but neglect the cuff of his coat, he may still convey the deadly poison to every patient whose pulse he feels during the day.—*Report*, page 46.

And again, page 47.

'Strictly, contagion, as the word implies, is capable of being communicated only by actual contact; while the influence of infection, as far at least as regards the diffusion of the exhalations of the sick into the surrounding atmosphere, is represented to be limited to the distance of a very few yards.

It appears to us, therefore, and

we cannot conceive a difference of opinion upon the point, that with this distinctive definition and limitation of quarantine regulations to contagion, the primary aim of a report impugning the principle of quarantine, should have been to prove either the non-existence of such a thing as communicability of disease by contagion, or the inadequacy of any regulations whatever to prevent such communicability. Annihilate contagion, or prove the impossibility of its prevention, quarantine is dead for ever. Accordingly, all the opponents of quarantine are necessarily non-contagionists; their arguments and evidence are directed to the explosion of the doctrine of contagion, as contended for by the supporters of quarantine; and it is impossible to imagine to what else they could be directed. The Board itself says most truly, in the letter in the Appendix, addressed to the Privy Council:

The only theoretical ground on which the precaution of quarantine can be considered necessary or justifiable with reference to any disease is, that it is of a contagious nature. — *Appendix*, page 142.

What, then, shall we say to the following passage in the Report?

Quarantine is based, as has been stated, on the assumption that epidemic diseases depend upon a specific contagion; but the question of contagion has no necessary connexion with that of quarantine (!!). The real question is, whether quarantine can prevent the extension of epidemic diseases, whatever may be their nature, whether contagious or not. If it can, it is valuable beyond price; if it cannot, it is a barbarous incumbrance, interrupting commerce, obstructing international intercourse, perilling life, and wasting, and worse than wasting, large sums of the public money. But if the power of protecting the country from the introduction and spread of disease, whether contagious or otherwise, claimed by quarantine, be really possessed by it, this must be proved by other considerations than those which establish the contagiousness of disease: it is a mere matter of evidence and experience, and consequently the disputed point of contagion should be placed entirely out of view in this discussion, and the whole question should be argued on the broad ground, whether or not quarantine is a public security, or is capable of affording practically any useful result. —*Report*, page 17.

We despair of thoroughly comprehending the whole of this passage, and our incapability will not perhaps be deemed surprising, when independently of other contradictions to it, there lies before us a *Report on Quarantine*, of 128 printed octavo pages, throughout the far greater portion of which contagion and quarantine are specifically treated as bearing upon each other; and we defy any reader, in perusing any part of the work, to get rid of the idea of their indispensably necessary connexion. We guess that the Board means to hold as established, that whereas all disease is communicable only by 'epidemic atmosphere,' against which quarantine is avowedly ineffectual, contagion need not be taken into consideration at all; but can even this assumption drive contagion out of the discussion? Is it conceivable that while there is in the world such a thing as contagion, it can be left out in an inquiry tending to abolish a system founded solely on its existence, real or presumed? The idea appears to us a contradiction in terms.

One of the most obvious and embarrassing of the evils of the system of amalgamation of diseases, and neglect of distinction of terms adopted in the Report, is the impracticability thereby created of examining and exposing observations and evidence which, as applied to one epidemic — influenza, for example, and, to a certain point, cholera—we might agree to and admit, but which, as applied to the others, we more or less strongly repudiate and deny. In cases of influenza or cholera, where the non-contagious principle is either established by experience, or approaching to confirmation, the utility of quarantine may reasonably be questioned; and we should have pleasure in assenting to the sufficiency, though in different degrees, of 'sanitary measures' for the prevention or extirpation of these diseases; but it does not follow that because such sanitary measures, always excellent in themselves, are effectual against one or more epidemics, quarantine is ineffectual or can be dispensed with as to all. Here, indeed, there is no necessary connexion; to maintain, as this Report loudly and ela-

borately does, that quarantine is to
be entirely abolished as ineffectual
against all diseases alike, is to maintain that prevention of contact—for
that is the strict and true meaning
and intent of quarantine—will be ineffectual against small-pox, measles,
psora, and syphilis, and that pure
air, water, drainage, light, and elevated dwellings and cleanly habits
render the human body impervious
to the communication of disease by
touch. One medical authority, the
late Dr. W. Fergusson, who would
have been a powerful supporter of a
great portion of the Board-of-Health
doctrine, asserts that these conditions absolutely aid and facilitate the
conveyance and diffusion of scarlatina, one of the Board's amalga-
mated diseases ; and that purity of
atmosphere adds to the virulence of
some infections.* But without impugning the value of ' sanitary measures,' than which nothing is more
strenuously to be deprecated, let us
try conclusions between them and
quarantine, even on the ground of
this Report, where they are strongest,
and quarantine is powerless.

In page 56, the Board, after stating
the power of the human body, even
in health, to corrupt the air, and
that the breathing of such air, holding in solution, as it does, quantities
of noxious animal matter, may
poison the blood to such a degree
as to produce fever, proceeds—

But if the exhalations from persons in
health are capable of producing this result, what must be the danger of breathing the air of a close room, in which
numbers of persons are crowded together, labouring under such diseases as
typhus, plague, and yellow fever ? The
predisposed or susceptible cannot, as
has been stated, breathe such a pestilential atmosphere, even for a short
time, without the most imminent risk ;
but if they continue to breathe it uninterruptedly night and day, and perhaps
in a state of anxiety and exhaustion, is
it necessary, should they be attacked
with the prevailing malady, to resort to
the supposition of contagion to account
for the event?

We think we could make out a
case of discrepancy, at least in degree, between this statement and
that in page 51, where the dreadful
consequences are pointed out,· *if*

emanations from the living body
formed permanent and powerful
poisons, but our object is to show
that in the imagined case, whether
we are ' to resort to the supposition'
of contagion or infection to account
for the event (for to one or other it
must be ascribed), a judicious quarantine or *prevention* system would
infallibly have rendered it impossible. The ' close room' would have
been interdicted, and even suspicion
of any of the dreadful diseases mentioned would at the outset have prevented any accession of persons ;
and if fatally congregated, they
would have been isolated, separated,
and attended till cured, and the pestilential atmosphere would have been
so restricted or purified, that external conveyance of disease would
have been arrested. In like manner,
in the real case of cholera in the
Market Drayton Union, in 1849,
specified in the registrar's report,
and cited in this Magazine of December in that year, it is obvious
that the healthy condition, the perfect sanitary measures established
in that place were insufficient to
prevent the deaths of seven of its
inmates, from the ' introduction'
into it of a diseased pauper from
Wolverhampton, which introduction
or communication of the diseased
with the healthy, a quarantine regulation would have effectually
barred. The result seems to be,
that sanitary measures, powerful as
they are, and always wise and salutary, are no more sufficient of themselves than quarantine is of itself to
prevent infection or contagion of all
diseases.

But it is time to come to what,
amid all avoidances and amalgama-
tions, is undoubtedly the real question at issue, not perhaps *in terms*,
but necessarily pervading the whole
of this Report—namely, the contagiousness or non-contagiousness of
plague, and consequently the efficacy
or non-efficacy of quarantine against
plague—oriental plague—known to
the world from Thucydides down-
wards. Originating in Egypt and
Ethiopia, where, though it is never
entirely extinct, its epidemic ravages are periodic, it devastated
Attica in the times of Socrates and

---

* *Notes and Recollections of a Professional Life*, pp. 101, 102.

Pericles (who died of it), and in the sixth century of our era nearly depopulated the earth. The chief towns of Italy suffered frightfully from its visitations in 1349, London in 1665, Marseilles in 1720, Messina in 1743, Moscow in 1771, and Malta, Gozo, Corfu, and Cephalonia (British possessions), in 1813, 1814, 1815, and 1816. Contagion was its inseparable, and, down to 1720, its unquestioned character; but in that year doubts of its contagiousness for the first time arose, and were published by some of the French physicians at Marseilles. The celebrated Dr. Mead, who, we are told by Dr. Rankin, cited in the Report, ' studied plague profoundly,' published (1720) his *Discourse concerning Pestilential Contagion*, a concise but consistent and well supported exposition of the doctrine of contagion and infection, and of the efficacy of quarantine for their prevention and extirpation. His work called forth a number of answers in the shape of Explanations, Examinations, and Remarks; and it is truly curious to read in one of them—*A Discourse of the Plague*, by Dr. George Pye—a clear enunciation, almost in the terms of the Report before us, of the doctrine there maintained, of the impossibility of transmission of plague by communication of person or material, and the consequent utter inutility and even danger of quarantine. Dr. Mead, in a subsequent edition (the 8th, 1722) refuted the objectors, and adhered to his doctrine, always, however, condemning many of the obvious abuses of quarantine, such as shutting up houses, and abandonment of sick. The controversy seems to have died away, at least to have slept for a century, during which quarantine, which we need hardly say is perennial, and independent of the existence of plague, flourished unassailed, although the question of conta-

giousness of particular diseases often gave rise to much medical discussion. In 1815, however, the then Levant Company sent a physician, Dr. Charles M'Lean, to Constantinople for the express purpose of inquiring into the nature of the dreadful epidemic, and in 1817 he published, in a small pamphlet (afterwards extended to two volumes), the result of his mission. He utterly repudiated the idea of contagion at all in any disease whatever, except small-pox and measles; asserted that it originated in a mere ' pious fraud' of Pope Paul the Third, to remove the sittings of the Council of Trent to Bologna* (a notion which he found but did not acknowledge, in one of the anonymous answers to Dr. Mead in 1722), and he denounced quarantine in the violent and virulent strain which seems to be natural to its opponents. His practical knowledge of plague strangely contradicted his theory (though of course he did not admit it), for he had scarcely entered the pest-house at Constantinople, when he was himself seized by the pest! His confident tone, however, in the face of the then recent narratives of Sir A. Brooke Faulkner and Dr. Tully, of their personal knowledge and treatment of plague at Malta and the Ionian Islands, drew very great attention to his work, and we doubt not it originated the Committee of the House of Commons of 1819, to inquire into the subject.

The Report of that Committee, however, after examining Dr. M'Lean and numerous witnesses at great length, and receiving reports from the quarantine stations of England, was in substance, that no sufficient evidence had been produced of the non-contagiousness of plague, or of the inutility or inefficiency of quarantine. Another committee was appointed in 1824, before which the examination of witnesses was re-

* Quarantine seems to have originated at Venice in 1423, when a lazzaretto was built on the occasion of a plague which, between August and December, carried off 15,300 of the inhabitants.—*Daru.* The Decameron showed Dr. M'Lean that isolation for prevention of contagion was practised nearly a hundred years before, but he seemed to doubt its authenticity, because there was no evidence of the date of its being first printed. Even if the silly interpretation of Paul Sarpi (*History of the Council of Trent*, book ii. cap. 96 and 97) were correct, it proves that contagion could not have been a new idea then broached for the first time; it was known to the ancient Greek physicians—to Aristotle, Galen, Lucretius, Tacitus, and Virgil —as well as to the middle-age Italians.

newed, and a reference made to the College of Physicians, whose answer —we believe unanimous—was decidedly adverse to the doctrine of non-contagion, and to any interference with the principle or existing practice of quarantine.

It was in this year that the *Westminster Review* was established, and its fifth and sixth numbers attracted very great attention from elaborate argumentative articles on contagion and quarantine. Contrary to what we have shown to be the framework, and, we think, the flaw of the present Report of the Board of Health, these articles carefully divide diseases according to their ascertained specific nature, and reason against contagion of plague (upon which, *of course*, they say 'the whole system of quarantine laws depends') on the grounds of its non-admissibility into the category of epidemics which they characterize as capable of diffusion by contact or close approximation. The articles display comprehensive knowledge of the subject, but, as usual with partizans of any new and seeming philosophic or philanthropic theory, they omit or overlook, positive in their over-charged exhibition of comparative evidence. Their tone, moreover, is much too assuming and confident in treating a question upon which the wisest and most experienced of men held totally opposite opinions. In the meantime, the British Government, with the laudable view of relieving commerce from the fetters of quarantine, relaxed its laws so far as to allow pratique to vessels and cargoes from the East bringing a clean bill of health. In the words of the *Westminster Review*, they removed forty-six of forty-seven of the evils of quarantine; but alas! for the relief of commerce—nearly every power on the Continent simultaneously placed England and her European dependencies in quarantine! Marseilles, Genoa, Ancona, Trieste, Naples, apparently without intercommunication, closed their ports to English vessels under various periods of detention, till the order was recalled!

A new, and to that period unknown authority, now appeared in the controversy, in the shape of a dispatch (printed and laid on the table of the House of Lords, 17th June, 1825, on the motion of Lord Lauderdale) from Sir Thomas Maitland to Earl Bathurst, dated 8th April, 1819, 'on the subject of the plague.' It was published *in extenso* in the newspapers, and it is really not saying too much that, at least as to the only instances of plague in Christian Europe within the memory of man, it settled the question as to its communicability by contact alone. Sir Thomas carefully eschews 'any theoretical or medical discussion on the character or nature of contagion or infection,' and 'confines himself entirely to facts,' and such an overpowering body of them, combined with such closeness of reasoning and deduction, certainly never was exhibited in the same space of writing. This was followed by an elaborate article in the *Quarterly Review*, (vol. xxxiii. 1825,) in direct answer to and refutation of the *Westminster*, written with equal confidence but far greater power, and with a vast preponderance of evidence on the other side; and as a close to the contest for the time, the *Edinburgh Review*, in an article (September, 1826,) on the parliamentary history of the session, signified its opinion in the following words, which we quote with especial reference to the very different view of the question taken in the last number, in treating of this Report of the Board of Health:—

The dissertation on the quarantine laws possesses very great merit indeed. The question of contagion is discussed in a most masterly style, and the demonstration is so complete as to set at rest, we should think, for ever, the doctrines which have been so idly ventilated on this momentous subject. It seems hardly credible that men should have been found to recommend a remission of the quarantine regulations upon the ground of their belief in the new theory, which affirms typhus and plague to be entirely epidemic, and not capable of communication by approach, or even by actual contact. Their advice was grounded upon the expense and inconvenience occasioned to commerce by these regulations. They never seem to have reflected on the possibility that this theory might prove unfounded, and that its overthrow would be effected by the infliction of a wide-spreading pestilence. But, besides that, all the facts triumphantly demonstrate its fallacy. Commerce, it should seem, has already suffered no little embarrassment from the bare promulgation of the doctrine. The concluding remarks of this admirable discourse are well deserving of attention. — *Edinburgh Review,* September, 1826, p. 475.*

We do not find any further public notice of the subject, controversially, till 1838, when Dr. Bowring published a letter addressed to the British Association for the Advancement of Science, then at Newcastle, in which he repeated the assertions and reiterated the arguments against quarantine, founded, as every argument against it must be, on the non-contagiousness of plague.

Dr. John Davy, a physician of great experience and practical knowledge of epidemics in the Mediterranean, devoted a chapter of his interesting work (1842) on Malta and the Ionian Islands to observations on quarantine, in which he treats the subject in a painstaking and impartial spirit. He started as a contagionist in 1824, but was shaken by the array of counter-evidence which he met in his inquiries in the East. Still, he was only for a qualification of quarantine regulations, and would have witnessed with regret any alteration in them not preceded by inquiry. In the course of writing his observations, however, he heard of an instance of such unequivocal communication of the disease at Constantinople by mere contact, that his doubts were finally removed, and he was satisfied of its simple contagiousness, and consequently of the indispensability of quarantine.

Whatever side of the question may be adopted by any person desirous of enabling himself to judge between the two, by an impartial examination of the evidence and arguments on both, there will be no difference of opinion in any class of inquirers as to the awfully-important interest involved in the issue. No language can adequately express it. If there be such a thing in the physical world as communication of disease by contact,—and

that there is, every living man, even to the hind, who sees it in his flock of sheep or goats, is as well persuaded as he is of his existence—and if such communicability has been proved even once in the disease called plague, against five hundred times that it has been disproved in other instances, is any sacrifice, consistent with the maintenance of human society, too high to be made to prevent the contingent *possibility* of the results of such a calamity? The evidence on the non-contagion side is necessarily negative and general, while that on the other is positive and specific; and this alone might deter abolition of an establishment which, whatever its defects, barbarities, and abuses, avowedly prevents the one medium of communication, (disputed, if you will,) namely, touch; but what will be said when, not only in the midst of the negative instances there are numerous cases of positive contradiction to them; — witness Dr. M'Lean, the death of Dr. White, and others, *from inoculation,* the French army in Egypt, the Russian experimentalizing physician at Alexandria, and very many others in that country —but that in Christian Europe the instances of non-contagiousness are the mere exceptions that form the rule. Even if they were the more numerous, is there anything in this subversive of the principle of contagion—anything to justify unrestricted communication? If so, our mothers and nursemaids may cease their precautions against small-pox and measles, and our high-fed ladies and gentlemen against psora and other cutanea, for assuredly the instances in which contact does not communicate these and other worse contagious diseases, are at least equally numerous as those in which it does not communicate plague. Further, even if the guiding principles of human judgment admitted of an equality of weight to negative as to positive testimony, the latter in this question of contagion outweighs the former both in quality and amount in an enormous proportion;

* 'Quarantine is a system utterly powerless to arrest the progress of epidemic disease, but most powerful to multiply its victims and aggravate its horrors.'— *Edinburgh Review,* October, 1852.

—the accumulation of it in Europe for centuries, down to 1816, is overwhelming, while that on the other side, mere theory in Dr. Mead's time, is now limited in its facts to situations where, besides the disease being endemic, and consequently not under the same law of propagation as where it is epidemic and exotic, the attainment of accuracy is, from the nature of the governments, next to impossible. The opinions in favour of non-contagion are limited to some half dozen medical men, who, were they entitled to ten times the respect which we willingly allow them, are utter insignificance against the whole medical body of England,* collectively and individually—to say nothing of general officers, consuls, practitioners, and private observers in foreign countries.

The non-contagionists may say that this mass of evidence has not been sifted, investigated, submitted to their process of annullation, as was very ably, but in our opinion unsuccessfully, done by the *Westminster Review*, but they cannot and do not deny its existence; and yet, in a Report pronouncing dogmatically and authoritatively the absolute, immediate, and *entire* abolition of an institution, of which the one sole and exclusive ground has for four centuries been, and still is, the principle of contagion thus proved, not one word of notice, nor the slightest allusion, is from beginning to end made that there ever was, or that there is any evidence whatever except that *against* it, with which the Report is loaded, applicably and non-applicably, to the exclusion of everything in its favour! This is most unfair and unwise; but how shall we characterize an attempt to pervert in favour of their principles the testimony of about one half of their strongest opponents! We say, that any reader not possessed of previous information, and not intending to inquire further than the Report itself, must unavoidably conclude, from the citations of evidence on page 63, that the medical witnesses there named were

as much anti-contagionists as the Board itself—not indeed from the words cited, for they refer to facts which nobody ever questioned—but from the way in which the witnesses are introduced, and from 'their being *introduced at all.*

It would lead us much beyond our limits and beyond our sphere to enter into discussion of the theory of mere tainted atmosphere being, conjointly with predisposition or separately, the medium of communication of plague as of epidemics; but if so, and if quarantine should thereby, as we admit it would, be proved to be useless as a preventive, what better would be the sanitary measures that are to supersede it? Allowing all that is asked for them in warding off and dispelling epidemic, shall we be told that the atmosphere will respect them, as the destroying angel did the houses of the Israelites—hovering over but not alighting on square acres of cleansed, drained, ventilated, and purified lands or dwellings?—or, even admitting this assumption of exemption to such places, of what avail would they be in yellow fever, for example, which is purely a disease of place, and, as we are told in the Report on it by this Board (7 April, 1852), sometimes attacks the upper and not the lower part of a house, sometimes one end of a floor and not the other, sometimes one side of a ship only! To argue, however, that because sanitary measures cannot extend to such cases, they are not to be inculcated and enforced, or that they ought to be discontinued because expensive, is analogous to arguing that because quarantine cannot prevent the approach of pestilential *contagion* (which we need not say is not proved) therefore quarantine must be abolished.

We are ignorant how far this Report may have originated the idea of the National Sanitary Conference, which met in Paris in July, 1851; but we learn that it was translated into French and Italian, and submitted to the delegates from the twelve European powers —Austria, France, Spain, England,

---

* Of twenty physicians examined by the committee of 1819, only two, Dr. M'Lean, the *fons et origo*, and Dr. Mitchell of Edinburgh, were non-contagionists. We are really at a loss to name more than the remaining four that we have allowed.

Greece, Naples, Portugal, Rome, Russia, Sardinia, Turkey, and Tus-, cany. Lord Shaftesbury, one of the members of the English Board, informed the House of Lords on 28th May last, that the general principle of the adoption of sanitary measures (we wish they had been more definitely described) had been agreed to by the conference. The modifications of quarantine, however, which they recommend are exceedingly slight when contrasted with the total abolition so vehemently urged by the English Board. With the exception of restricting quarantine to the three diseases, cholera, yellow fever, and plague—in the last of which they make no diminution of period of detention,—the mitigations are scarcely more than each state frequently assumes the power of making for itself upon representation of special cases. But comparatively insignificant as they are, it seems from Lord Malmesbury's speech in the House of Lords, on 18th November last, that four only of the continental powers, Portugal, France, Sardinia, and Russia, will sign the Convention proposed for carrying them into effect; and thus this most momentous question stands where it did, with the obstacle to partial amendment of quarantine created by the dread of its entire abolition.

We have read the Report on Yellow-fever, and its very interesting Appendix. The question there treated is much more of a professional and technical nature than that in the preceding Report, but we observe too much of the same partizan spirit in the collection of evidence and prominence of opinion on one side only. It is from the documents in the Appendix that we learn the opinions and evidence on the other; and it appears to us that although, happily for this country, the existence of yellow fever seems incompatible with its temperature, its non-importation into the warmer climates of Europe, or even into England during very hot months, is by no means so satisfactorily established.

NEGLECTED HEALTH.

TELL him of an intent that's coming towards him.' The British citizen was told on various occasions early in the present session, that there were six or eight sanitary measures to be made payable to him in the course of a few months. Bills were, indeed, duly drawn, but they have all been most unduly withdrawn. For, to finish the quotation we had just begun, ' Promising is the very air o' the time ; to promise is most courtly and fashionable : performance is a kind of will or testament, which argues a great sickness in his judgment that made it.' If this be true philosophy, the judgment of the House of Commons upon matters that concern the public health is very sound indeed. The end of the session brings our patience to an end. We have been quiet. Trusting in those who should know what is good for us, we have heard, seen, and said nothing ; but now we must speak.

We will not pain ourselves by uttering the names of the eight or nine measures, great and small, more or less bearing upon the improvement of the public health, that we have seen, during this spring and summer, perishing before their prime. We were friends to them, and they are lately dead, all barbarously murdered in the House of Commons. Surely it was not the time for a national assembly, far removed from barbarism, to declare that a time of war—a time when the rich of necessity must suffer more than usual pressure, and the poor be more than ever crushed—was not a right time for removing burdens on our social state. Deliberations on the conduct of the war have formed a very small part of the business of Parliament ; no topic of debate was less welcome to ministers, or, except as touching a few points, less relished by the country. The war has not thriven or gained weight an ounce for having eaten up the other business of the session. Let some German critic, with a German constitution able to endure the work, read the debates of the year through, and he will find that, allowing to war-topics all the hours they occupied,

there remained an abundance of time spent in declaring there was no time. His decision will be, that it took as much strength to push on one side the work of the country as would have sufficed to push it to a useful extent forward.

We believe that an abuse of the privilege of faction is in some degree responsible for the late stoppage of all domestic legislation ; but whatever may be the cause or causes of it, we do not believe that statesmen have been justified in excusing their own inaction by the sluggishness of public interest in any other than the leading topic of the day. The filth that swims in his back-yard and oozes through his bedroom floor is infinitely nearer to the poor inhabitant of Rotherhithe or Bethnal Green than the corruption of the Russian Government. The labourer who has been earning his own bread for years, and in some chance week (fallen, perhaps, under the pressure of war times) needs parish aid, is thereupon, by the unamended laws of poor removal, carried away, and set down naked with his household in some place where he finds the legal fiction of a settlement, but no home, and no face of friend or place of work. This man thinks more of his boys and girls in the workhouse than of the ships in the Baltic ; he turns his face to Westminster for help—it might as well be turned to Mecca. But these men, and millions in the same or some other way not less concerned in the measures that have been ostentatiously neglected during the past session , these, it may be, are not the people who express the public interest in one thing or another. It has often been said, that if eels and lobsters were not dumb, but could express their sufferings by shrieks, they never would be skinned or boiled alive. Something of the same kind may be said of the dumb classes in society ; there is no active desire to give them pain, or to prolong any pain they feel, and there is some heed paid to their sufferings, but not enough. The tongue being an unruly member, lawgivers legislate for that. At present it appears to them wisest to do nothing. A sergeant of the old school in some French caricature drills his troop, and when he has got the men fixed in a row like statues, cries to them with enthusiasm: 'Immobility's the finest movement in the exercise!' While the public was crying out upon Lord Aberdeen for having in this spirit dealt with the Russians, it was much more evident and certain that in this spirit the whole Parliament was dealing with ourselves.

We will take, however, the grave omissions to which we refer as lapses in duty natural to men troubled by an unaccustomed care. We are not used to have a war upon our path, and may be allowed at first sight to form wrong impressions about the extent to which it is to be considered an impediment to social progress. We have yet the benefit of sanitary laws made in preceding years. The German critic whom we have already invoked would, indeed, find upon close study that there is not one of them wholly sufficient for its purpose—not one that does not either exist now in the form of an Amended Act, or else await some necessary emendation. Boards have been so created that they could not do what they might, and might not do what they could. Parliament has put into the midst of them the leaven of unpopularity: it has worked, they have become unpopular, and then they have been officially snubbed or officially thrown over.

Bodies of law have been created without legs to carry them along, lumps that, like the Interments Act, are able to arrive at nothing. We are not half so much surprised at the unpopularity of the Board of Health, considering the work it had to do and the powers given for the purpose, as at the fact that it really is able to show a large amount of work accomplished. It has rescued thousands of men from death by cholera, has taught more than a score of towns how to be wholesome: it has underbid dirt in the market by proving that cleanliness is cheaper, not in any indirect way by its consequences, but directly, scheme against scheme, clean sewerage against stink, constant supply of good water all over the house against an intermit-

tent supply of bad water in the scullery. An extensive amount of accurate sanitary knowledge has by the same agency been diffused, and two or three new and important principles have been established, though they have not yet all conquered the hostility of vested interests. This Board was sent into the world almost without any other tool or weapon than its tongue; it has used that well, and we complain of its much talking. It was set to a task of innovation, bidden to tread on a whole army of toes; the owners of the toes cry out, and so we all cry shame on such a Board of Health for having made itself unpopular. Where there is so much cry, there must be some wool, we say; there cannot be all this smoke and no fire. Certainly not; but the fire may be one that, if wise, we should be in no hurry to quench. When we see much smoke after the kindling of a necessary fire, we do not throw cold water on the coals we have been lighting, but rather, if we must do something, aid them with an extra faggot, or give them a little helping breath out of our bellows. It is in the first kindling, the freshness of the coal, that we get more than a common show of smoke, but let the fire burn up, and it will soon wear a more cheerful aspect. That was not the philosophy of Lord Seymour (whom no labourer for public health has ever blessed as an ally), or of Sir Benjamin Hall, when those gentlemen marked a session that had done no good to the sanitary cause with a strong effort to do it harm. It may be true that Dr. Southwood Smith and Mr. Chadwick are themselves responsible for some part of the unpopularity attaching to their office. We do not know that they are. We know that in the mere fulfilment of their duty they must have affected many prejudices, wounded many interests, and incurred inevitable odium which it is an honour to have deserved. No doubt they may have had their faults, but we know very well how much good service they have done, and if we felt, as we do not, that we could point out how it might have been done with a better grace, we should be chary, even then, of censure. For why should we throw stones into the garden out of which we gather flowers?

After all, now that we touch upon the Board of Health, we, for the first time, feel ground under our feet in a consideration of existing sanitary prospects. The Board's term of office now expiring is to be renewed provisionally for a year or two, until 'something may turn up;' and, in the meantime, to be subjected to the full control and supervision of the Home Office, which shall have power to dismiss any of its members. The influence of a department of the Government may, therefore, be used in backing with its weight all the just wishes of our sanitary councillors;* while the duty of the State, to concern itself actively with details of sanitary discipline, will at the same time be suggested rather more practically and distinctly than it hitherto has been. On the other hand, the spokesmen for the vested interests rejoice in the control to which too energetic leaders of the struggle against filth and pestilence are to be subjected, and are not without hope that ere long those sanitary champions may be sacrificed to meet the humour of a public that is so frequently ungrateful, because unreflecting.

Our public, however, is a very sensible and kindly one when it does think. A section of it is already thinking busily about our weak defences against filth and fever; and there is surely just now more than enough matter for the cogitation of us all. While we write, we are told of five thousand people killed in a fortnight at Jamaica by the cholera, and of the ravages of the same

plague at Marseilles, where nearly two hundred deaths have occurred in a single day, and where the inhabitants, until restrained by a decree, were taking flight by troops into the open country. The terrible disease has already sent forward announcement of its probable arrival in strong force among ourselves. Deaths by cholera have occurred here and there. Cholera broke out lately in a ship at Liverpool; it has been gaining strength at Glasgow; it has already appeared, and is now rapidly increasing, in London. It is hardly possible that we shall escape a severe visitation for the present season; the hot summer weather has but recently set in, our river banks and the great fetid pools under our feet, are only now beginning to reek out their poison in a concentrated form, and it is difficult not to fear that we are now again on the verge of an immense calamity.

When this possibility was distant, thought was taken for it by a writer whom the public honours, because they have been none but just and noble thoughts to which he has given permanence in sterling English. This gentleman, author of *Friends in Council*, printed some months ago for private circulation, a small work entitled *Health Fund for London; Some Thought for Next Summer.* Its immediate purpose was to suggest a combination of the strength of private men determined to do something; however little it might be, yet to get something actually done; for the abatement of the evils out of which all pestilence arises. Let them, it was urged, subscribe a sum of money, and administer it in

---

* Whilst these sheets were passing through the press two incidents have occurred calculated greatly to dishearten all friends of sanitary progress, and especially to disappoint the hopes which had been formed of Lord Palmerston's activity in the cause. First, in a debate on the Public Health Amendment Bill, Lord Palmerston, while in the very act of claiming to be the representative of the General Board of Health, took occasion to make a very sarcastic and ostentatious disclaimer of having read the important *Report*, in which that Board had just endeavoured to relate its achievements and justify its policy, this *Report* being at the moment under discussion in the House. And, secondly, within the last day or two, after introducing the ' Nuisances Removal Amendment Bill,' one of the most important endeavours for sanitary legislation which late years have witnessed, Lord Palmerston, on the first show of opposition, declared himself ' the last man in the world to give unnecessary trouble,' and accordingly withdrew his bill. If the country is to have its sanitary affairs properly administered, this must be under the auspices of a minister who is superior to flippant vanity and selfish indolence—of a minister who will take the trouble to read that for which he claims to be responsible, and will be content to struggle with some obstacles when the lives of millions are at stake.

the form of concentrated help to some one filthy district, so that it might be cleansed, and become on a pretty large scale, what on a small scale the Model Lodging-houses are already—irresistible evidence in favour of the right use of air, water, and drainage. Recent reports of the result of the working of those model lodging-houses that have been now a sufficiently long time established, show that although they are erected commonly in the midst of the worst London neighbourhoods, and have stood the siege of cholera, by which they were on some occasions hotly surrounded, yet in no form has pestilence hitherto crossed one of their thresholds. The low rate of even ordinary mortality in these buildings is so positively startling, that we dare not quote it until more experience shall have confirmed the opinion it suggests. The Health Fund, then, was proposed, in order that, as nearly as possible, not a house only, but a district, might be made in this way pestilence-proof.

The idea so proposed fell upon good soil, and aroused much active and sincere desire for co-operation, but for reasons that need not here be specified it has never yet been actually carried out. The pamphlet of which we speak did nevertheless much good in its own sphere by the infusion of new vigour into the general discussion about matters of hygiène, and it contained many wise thoughts pointing forward to the legislative and administrative powers that it will be best to seek for sanitary purposes.. We agree so thoroughly with the main principle affirmed under this head in the little tract, that we will venture to quote from it a passage bearing most directly on our present argument :—

In the first place (it is said), the management of such a thing as the public health should not be dependent upon the spare time of Parliament, or be subject to the interruptions caused by the recesses of you legislators. The waiting from the close of one session to the beginning of another, [and we have now to add, from the beginning of one session to the close of the same,] for such sanitary measures as may suddenly be required, is a palpable defect, a manifest failure. It shows at once how ill such things are regulated. Any particular evil which occurs should be

remediable, either by a municipal body, or a Department of the State. How contemptible a thing it is, that there should be great public works of the first necessity required ; and that mere offsets of authority — powerless, moneyless commissions—should be the only bodies to appeal to for orders in such a pressing matter. There should be a great Department of Public Health, distinct from that of justice. Many matters, not now thought of, should come under the jurisdiction of this Department. To prevent the adulteration of food, for instance, should be one of its duties. It should turn science to account in every way. It should encourage and enable scientific men to work at matters connected with the public health.

This we believe to be a view of the question to which it is important that attention should be steadily directed. The peculiar connexion that is to exist, *ad interim*, between the Home Office and Board of Health may be used as a preparation for some definite and well-developed measure, that shall establish, finally, the care of public health, as an essential portion of the business of the nation. In this event it will be seen that the direction of it is to be entrusted only to the highest class of public servants. It is not a trust to be disposed of at the option, or, at best, mismanaged by the discordant action of ten thousand small municipalities or parish vestries. Let the deadliness of the poison steaming from a cesspool or a sewer-of-deposit once be fairly recognised, and nobody will be disposed to assert that a due regard for popular institutions makes it proper for a corporation or a vestry to maintain it in existence. No local board should be entitled to declare that a murderous piece of brick and mortar shall not be summarily dealt with, and that the state is not, unless the vestry or the corporation pleases, to take thought for the protection of lives visibly in danger. Municipalities have no more right to exercise their mercy on a cesspool than to save from the prison or the gallows any other sort of Greenacre. Not even a vestryman, if he be a fishmonger, may offer for sale, as food, stinking turbot ; is there reason why he should have right, if he be a house-owner, to offer for tenancy a stinking habitation? For nobody can doubt which is the more fatal bargain of the two. The time will surely come when not a man in England will be blind to the fact, that there should be no option left with any one, as to the performance or neglect of the main duties that belong to public hygiène. They are matters of life and death, for which the greatest of our representative institutions, namely, the State, alone can take thought in a proper manner. It is a matter also that nearly concerns national morality. An old French poet, François Villon, who sank deep in all the filth of filthy times, and wrote much reckless levity, but now and then moaned like a fallen angel in the midst of his defiant revelling, uttered the despair not of himself only, but of a host, when he exclaimed—

Ordure avons, et ordure nous suyt ;
Nous defuyons l'honneur, et il nous fuyt.

The most surprising part of the whole subject is the speed with which health and honour are recovered, when once ordure has been thoroughly turned out of doors. This point of the case is really a hindrance in discussion, by its very strength. Proper sanitary care tells so amazingly upon a population that we get on faster in a controversy when we let our facts alone. The Board of Health states the results it has produced, and men at once cry out on hot-headed enthusiasts, who prove too much. When facts are to be dealt with, in the present state of human cautiousness, (cautiousness not to be discouraged,) half as good a case for sanitary discipline would make twice as certain an impression. We have for this reason abstained, hitherto, from figures, but we cannot refrain from allusion to the evidence of one witness, who has no connexion with the Board of Health, and cannot be said to have a crotchet of his own to prove. In a very pithy and business-like second report, recently issued, on the operation of the Common Lodging-Houses Act, Captain Hay states that among thirty thousand tenants of registered lodging houses, places infested formerly by pestilence, and now, to a certain moderate extent, cleared of filth by the operation of a tolerably easy law, among those thirty thou-

sand people there were, in the twelvemonth, only ten cases of fever. An improvement has, at the same time, taken place in the character and habits of the lodgers, almost commensurate with this improvement in their physical condition. The supervision extends now only over common lodging-houses, no protection is afforded to the occupants of other dwellings.

Every man knows that arsenic is poison ; to administer it, therefore, in a dangerous or fatal dose, is to commit a felony. When every man has learned that filth in certain forms is poison, ought it to be left to his discretion, or to the discretion of his parish, whether dangerous or fatal doses of it are to be administered to any neighbour ? We do not, in what we have been saying, diminish the office of any local body. In grave matters it is for the State to ordain what must be done, and by local self-representation, each little community—perhaps by means of Local Boards of Health—may decide for itself how to do it.

A scheme of representative self-government especially designed for the metropolis, and bearing largely upon the advancement of the public health, has been suggested in a thoughtful and ingenious pamphlet by Lord Ebrington. To this we may refer readers who desire to see justice done to the great principle of local self-representation, without hurt to any public interest. Due provision is made by the plan for securing certain weight in each Council to the nation at large, as represented by its government; and we accept many of Lord Ebrington's ideas, though we attach little importance to one of the arguments on which he bases them. He thinks it necessary to take care lest a metropolitan government, with too extensive and independent powers of control, should become at any time an *imperium in imperio*, and be a source of danger to the central government. He points to the great prominence given already by large vestries to political discussion and the composition of memorials On any such account we own that we have no fear. Only the lessening of public liberty could make a London revolutionary junta possible. Govern-

ment never can be more under
London influence than it is now.
The most comprehensive representation of the municipality of London
could not carry more weight than
exists already in the columns of the
London press, and in the free expression of opinion by all citizens.
The town is by a great deal too
large for any narrowness of local
feeling; it is practically a great
British province, in which are found
represented the interests of the
nation here and in all quarters of
the world. A government with
which the whole metropolis contended, would exist in opposition
to the will of the whole nation. If,
however, the municipality were no
more than a representation, having
local feeling for its animating soul,
there would be no need to protect
the State against it. There is no
need to look for danger from im-
proper steps that may be taken by
the little parliaments we cherish
and desire to cherish always, however true it may be that, like
greater parliaments, they indulge in
occasional absurdities. Lucian tells
of a king of Egypt who taught
monkeys to dance. They danced
correctly, and with a profound
gravity, until some citizen threw
nuts among them. Now there
are many little matters that are
nuts to the members of a town
council or vestry, and whenever
public liberty may be in danger
from steps taken by any such body,
we will undertake to get up in that
town council or vestry, and to save
the country. We would propose
such a halfpenny rate—but no, why
need we reveal the nostrum? If we
speak lightly of our small self-repre-
senting bodies, let it be remembered
that men laugh with the most freedom at what they love. Were the
true rights of municipalities endan-
gered by denying to them uses they
were never meant to serve, we
should be very serious in their defence. But as it is, while we declare
our belief that in their worst form
they care, as they should do, infinitely more for their own quarrels
than for those of anybody else, and
that under no possible circumstances

could they in this country ever
assume a revolutionary character,
we must object to all confusion of
departments. There is a fable about
a man who quarrelled with his hair-
brush, and, setting it aside, elevated
three old servants, blacking brushes,
to the vacant situation. Admirably
had they performed the not unim-
portant duty formerly entrusted to
them, but when the change was
made, their owner did not find much
reason to congratulate himself.

We have touched very lightly and
briefly on the points to which it has
seemed to us most expedient to call
attention, and have made no attempt
to enforce our argument by an array
of sanitary facts. But upon these
facts it is nevertheless requisite
that men should dwell with an in-
cessant patience. Whoever will go
with the clergyman or parish surgeon
of any wretched district in this
country, using his own eyes and his
own nose, though he will not see in
one visit a tenth part of the pollution
that exists above ground, and will
have imagined most imperfectly the
horrors that lie underneath the soil,
will yet come away eager to be at
work, and make his heavy heart a
little lighter by some effort to be
helpful. The next best thing to
actual inspection for an acquisition
of some knowledge of the truth, is a
reading of the evidence of faithful
witnesses. The reports of the inspectors who have been invited in
various places to make the preliminary inquiry that is requisite before
there can be any question about an
application of the Health of Towns
Act are worth reading with care.
They show not only what terrible
neglect of all the ordinary means of
health is common, but also—as at
Swindon, for example—what angry,
dogged opposition may be made by
selfishness and ignorance together,
even against changes that one might
think would be dictated by the
simplest sense of decency. A
vigorously-written summary of the
chief sanitary events of the metropolis exists in the well-known reports of the City Officer of Health,
which are now collected.* Mr.
Simon's excellent reports in their

---

* *Reports relating to the Sanitary Condition of the City of London.* With
Preface and Notes. By John Simon, F.R.S., Surgeon to St. Thomas's Hospital, and
Officer of Health to the City. London: John W. Parker and Son. 1854.

present form are likely to do as
much good service in the future
as they have done already in the
past, as official documents suggesting
lines of action to a public body, or
as matter for the newspapers. They
have become now a possession to
the student. There are several
things pointed out by Mr. Simon in
the preface to his volume upon
which we find that we have already
touched. Other topics—as the adulteration of food and the serious and
extensive falsification of drugs, both
evils upon which there is now no
adequate check—have escaped our
mention. Men are plunged into
disease by want of proper sanitary
care over the town, and the best
doctor is defied often to drag them
out of their disease, for want of
proper supervision exercised over
the druggist's shop:—

It is notorious in my profession, (Mr.
Simon writes), that there are not many
simple drugs, and still fewer compound
preparations, on the standard strength of
which we can reckon. It is notorious
that some important medicines are so
often falsified in the market, and then so
often mis-made in the laboratory, that
we are robbed of all certainty in their
employment. Iodide of potassium, an
invaluable specific, may be shammed to
half its weight with the carbonate of
potash. Scammony, one of our best
purgatives, is rare without chalk or
starch, weakening it, perhaps, to half
the intention of the giver. Cod-liver oil
may have come from seals or olives. The
two or three drops of prussic acid that
we would give for a dose may be nearly
twice as strong at one chemist's as at
another. The quantity of laudanum
equivalent to a grain of opium being,
theoretically, 19 minims ; we may practically find this grain, it is said, in 4·5
minims, or in 34·5. And my colleague
Dr. R. D. Thomson, who has much experience in these matters, tells me that
of calamine—not indeed an important
agent, but still an article of our pharmacopœia—purporting daily to be sold at
every druggist's shop, there has not for
years, he believes, existed a specimen in
the market.

Mr. Simon urges very strongly
the necessity of dealing with the

great subject of our sanitary condition, by comprehensive and scientific
legislation, ' that it should be submitted, in its entirety, to some
single department of the Executive,
as a sole charge ; that there should
be some tangible head, responsible
—not only for the *enforcement* of
existing laws, such as they are or
may become, but likewise for their
progress from time to time to the
level of contemporary science, for
their *completion* where fragmentary,
for their *harmonisation* where discordant.'

The department of a President of
the Board of Health, sitting in Parliament, should be, ' in the widest
sense, *to care for the physical necessities of human life*,' and we regret
that we have only space to quote the
conclusion of Mr. Simon's able summary of the duties for which such a
Minister of Health should be responsible :—

Into the hands of this new minister—
advised, perhaps, for such purposes by
some permanent commission of skilled
persons, would devolve the guardianship
of public health against combined commercial interests, or incompetent administration. He would provide securities
for excluding sulphur from our gas, and
animalcules from our water. He would
come into relation with all local Improvement Boards, in respect of the
sanitary purposes of their existence.
To him we should look to settle, at least
for all practical purposes, the polemics
of drainage and water supply; to form
opinions which might guide parliament,
whether street sewers really require to
be avenues for men, whether hard water
really be good enough for all ordinary
purposes, whether cisternage really be
indispensable to an urban water-supply.
Organisations against epidemic diseases—questions of quarantine—laws for
vaccination, and the like, would obviously
lie within his province ; and thither perhaps also his colleagues might be glad
to transfer many of those medical questions which now belong to other departments of the executive — the sanitary
regulation of emigrant ships, the ventilation of mines, the medical inspection
of factories and prisons, the insecurities
of railway traffic, *et hoc genus omne.*